ROCKE ROBERTSON

ROCKE ROBERTSON

SURGEON AND SHEPHERD OF CHANGE

Richard W. Pound

McGill-Queen's University Press

Montreal & Kingston · London · Ithaca

Legal deposit first quarter 2008
Bibliothèque nationale du Québec

Printed in Canada on acid-free paper that is 100% ancient forest free
(100% post-consumer recycled), processed chlorine free

McGill-Queen's University Press acknowledges the support of the
Canada Council for the Arts for our publishing program. We also
acknowledge the financial support of the Government of Canada
through the Book Publishing Industry Development Program (BPIDP)
for our publishing activities.

Library and Archives Canada Cataloguing in Publication

Pound, Richard W.
Rocke Robertson : surgeon and shepherd of change / Richard W. Pound.

Includes bibliographical references and index.
ISBN 978-0-7735-3374-5

1. Robertson, Rocke, 1912–1998.   2. McGill University – Presidents – Biography.
3. McGill University – History – 20th century.   4. Surgeons – Canada –
Biography.   5. Montreal General Hospital – Biography.   6. University of British
Columbia. Faculty of Medicine – Biography.   I. Title.

R464.R59P68 2008   378.714'28092   C2007-906264-4

Set in 10.5/13.5 Minion Pro with Copperplate Gothic
Book design & typesetting by Garet Markvoort, zijn digital

CONTENTS

ACKNOWLEDGMENTS

I want to thank members of Rocke Robertson's family, Stuart, Ian, and Bea, for their assistance in checking facts and locating materials and for the care they have taken in the organization of the family records, all of which made the task of highlighting the important aspects of their father's life – personal, professional, and family – far simpler than if one had had to sort through a mass of uncatalogued materials. From the farther reaches of the Robertson family, Jay Eberts was most helpful in assisting me to cross-check some facts and to produce a photograph of one of Robertson's principal mentors.

At McGill I had plenty of assistance locating and accessing Robertson's administrative record and digging into much of the background to the events during his tenure as principal. The McGill Alumni Association was kind enough to locate sufficient funds to engage some archival assistance, and I am grateful for the help provided by Johanne Pelletier, Gordon Burr, Tina Witham, and Sarah Jensen, as well as by Peter McNally.

Nothing having to do with any aspect of the history of any portion of McGill could be contemplated without going to the ultimate "source," Stanley B. Frost, to whom I express both my thanks and admiration for his prodigious contributions.

Special thanks go to David Mulder, one of Robertson's recruits and one of his successors as surgeon-in-chief at the Montreal General Hospital. He undertook a review of Robertson's many surgical and other publications and was able to evaluate their significance, something far beyond the ken of a tax lawyer, without which a knowledgeable assessment of Robertson's important contributions to surgical and medical scholarship would have been difficult, if not impossible.

INTRODUCTION

There is probably no genre of work that permits the writer more opportunity to learn, in the course of writing, than biography. No matter where one picks up the thread of a subject's life – beginning, middle, or end – there lies ahead a fascinating journey of exploration, of discovery, of sorting out the essential from the routine, of determining the influences that led the subject in one direction or another, and finally, of drawing conclusions about the life and contribution. The outcome can never be certain – nor may it be what might have been expected at the outset of the journey.

This is not intended to be a history of McGill University during the time of Rocke Robertson's term as principal. That will become the task, in due course, of those responsible for charting the history of the institution. Of course, some elements of this history, particularly during some turbulent and troublesome years, are inseparable from the man on the spot, and they are portrayed largely through his eyes as he lived the experience, but the account of these elements can, from this perspective, represent at best a partial appreciation. In some respects, Robertson was too close to many of the events and too personally affected by them for his judgment to reflect the balanced view that will be provided by history. On the other hand, he was there, at the centre of the changes that occurred, where the pressures exerted on him and on the institution were the greatest, and he had a personal view of events and of these pressures, which cannot, and should not, be dismissed. In the course of managing the huge, often disruptive, changes that occurred, he gained his achievements without losing his personal stature or allowing his principles to be dictated by the conduct of others. These achievements are important elements in his story and a measure of his integrity.

While his position as principal of McGill University was the peak of his career, he did not arrive at McGill without a past. It was this past that had attracted the university and encouraged it to recruit Robertson for the office. During a relatively brief stint as surgeon-in-chief at one of its teaching hospitals, the Montreal General Hospital, and as head of the Department of Surgery in the Faculty of Medicine, he had brought about extensive changes in the mutual reinforcement of academic and clinical medicine, demonstrated superb skills in clinical teaching, recruited a generation of outstanding academics and clinicians, and fundamentally reorganized the surgical services of the hospital. These were transformative changes that took the hospital from its comfortable role of a hospital with competent surgeons into a completely revitalized teaching hospital with state of the art techniques and a commitment to research and experimentation, aligned with the academic mission of the Faculty of Medicine and its exploration of new ideas and techniques. It had been an extraordinary performance that generated attention in Canada and internationally.

Robertson's ability to bring about change, too, had not come about by chance. He was well educated at McGill and was in the process of adding to his qualifications, which would undoubtedly have led to a successful career as a surgeon, when the Second World War broke out. He enlisted in support of his country but with the objective of saving, rather than taking, lives. The learning curve for a young surgeon, especially one with very limited operating room experience, was extraordinarily steep, exhilarating in some respects but terrifying in others, as he had to perform operations for which he had no training. This would have been bad enough under the best of conditions, but in a field surgical unit, close to the fighting, it is hard to imagine the difficulties he and his colleagues faced and to share their frustrations of knowing that, with proper training and full technical support, some of the outcomes might have been different. In the process, however, he did have the chance to be at the cutting edge of some of the new developments in medicine, especially the introduction of penicillin, and to see the impact of the new miracle drug on some of the war casualties he was treating. Despite the many handicaps under which they operated, it was nevertheless an experience that led him to observe how medical treatment, especially for trauma, could be organized and delivered as efficiently as possible. Like many war surgeons, he knew that the shorter the interval between the injury and the necessary medical intervention, the greater were the chances of survival and recovery. This was empirical knowledge that he brought back to civilian practice and that he was able to apply wherever he worked and taught. He also knew how important it was to understand the causes and to manage the spread of infection in hospitals, leading to his important influence in both fields.

His energy and ability led Robertson to take on complex organizational challenges after the war, including studies in hospital administration, in emergency services, and in hospital infections, as well as longer term experiments in several aspects of surgery. He was very much involved in the establishment of a new faculty of medicine at the University of British Columbia, was one of the initial professors in this faculty, and was deeply involved in the development of its academic program. He was very active in his early civilian years with the Royal College of Surgeons, the beginning of a lifelong connection with the work of this organization, where he developed an extensive network of colleagues and friends – just as he did when he was a member of the University of British Columbia's Faculty of Medicine. Although from the outside he may have appeared to be a "natural" leader, it was a combination of hard work, a willingness to listen, an ability to organize and communicate his thoughts, and a capacity to recognize and recruit talented people and encourage them to realize their potential that may have made it look easy to a casual observer.

I was exceedingly fortunate to have access to both McGill and Robertson's personal records, all in excellent condition and well organized, which rendered the task of making sense of Robertson's life much simpler than it would otherwise have been. One of these records was his diary, which he kept with considerable determination during significant parts of his life: his days as a McGill student, the war, and particularly his time as principal of McGill. The use of diaries for purposes of biography varies greatly. Some diaries are written with a distinct view as to how the author wishes to be perceived by history (à la Churchill: "History will be kind to me for I intend to write it"), some are little more than mundane accumulations of the details of daily activity, some are therapeutic, and others can be deeply reflective. Robertson's diary entries tend to fall into the middle two categories and were useful principally for cross-checking times and dates. They also provide occasional glimpses – not much more than glimpses – into the low or discouraging points of his life. There are no deep insights, and generally his personal observations about himself and his achievements tend to be understated and clothed in more doubt as to his capacity than he likely felt. For the period when he was principal of McGill, the diary reads as though he knew that it would be read some day (he delivered a copy to McGill when he retired) and did not want to be perceived as having been too full of himself.

Undertaking this work has been an interesting and enjoyable experience, and I hope the reader will take away an understanding of an able and fundamentally gentle man whose deep sense of personal values provided a moral matrix that sustained him throughout a fascinating and often stressful life. It was a life of learning and service, the advancement of medicine, the defence of his country, the advancement of higher education generally, the defence of the position of the English-speaking minority in Quebec, and the shepherding of massive changes in the governance of a publicly funded university. There is no recognition he received that he did not fully earn and many others that he might well have deserved. He wore his honours well and had the additional satisfaction that he had never sought them. He did his duty, did his best in the circumstances, and needed nothing more than the internal peace that came from this knowledge.

Rocke Robertson was a man for his season.

Richard W. Pound
Montreal
September 2007

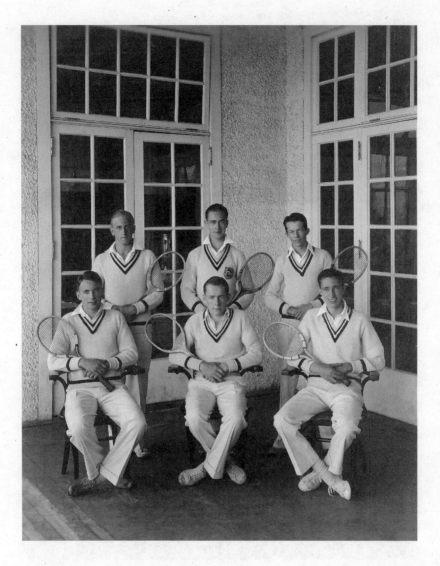

H. Rocke Robertson as a member of the Brentwood College tennis team. David O. Wootten (back left), Ross Hanbury (front centre), H. Rocke Robertson (front left). McGill University Archives (MUA), photographic collection, PR044096

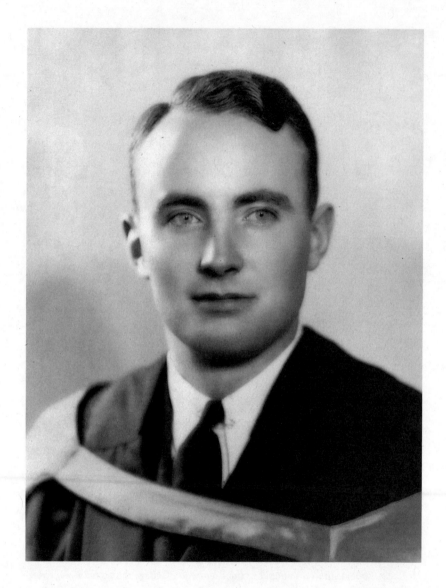

Rocke Robertson at his graduation from McGill University. MUA, *photographic collection,* PA044157

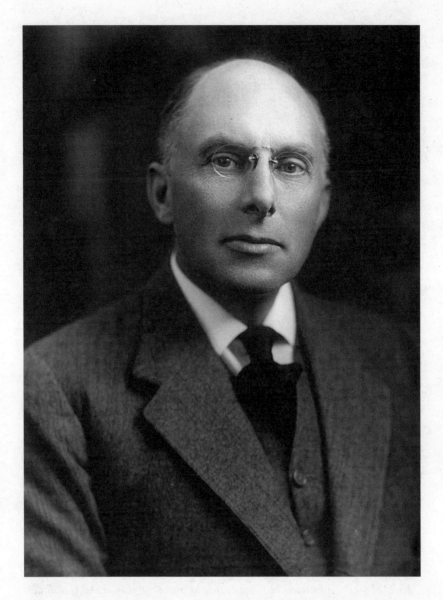

"Uncle Ted," Edmond Melchior Eberts, 1921. McCord Museum of Canadian History, Notman Photographic Collection 11-241905

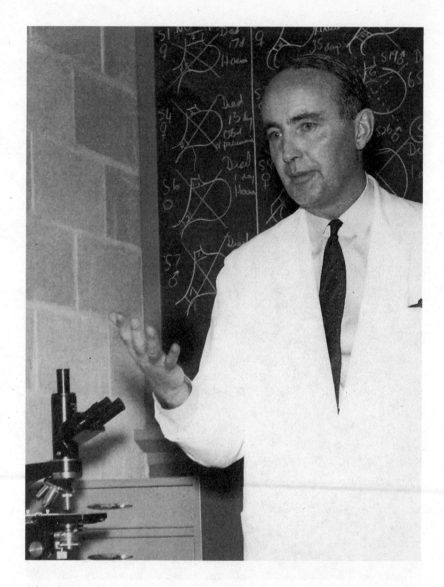

(above) H. Rocke Robertson with microscope at the Montreal General Hospital, 1960. MUA, photographic collection, PU044121

(facing page, above) Montreal General Hospital emergency ward, as designed by H. Rocke Robertson, c. 1960. MUA photographic collection, PA044125

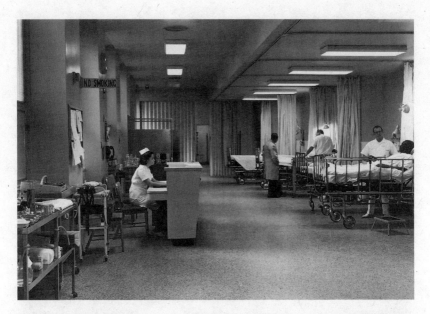

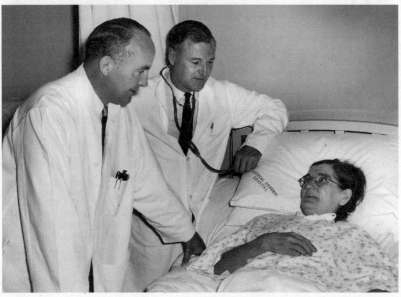

Douglas Cameron, physician-in-chief at the Montreal General Hospital, and H. Rocke Robertson, surgeon-in-chief at the Montreal General Hospital, with a patient, 1960. MUA, photographic collection, PR044122

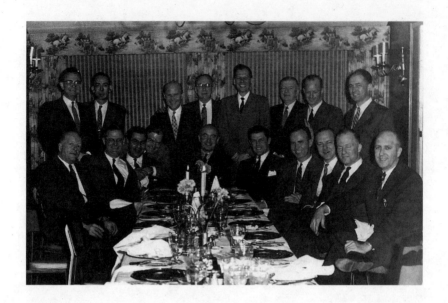

(above) A dinner for some of the members of McGill's Department of Surgery
at Ruby Foo's, c. 1960. Front row, left to right: Ray Lawson, Fraser Gurd, Eddie
Tabah, Arnold Jones, H. Rocke Robertson, Harry Scott, Larry Hampson, Jim
McCorriston, John Palmer, Doug Munroe. Back row, left to right: Don Ruddick,
Bob Estreda, Shorty Long, Cam Dickinson, John Moore, Don Webster, Alan
Thompson, Tony Dobell. MUA, photographic collection, PR044200

(facing page, above) H. Rocke Robertson, Sir James Peterson Ross of Saint
Bartholomew's Hospital, London (visiting professor at McGill University), and
David Wanklyn, president of the Montreal General Hospital, April 1962. MUA,
photographic collection, PR044124

(facing page, below) H. Rocke Robertson, new chairman of the Alma Mater
Fund, studies a fifteen-year chart of the fund with retiring chairman A. Deane
Nesbitt, spring 1962. MUA, photographic collection, PR044081

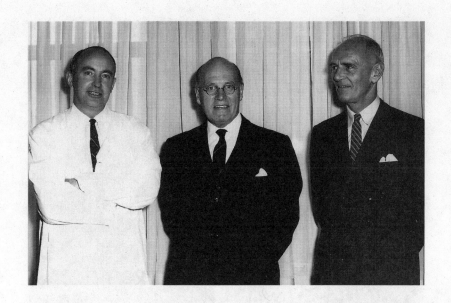

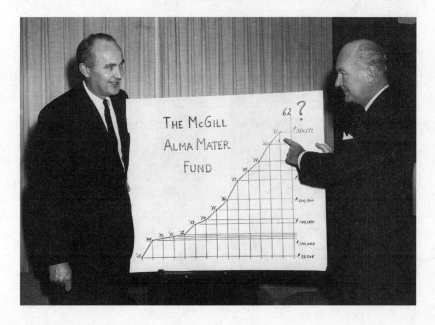

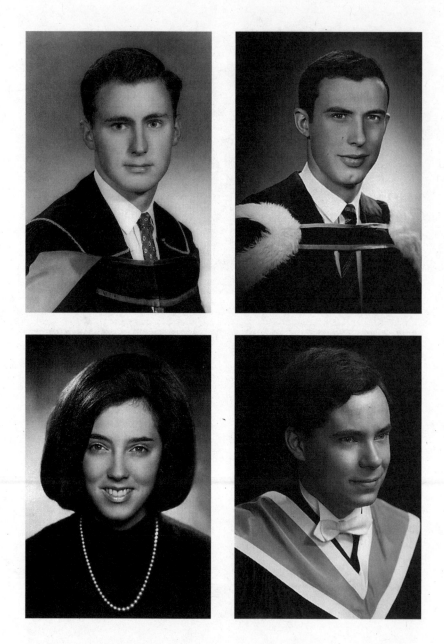

Robertson's children: Thomas (Tam), Ian, Beatrice, and Stuart.

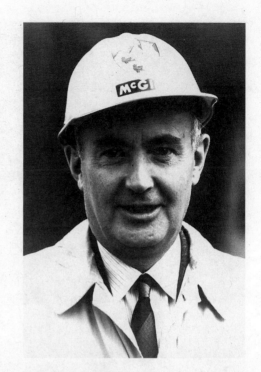

(above) H. Rocke Robertson wearing a construction helmet at the sod-turning for the University Centre, April 1964. MUA, photographic collection, PR036320

(below) Principal H. Rocke Robertson delivering a speech, c. 1965. MUA, photographic collection, PR036303

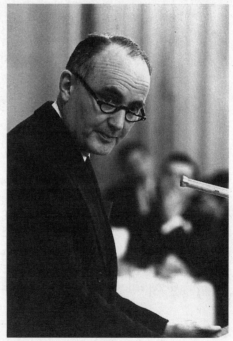

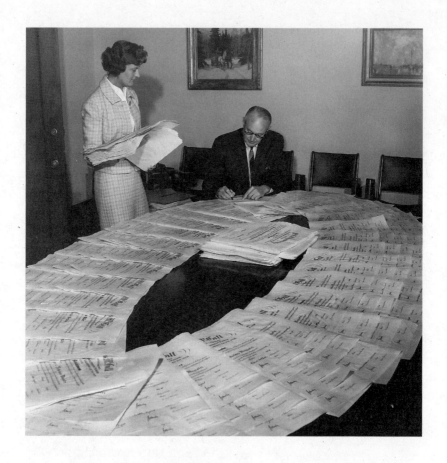

*(above) Principal H. Rocke Robertson signing degrees with secretary,
Mrs S. Ruthven, c. 1965. MUA, photographic collection, PR044136*

*(facing page, above) Hugh MacLennan, McGill professor of English and author;
Donald O. Hebb, McGill chancellor and professor of psychology; H. Rocke
Robertson; Robert E. Bell, McGill principal; and Roslyn Robertson, October 1970.
MUA, photographic collection, PR044002*

*(facing page, below) Montreal General Hospital surgeons-in-chief: Alan
Thompson, Fraser N. Gurd, H. Rocke Robertson, David Mulder, c. 1984. MUA,
photographic collection, PR044199*

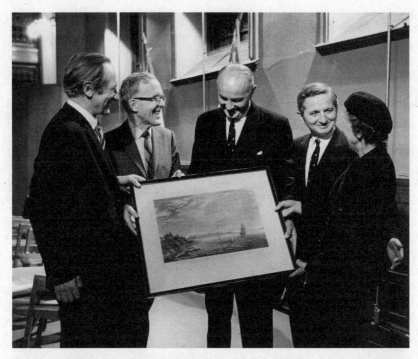

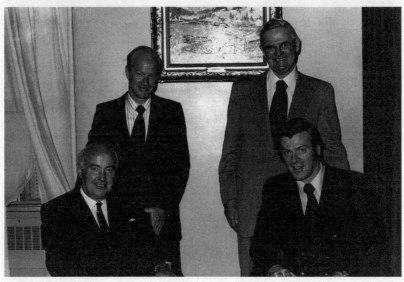

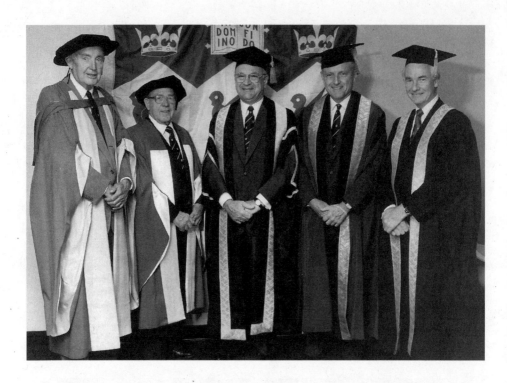

(above) Convocation photos with H. Rocke Robertson, Stanley Frost, Chancellor Albert Jean de Grandpré, chairman of the Board of Governors Hugh G. Hallward, and McGill principal David L. Johnston. MUA, photographic collection, PR044128

(facing page) H. Rocke Robertson and Beatrice Roslyn "Rolly" Robertson at their fiftieth wedding anniversary, 28 June 1987. MUA, photographic collection, PR044047

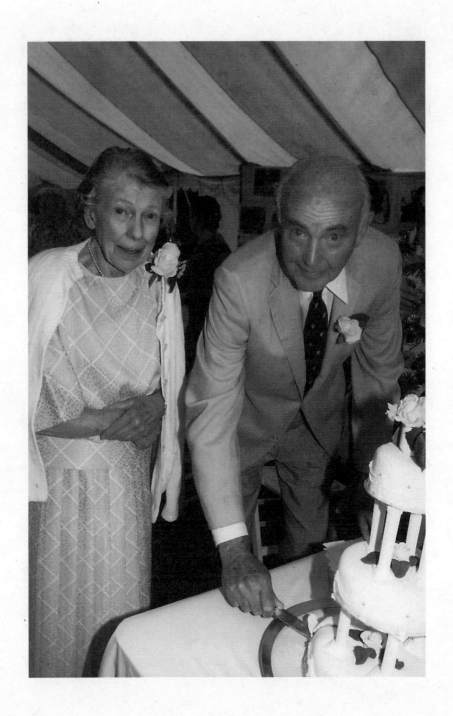

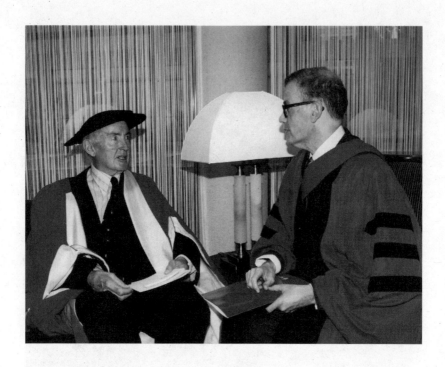

H. Rocke Robertson with new McGill principal Bernard J. Shapiro, 1995. MUA,
photographic collection, PR044130

ROCKE ROBERTSON

FAMILY BACKGROUND AND TRADITIONS

Harold Rocke Robertson was born in Victoria, British Columbia, on 4 August 1912, the youngest of four children born to Harold Bruce Robertson and Helen McGregor Rogers. Some fifty years later, he would become the tenth principal and vice chancellor of McGill University in Montreal, his alma mater, during one of the more tumultuous periods in the existence of the institution. This work surveys a portion of his life.

THE ROBERTSONS

Robertson's family traces its Canadian connections to his great grandfather, Alexander Rocke Robertson, a medical doctor born in Peebles, Scotland, in 1801 and schooled at the Edinburgh Royal Academy of Surgeons, graduating in 1826.[1] After joining the Royal Navy, he served as a surgeon on British war ships, which at the time were all sailing vessels.[2] Upon leaving active military service, he arrived in Canada in 1830, where he was posted, still as a military doctor, in Chatham, Upper Canada, a professional status that saved him the requirement of obtaining a Canadian licence. In this position, he was Chatham's first medical doctor. Although he was then out of direct military service, the times were nevertheless tense, especially with regard to the United States, which had been generally unsatisfied with the outcome of the War of 1812–14. Its expanded navy, although no match for the British on the high seas, was particularly aggressive in what were perceived or claimed as American waters. Chatham was a significant military post, given its proximity to Detroit and access by both land and water. But since there was no active war in progress and because there was a need for medical practitioners, Robertson was allowed to open a medical clinic and pharmacy.

In 1839 Robertson married Euphemia Eberts – the younger sister of the landlords of his medical clinic, daughter of local soldier and trader Joseph Eberts[3] and his wife, Ann Baker[4] – and they had nine children. The second of these was named after his father, but unlike his father, he opted for a career in law.

GRANDFATHER ROBERTSON

The younger Alexander Rocke Robertson was born in Chatham in 1841. He attended the local public school, then went to Caradoc Academy near Windsor and, later, to Upper Canada College in Toronto. Even before he was sixteen, he entered the law offices of Alexander D. McLean in Chatham and had completed his articles before he was old enough to write his Bar examinations, which could be written only when a candidate had attained the age of majority, then twenty-one years. While waiting to write the examinations, he worked in the Toronto offices of Prince and Blain. He was called to the Bar, in what had by then become Canada West, on 1 October 1863 and practised for six months in Windsor in partnership with S.S. Macdonnell before leaving the relatively comfortable eastern part of the country on 31 March 1864 for the separate colonies of British Columbia and Vancouver Island. He had been asked by his uncle, John William Waddell (mentioned later), who was returning to the West after an initial venture there, to accompany Waddell's wife and children on the trip. Waddell convinced him that there was a great future in the West. One description of Robertson contained in the Eberts family history recounts: "From early youth he was noted for steadiness of purpose, suavity of manner, and a bright and happy disposition. Standing over six feet in height, his fine features always lit with smiles, he captivated strangers and friends alike by his imposing presence."[5]

There is every evidence that he was extraordinarily highly respected in the community. No less than the Municipal Council of Windsor passed a resolution wishing him success: "The Council cannot allow a young Gentleman of such high character and promise, born and educated in this part of the Province, to depart for so distant [a] portion of the British Empire without their appreciation of his excellence and worth, nor without expressing to him their wish for his success in a more extended and profitable field for the exercise of his abilities."[6]

In addition to such a glowing testimony, he was presented with a silver watch and an address of regret at his departure, signed by a group of law-

yers, doctors, bankers, newspaper owners, clergymen, and other prominent citizens, in which he was highly praised.

It is not clear why he would have chosen Vancouver Island, as opposed
to the mainland, but perhaps he did so because Victoria was the principal business city at the time. The move itself was more easily imagined than accomplished since there was no railway linking central and
eastern Canada with the West Coast. This was an initiative that would
not come to fruition until post-Confederation, when the new country
became concerned that unless such a railway existed to link the West to
the East, there would be little to prevent northbound expansion of the
United States, whose population had by then reached the West Coast and
which cared little for a line drawn on someone's map along the forty-
ninth parallel. Added to the difficulty was the nightmarish Civil War in
the United States, then still in fratricidal progress. The way to the West
was by train to New York, followed by a hazardous voyage by sea in an
ironside side-wheeler, the *Champion*, one of the Vanderbilt Line. Ships
of the Confederate states regularly laid in wait for federal vessels passing down the East Coast of the continent, which led to the *Champion*
being convoyed for part of the way by the *Neptune*, a federal warship.
The vessel nearly foundered off Cape Hatteras, but it survived and they
eventually landed in Aspinwall (now Colón), Panama, after a call in at
the Bahamas. An overland train brought the travellers to Panama City,
where they sailed on the *Constitution* via Acapulco to San Francisco.
After seven days, they boarded the steamer *Sierra Nevada* and travelled
via Portland, Oregon, to Victoria, docking at Esquimalt on 14 May 1864,
some six weeks after leaving New York.

Victoria, the present capital of British Columbia, had its beginnings as
an outpost of the British Empire. It had first been established as a fort by
the Hudson's Bay Company, construction of which had commenced in
the summer of 1843. Joseph Pemberton had surveyed the land around the
fort (now including Esquimalt and Saanich) and had laid out the township of Victoria in 1851, which was incorporated as a city in 1862. Prior
to the opening of the Panama Canal in 1914, Victoria was arguably the
farthest point of the empire, reachable only after long voyages around the
Cape of Good Hope if one headed east or around the treacherous Cape
Horn on the westerly route.[7] It was a rough and tumble town, gradually
hacked out of the primeval forests, and those willing to risk their lives
and fortunes on the new frontier shared a mutual self-interest in building the community. By June 1863 a legislative council had been appointed

for British Columbia, the first session of which opened at Sapperton in January 1864. In July 1863 an Imperial statute had defined the boundaries of the colony.

The two colonies of British Columbia and Vancouver Island were combined into a single political unit when the Act of Union, passed in the Imperial Parliament in August 1866, was proclaimed three months later in November. Within days of the enactment of the British North America Act on 8 March 1867, there was action in the British Columbia Legislative Council promoting the idea of union with the new confederation, partly to prevent annexation by the United States[8] and partly to try to get relief from the financial troubles experienced in the colony.[9] The Robertson family and many of its connections would play an important role in the development of Victoria and the process of incorporating the colony into the new country gradually taking shape to the east of the Rocky Mountains, which would eventually reach and embrace the Pacific boundaries.

Upon his arrival in Victoria, Robertson found that the colonial Bars were closed to barristers from other parts of Canada, a territorial imperative that would take more than a century to wither away.[10] He nevertheless applied himself to obtaining a local qualification, while making ends meet as a $25-per-week editor of the *Victoria Daily Colonist*, and passed the Mainland Bar in November 1864, thus becoming entitled to practise in British Columbia. The judge presiding at his induction was reported as "expressing the hope that the Bar would have no occasion to regret the step."[11] These were the days following the gold rush that had started in 1858, which had dramatically changed the dynamics within the colonies, with the arrival of thousands of new non-natives resulting in tensions between themselves and the existing population, on the coast and in the interior, as the gold and fur cultures clashed.[12] A good deal of his legal work, in addition to that in New Westminster, was to be found at Yale, in the Cariboo region, then filled with a volatile mix of successful and desperate fortune seekers. After the colonies of British Columbia and Vancouver Island were merged on 17 November 1866 (although maintaining their separate court systems), he also obtained admission to the Vancouver Island Bar.

After practising for three years Robertson had accumulated sufficient means to return to Chatham, where, on 3 March 1868, he married his first cousin, Margaret Bruce Eberts, to whom he had been engaged, and they returned to Victoria. Almost immediately, he was appointed Crown prosecutor at the Yale assizes, and a year and a half later, at the age of twenty-nine, on 10 November 1870, he was elected the fifth mayor of the city of Victoria, in which office he served for a year. This was not an office that he had wanted; when first approached to stand for the mayoralty, he had declined, preferring to devote all his energies to his profession, but he later acceded to the pressure. The comment in the local media was quite laudatory: "It is seldom that so young a man [twenty-nine] has been placed in so exalted a position, but then it is not often that so young a man is possessed of those sterling qualities which fit Mr. Robertson for the position."[13]

He was active in support of Victoria, as opposed to its determined rival, New Westminster, becoming the capital of British Columbia – a hotly debated question of the day. Newspaper accounts in the *Daily Colonist* of his involvement in this debate give some indication both of the struggle and of the enthusiasm with which Robertson engaged in it:

> Mr. A. R. Robertson came forward – saying that he conceived it to be the bounden duty of every citizen to do what he could for his adopted country. Boldly and deliberately he said he would assert that with the exception of the few who had interests in New West-minster, the miners to a man were in favor of Victoria as the capital (applause). It was impossible that there could be two large cities; and if we wished to build up one we must concentrate our exer-tions to build up Victoria (renewed applause). If New Westminster were made the capital another blow would be struck at Victoria, without doing any permanent good. The naval station was here and must remain here. Mr. Robertson said that in weighing the rights of Victoria and New Westminster in the scale, the latter's rights to the capital were 'lighter than a feather shaken from the linnet's wing.' Mr. Robertson retired amid much applause.[14]

In 1871 British Columbia joined Confederation, a decision that he strongly supported. The *Daily Colonist* again described his participation at a "Let's Join Canada" meeting:

> Robertson – in an excellent and telling speech in favor of Confed-eration pointed out the means it would afford us of changing our

present unpopular form of government for one more in keeping with the spirit of the age – a government by the people that would enable the people to legislate for themselves and manage their own affairs. He further showed how it would be the means of attracting population and capital and of strengthening and perpetuating the bond that united them to England. The learned gentleman was loudly applauded.[15]

That September he was elected as a member of the first provincial legislative assembly for the electoral district of Esquimalt. He was appointed to Cabinet on 14 November, both as colonial secretary (later to be redesignated provincial secretary) and as the province's first minister of education, and became known as the father of the British Columbia school system, having introduced the legislation respecting schools.[16] Four years in the Assembly, one as part of the government and three in Opposition, following the defeat of the government in December 1872, proved to be enough, and he did not allow his name to be put forward for re-election to the Legislature or for election to the federal Parliament in a politically safe riding but returned full-time to his legal practice.[17] He was appointed in the first list of British Columbia Queen's Counsel in 1873 and, in 1879, was made legal agent in the province for the Dominion of Canada. On 26 November 1880 the thirty-nine-year-old Robertson, recognized as a leading counsel in the province, was appointed to the bench of the British Columbia Supreme Court, becoming the first Canadian-born justice in the province, assigned in July the following year to the Clinton judicial district near Kamloops.

The *Colonist* was horrified – not because he was unworthy of appointment but because he had had such a bright political future ahead of him:

Mr. Robertson is a young man, being under 40, with many years of what the Americans term 'go' in him. By the acceptance of this office he retires from the active pursuit of his profession, which has been lucrative, and is brought up against a dead wall. Literally, his road to further preferment is blocked. He is shelved at an age when the faculties and energies of most men – and his certainly – are still in the gristle, so to speak, of great expansion and development. We have looked upon Mr. Robertson as one of the coming political lights of the country – with at least 20 years' capacity for the hardest kind of work by him. The acceptance of the position, we fear, is a mistake which he will regret.[18]

His career was cut tragically short when he injured a knee while bathing in the North Thompson River near Kamloops – in the Clinton judicial district to which he had been assigned and where he would eventually have moved his family – and then re-injured it by striking it against a carriage brake. He returned to Victoria for treatment of the extremely painful swollen and inflamed leg, probably leading to blood poisoning. The treatment culminated in unsuccessful surgery and his death shortly thereafter on 1 December 1881.[19] There was a public outpouring of grief and much recognition that the life of a remarkable individual, so obviously destined for greatness, had been cruelly cut short while he was still at the beginning of his prime. His widow returned to Chatham early the following year with their seven children.

FATHER ROBERTSON

The fourth of these children, Harold Edwin Bruce Robertson, was born in Victoria on 26 February 1875. He, too, followed a career in law. He graduated in 1894 with honours in arts from Trinity College, University of Toronto, studied law at Osgoode Hall, and was called to the Ontario Bar on 4 June 1897. He then headed west, like his father before him, and was admitted to the British Columbia Bar, after a qualifying residence of six months and after passing the required examinations, on 19 January 1898. He took up practice in Victoria with his elder brother Herbert. When Herbert went to the Yukon in September 1898, Harold continued the practice alone, until joining up with George Henry Barnard in 1906. Harold married Helen McGregor Rogers from his hospital bed (confined there by a bout with diphtheria, from which he speedily recovered) on 3 June 1903 in Peterborough, Ontario, and they returned thereafter to Victoria.[20] He was very active at the Bar and was a bencher from 1918 until 1933. He was appointed as King's Counsel on 30 January 1922, the only Conservative on the list, and was a partner of the firm then named Barnard, Robertson, Heisterman and Tait. By this time, he had been identified in the *Vancouver Daily Sun* as one of the ablest of the younger generation of lawyers in the province. He appeared before the British Privy Council on several occasions, both as a junior and pleading himself. He was involved in many civic projects, including serving on the board of the Provincial Royal Jubilee Hospital. The City of Victoria appointed him as city counsel to represent it in all court cases, for which he was entitled to the princely sum of $125 per month, with possible extra remuneration for out-of-town cases. In addition to Harold's very successful law career, the couple had four children, of whom Harold Rocke Robertson, the subject of this work, was the youngest.

In 1925 Harold Robertson moved the family to Vancouver, where he was a partner in a firm eventually known as Robertson, Douglas and Symes. It was clear to the legal community and appreciated in the community at large that Harold, respected as a fine lawyer and a kind and intelligent man, was on his way to the bench, and in 1933 he was appointed, as his father had been before him, to the Supreme Court of British Columbia.[21] His name had been brought to the attention of Prime Minister R.B. Bennett by E.P. Davis, the senior partner of the Vancouver firm of Davis, Pugh, Davis, Ralston and Lett, who pointed out, by way of background, that the province had not been very lucky in the appointments to the bench made by past governments and that members of the Bar at large were hoping anxiously for a change in this respect now that Bennett was in power. Davis reminded Bennett that he had been practising for forty years and knew the capacity and ideas of different members of the Bar and thus which of them would constitute good appointments to the bench. Understanding that there would soon be vacancies on both the British Columbia Supreme Court and Court of Appeal, Davis urged that W.E. Burns be appointed to the Supreme Court and Robertson to the Court of Appeal.

Machinations dragged for the better part of a year as matters with the existing judges matured, and it appeared, to those "in the know," that an appointment for Robertson was more or less assured but that it would likely be to the lower court, provided that he would live in Victoria. The latest news was conveyed by telegram on 13 April 1933 from his former partner, now a senator, George Henry Barnard, who said that he would wait in Ottawa instead of returning home if he could be of help. Robertson cabled back the next day, saying that his position of having a strong preference for an appointment to the Court of Appeal was unchanged and that living in Victoria would be too expensive, as he would probably be unable to sell or lease his family's Vancouver home on Marine Drive. He urged Barnard not to stay in Ottawa on his account: "Come home early and don't swear."[22]

George Henry Barnard was "Uncle Harry" to Robertson's children, and his wife was "Aunt Bonnie." The Barnards had no children of their own. Harry had been a partner of Robertson and a great friend. He had been a mayor of Victoria and a member of Parliament (1908–17) before becoming a senator (1917–45). He practised law from time to time but had never had to work too hard for money, having inherited handsomely from his parents. It was his father who had run the famous Barnard Express to the Cariboo. A portion of Uncle Harry's fortune – one-fourteenth each – was passed to the Robertson children after the death of Aunt Bonnie. Harry's greatest claim to fame had resulted from the role he had played in the acquisition of two submarines at the beginning of the First World War. It was an interesting background since at the outbreak of the war Canada, and particularly Victoria, had no means of defence. It appeared that German warships had been sighted in the Pacific and that they were preparing to cease raiding merchant ships and to move north to attack Vancouver and Victoria, now that Canada was on the official list of Germany's enemies. There were, as it happened, two submarines in the Bremerton dockyards near Seattle that had been built for the Chilean navy and that were almost ready for delivery.

The situation was awkward for everyone involved. The Chileans wanted their submarines, the Americans were trying hard to appear neutral (even though an attack on Victoria or Vancouver would be perilously close to home), and the Canadian government, despite an obvious need for the protection and deterrence represented by having two operating submarines in the area, was overly cautious and would not authorize the acquisition. As mayor of Victoria at the time, Harry had played an important role in getting the purchase completed. It was one thing, however, to own two submarines and quite another to put together crews capable of operating them, although with some difficulty this was accomplished. Even more worrying was that there were no torpedoes. This lack, of course, was not mentioned in the course of the official ceremonies with which the submarines were put to sea in the hope that the Germans would learn of their launch and presume them to be properly equipped. In the result, the German admiral Graf Spee did not come close to the coast, whether out of concern for the existence of the submarines or for some other reason. In the event, the morale of British Columbia was greatly improved.

On 6 September 1933 Robertson's appointment to the Supreme Court was announced in Ottawa, and Robertson agreed to return to Victoria so that there would be a sitting judge of the Supreme Court present there. The Court of Appeal position went to William Garland McQuarrie, a former Conservative member of Parliament for New Westminster. Robertson's former partner H.G. Heisterman wrote the following day to congratulate him on his appointment:

> Since I have been practicing I do not know of any Judge's appointment which would give greater satisfaction to the Bar than your appointment, as in the past few months, since the vacancy occurred and speculations have been made as to the possible appointments, members of the Bar on both sides of politics have been unanimous in talking to me that your appointment would be the best one possible.
>
> I am sure it must be very gratifying to know the feeling of the Bar generally towards yourself. Personally I was sorry that you were not appointed to the Appeal Court as you were undoubtedly entitled to this appointment. I think, however, that the Bar from a purely selfish motive will be more pleased with your appointment to the Trial Bench than the Appeal Bench, as you know so much depends upon the Trial Judge, not only in his own Court, but upon his method of dealing with the evidence which to a large extent binds the Appeal Courts, and I know that the Members of the Bar will always feel that your decisions will be reasonable and bona fides.
>
> I, myself, think with appointments of Judges to the Bench – that the vacancies in the Appeal Court should be filled from the Trial Bench as I think it is invaluable to an Appeal Judge that he should have had this experience in considering the appeal which is brought before him, and I hope that in time, as a vacancy in the Appeal Court occurs, that you will be appointed to that Bench, and such an appointment to my mind shows that it is made from outstanding merit rather than from personal considerations.[23]

Public reaction to his appointment was particularly favourable, with extremely positive editorial coverage regarding Robertson's position and some arch comment to the effect that the particular appointment to the Court of Appeal continued the well-known association of this court with political personalities since practically all the members of the court had been leading figures in the political life of the province prior to their appointment.

Ten years later, on 5 July 1943, Robertson was elevated to the British Columbia Court of Appeal, ironically enough to replace McQuarrie, who had died at the end of May. It was, again, a popular appointment, perceived as based on merit and regarded in the media as an important step forward in improving the Court of Appeal. He was never elevated to the position of chief justice of British Columbia. This position had been awarded to Wendell Burpee Farris in May 1942, an appointment made by the Liberal justice minister, Louis St Laurent, prior to Robertson's elevation to the Court of Appeal. An editorial published by the *Vancouver Daily Province* at the time Farris was appointed made it clear that the natural best leader of the court would have been Robertson, by then a very experienced trial judge:

> Mr. Farris takes up his duties under a handicap. He has been actively engaged in provincial and federal politics. He has served his party faithfully, and there is no question that his appointment comes to him as a reward for his services to the party rather than in recognition of his qualifications for the chief justiceship.
>
> If qualification had been the touchstone, the senior puisne judge of the Supreme Court, Mr. Justice Harold Robertson, on the strength of merit and in the public interest, should have received the appointment.
>
> Preferment passes him by. The reward goes to the profession of politics rather than to the profession of the law – and that, in the interests of law and justice, is not desirable.[24]

Harold Robertson retired from the bench on 17 September 1955 at the age of eighty, in the same room where he had been called to the Bar in 1898, and died in Vancouver on 7 June 1961 at the age of eighty-six.[25]

By the time Rocke Robertson was born in 1912, Victoria was well established and increasingly comfortable with its role as capital city, a status conferred by proclamation in May 1868, a few months after the Legislature first met there in December 1867, replacing New Westminster, which had served as the capital since the 1866 merger of British Columbia and Vancouver Island. The population of the province hovered around the half-million mark, ten times what it had been forty years earlier. Business was thriving. The community consisted largely of people of British origin, with some Chinese and First Nations on the fringes. Victoria would eventually become almost a caricature of the British enclave in Canada, made famous by the cartoons of Len Norris in the middle of the twentieth century, published regularly in the *Vancouver Sun*. Not until Rocke Robertson was in his tenth year in 1922 did drivers in British Columbia change from driving on the left-hand to the right-hand side of the road. There were still annual summer visits of units of the Royal Navy, the presence of many cruisers, and on one occasion in the young Rocke's memory, the docking of the battleship HMS *Hood*. The naval visits were cause for great excitement and were celebrated with many sport competitions in cricket, lawn tennis, and track and field. A particularly special occasion was the early autumn of 1919, when the Prince of Wales, later to become, albeit briefly, King Edward VIII, visited Victoria.[26]

EXTENDED FAMILY

The Robertsons maintain a strong sense of family to this day, on both the maternal and paternal sides, and this family quilt had a profound influence on Harold Rocke Robertson throughout his life. The Scottish Robertsons were flanked on the paternal side by Austrian and French heritage, the dominant family being the Eberts, which had intermarried with the Hucques prior to the Napoleonic Wars. The Eberts and Robertson streams had joined when Alexander Rocke Robertson married Euphemia Eberts in 1839. The ties had been strengthened when his son Alexander Rocke Robertson married yet another Eberts, a cousin, Margaret Bruce Eberts, in 1868. The families have remained close for generations. Indeed, it was an uncle, John Waddell, married to a younger sister of his mother, who had encouraged the younger Alexander Rocke Robertson to move west in 1864.

On the other wing of the Robertson line are the Irish and Welsh traditions, the Rogers being of Irish descent and the Burritts of Welsh. Their streams merged with the marriage in 1863 between Henry Cassady Rogers (1839–1914) and Maria Burritt (1838–1913). Their daughter Helen McGregor Rogers (1880–1969) was the mother of Harold Rocke Robertson. Rogers had been born in the township of Haldimand, Upper Canada. At the age of fifteen, he joined the Peterborough Rifle Company and was in command of this corps during the Fenian raids of 1866–67 at the age of twenty-seven. He lived in Peterborough, where he was originally a merchant, until his appointment as postmaster, a position he held for some thirty-eight years until his retirement in 1909. In 1872 he organized and took command of the First Peterborough Troop of Cavalry, with the rank of major. The unit later became "G" Troop of the 3rd Prince of Wales Canadian Dragoons, a regiment he commanded for a time with the rank of lieutenant colonel.

Rogers married Maria Burritt, eldest daughter of Dr Walter Horatio Burritt of Smiths Falls, in September 1863. During her childhood, there had been a particularly hard winter, and several Indians came to the Burritt house for food, knowing that despite the scarcity of food for all, they would not be sent away empty-handed. Maria's mother went to get something together, leaving her in the cradle. Returning to the door, she found the cradle empty and the Indians carrying off Maria. She gave chase, pushed the woman carrying Maria to the ground, picked up the child, ran back to the house and barricaded the door. The Indians did not return. The mother was an intrepid soul who was reputed, while the doctor was off on his rounds, to have killed a wolf that was trying to get at the carcasses of two sheep hung in a shed behind the house. Maria suffered from asthma in later life and, even before Henry retired, was forced to move to Victoria for her health, living with her daughter Ethel, who had married George Henry Barnard, until she was joined in 1909 by the retired Rogers. They lived the balance of their lives in Victoria.

OTHER TRIBUTARY FAMILIES

In and around the direct lines were several other families, including Loewen (of Prussian origin), Smith (Upper Canadian), Barnard (Quebecois), and Waddell (Scottish), between which there were many marriages that produced a fascinating, if somewhat complex, family tree. It was a tree well nurtured by its members, each family conscious both of its own line and of the others with which it had been merged. The extended family was and remains very much aware of the main exploits and life stories of its members.

Johann Joseph Loewen (1832–1906), the son of Johann Loewen and Sophia Endress, was born in Ediger, on the Mosel River, then within the Kingdom of Prussia, and had sailed for the United States in 1848, settling in New York, until he left for California in 1856, where he was engaged in mining for two years. He left California for the Crown colony of Vancouver Island, arriving in Victoria on 4 July 1858. In Victoria he met and married Eva Margaret Laumeister (1842–1917), who had been born in Memingen, Bavaria. With his brother-in-law Frank Laumeister, he purchased a flour mill and distillery, but they were destroyed by fire in 1869. Three years later he founded the Victoria Brewery with Ludwig E. Erb. Joseph was active in the management of the business as a proprietorship until 1892, when it was reorganized as a corporation, Victoria Phoenix Brewery Ltd, of which he became president. The business grew in size and reputation, both for progressive methods and responsible business conduct.[27] Joseph was widely recognized as one of the pioneer settlers of Victoria and was active in development of the area prior to his death in 1906 at the family home, named Rockwood.

William Henry Smith (1826–71), born in Cornwall, Upper Canada, the son of a cobbler, became a progressive and self-made man. As had the elder Alexander Rocke Robertson, he married into the Eberts family, forming a union with Frances Jane Eberts (1826–84), the youngest daughter of Joseph Eberts and Ann Baker. Prior to the wedding, Smith had been the purser on one of the ships owned by Frances's elder brother William and after the wedding became captain of one of the vessels and continued to work for the Eberts family. He died in Owen Sound at the age of forty-five.

Francis Jones Barnard (1829–89) was born in Quebec City, and family lore has it that he was a direct lineal descendant of the Francis Barnard who had settled in Deerfield, Massachusetts, sometime prior to 1642. His father operated a hardware business in Quebec but died suddenly in 1841, leaving Francis to work at the age of twelve to support his mother and the rest of the family. In 1853 he married Ellen Stillman, also of Quebec, and they later moved to Toronto. There he suffered business reverses and left his wife and young family in the spring of 1859, bound for the Colony of British Columbia, where he first earned money by carrying cordwood to Yale and then sawing and splitting the wood. He later staked a gold claim, which he sold at a profit, and in the summer of 1859 he secured an appointment as a constable in the town of Yale. The next year he landed a position as purser on the steamer *Fort Yale* and, having put together a small stake of money, sent for his wife and children, who arrived in December 1860. On 14 April 1861 he narrowly escaped death when the steamer exploded just below Hope, killing the captain – who had ordered up excessive steam pressure in an effort to make up lost time against fast water – and several of the crew. Francis had been thrown clear and was rescued by some of the local Indians. In the fall of 1861 he started an express business, carrying letters and papers on his back, by foot, from Yale to the Cariboo, a round trip of 760 miles. The next year he established a pony express over the same route and later formed the Barnard Express Company, known as "BX," which was the longest stagecoach line in North America. In 1866 he was elected to the British Columbia Legislature for Yale, where he served until 1870. He was one of the prime movers and fathers of Confederation in British Columbia (as was the second Alexander Rocke Robertson) and served two terms in the federal Parliament for the riding of Yale-Kootenay starting in 1879, despite suffering a stroke in 1880 that left him partially paralyzed. He did not stand for re-election in 1887 and declined an offer of a senatorship in 1888 due to his ill health. He died the following year at the age of sixty.

His son Frank Stillman Barnard (1856–1936) was born in Toronto and moved west with the family when they left Toronto in 1860. His early education in Victoria was followed by a return to the East for further study at Hellmuth College, and then he joined Barnard Express as president from 1882 to 1886. He married Martha Amelia Loewen, daughter of Joseph Loewen, in Victoria in 1883. Frank was elected to the House of Commons as a Conservative representing the Cariboo from 1888 to 1896, after which he became one of the founders and later the managing director of the BC Electric Company from 1896 to 1899. In 1914 he was appointed lieutenant governor of British Columbia, in which office he served for five years. In 1919 he was knighted by King George V and admitted to the Most Distinguished Order of St Michael and St George with the class of knight commander, an order established for those rendering distinguished service in the colonies and in foreign affairs. The Barnard home in Victoria, called Clovely, was considered one of the most beautiful homes in the city. Frank died on 11 April 1936 at the age of eighty, less than three months after the death of the king who had knighted him. George Henry Barnard was his younger brother.

The Waddells had appeared in North America in the person of captain William Waddell (1778–1861), a Scot who had served in the Royal Dragoons. Serving under Wellington in Europe, he was seriously wounded during the Battle of Waterloo in June 1815, in which his hands and arms were severely crippled as a result of cannon shot. He returned to Edinburgh to marry Isabella Bell, to whom he had become engaged prior to the war. In 1834 he and his family, together with a large number of other officers on half-pay and their families, emigrated to Upper Canada. He settled at first in York (now Toronto), before moving to Niagara-on-the-Lake and then to Chatham, where he died at the age of eighty-three.

William Waddell's eldest child, John William Waddell (1818–70), came to North America shortly before the rest of the family, taking a position with Moffatt, Murray and Company in Montreal. In 1843 he married Nancy Almira Eberts (1820–1900), another daughter of Joseph Eberts and Ann Baker. After the wedding he worked as a purchasing agent in the shipping firm owned by his brothers-in-law William and Walter Eberts, living initially over one of the stores in the Eberts Block in Chatham. He later owned a lumber mill near the French River, as well as three ships built in his own shipyard, and served the public as high sheriff in the counties of Essex, Kent, and Lamberton in Upper Canada. Lured to British Columbia in 1862 by the gold rush, where he hoped to recover from business losses, he sent for the family in 1864, who were accompanied on the trip by the second Alexander Rocke Robertson. At one stage Waddell had been the western correspondent for the *Globe* newspaper. He returned with his family to Chatham a few years later and was drowned at Goderich in 1870 at the age of fifty-two.

CONCLUSION

The families were rich with exciting histories, some of triumph and some of tragedy, but all with distinction, one way or the other, and it was not surprising that the young Harold Rocke Robertson would absorb both the strong connections that surrounded the family and the sense that one was also expected to achieve, to keep up one's own end of the family and the next generation. Indeed, in the generations before him, there seemed to be a real "gene" that produced a drive to create, to open up, and to develop new things – a drive that acquired a sort of tradition but that was largely devoid of self-interest. This manifested itself in different areas of society, such as performing at social gatherings with the Victoria Amateur Band, in which his father played the violin, and running the Sunday School for children at the Church of St John the Evangelist in Victoria. The previous generations had possessed almost unbounded ambition, although it had nothing to do with being rich but instead was focused almost always in the direction of public or community service. This produced a profound sense of personal values among family members and a sense of a responsibility to assume leadership, to lead by example, and generally, to be leaders. For Rocke, the immediate example was of course his father (who had almost certainly been tremendously influenced by the remarkableness of his own father), and he saw himself – or more accurately, came to see himself as his understanding grew – as someone who should stand as his father had in public, not personal, service. It would become a hallmark of the emerging Rocke Robertson.

But as with Michelangelo's sculpture of David, it would take some time to chip away the unessential overburden and reveal the central character beneath.

COMING OF AGE, MCGILL
UNIVERSITY, AND MARRIAGE

Life at home for Rocke Robertson was comfortable by any standards. His father was a successful lawyer, and although money may have been tight in 1905 when he built the house at 510 St Charles Street in Victoria for the considerable sum in those days of $5,000, by the time of Rocke's arrival on the scene in 1912 the financial pressure was off and the house had acquired its name of Heatherdale. It was a large house, with a significant vestibule, drawing room with two fireplaces, big hall, library with another fireplace, sun room, nursery, dining room, pantry, kitchen, servants' quarters, four bedrooms and two bathrooms on the second floor, and upstairs at the back two more bedrooms, a long trunk room, and a veranda. It was built on a narrow but deep lot, measuring about 70 feet by 350 feet, that was well treed, mostly with oak, and that had enough lawn for some cricket and rounders of a sort for the boys. Daffodils were the main attraction, possibly because they were the only flowers that could survive a constant barrage of cricket, soccer, and tennis balls.

For the first eight years of his life, the family went regularly to its summer home at Shawnigan Lake, "The Pines," for the entire summer. Rocke recalled the swimming, boating, fishing, and treks through the woods – also going for the mail and getting the milk each day in the family launch, *Helen*, as well as the steady stream of visitors, capped with the special excitement of the Barnard visits (they always brought splendid foods, cakes, and watermelons). The place was sold in 1920, and thereafter the family spent summers at various places on Vancouver Island, on the Cowichan River, and at Qualicum Beach, the latter being ideal for summer vacations, with its superb beach, golf course, tennis courts, woods, streams, waterfalls, trout fishing (sea trout at the mouth of the rivers and brook and rainbow in the streams), and salmon fishing in the sea – altogether everything for which a young boy could possibly wish.

A special memory was a several-day expedition to Butler's Lake, with a drive to the base camp and then a nine-mile hike along a trail, carrying part of their gear, the balance of the food, and bedding loaded on pack horses, to the log cabin where they stayed. The cabin had not been occupied for some time prior to the visit, which required them to invest considerable effort to fix it up for inhabitation. The main purpose of the expedition was to fish, which they did with great enthusiasm. Rocke was too young to fish alone, so he accompanied his father, while the others set out on their own, some in boats, others along the river flowing out of the lake. When they reassembled at the end of the afternoon, they were embarrassed to find that they had brought in dozens of fish – each of them had thought that he had been extraordinarily lucky – which they could not possibly eat and which would undoubtedly rot long before they were to leave. The dilemma was solved the next day when they built a smoke house out of some logs and shingles and smoked the fish. They had smoked trout at home for several weeks thereafter.

Rocke's early writing efforts showed some flair, if little discipline, as may be seen from a letter that he wrote on 24 June 1921, not long before his ninth birthday, with original spelling and punctuation:[1]

Dear Dad, or people at Chenesiton house.

How are you getting along? And have you won any cases yet? I hope so. Today we went to the willowes beach. I had a swim with some other kids it was quite cold but not very. Tonight we lost my cricket ball, at least Alan did. it was lost just on top of a birds nest so we did not touch it. Aunt E. went out tonight to aunt Mables. We have had some of our exams and altogether I got 107/145.
must
     stop
        now
            Rocke.

P.S. something got my guine pig[2]

The elder boys, first Bruce and then Alan, had been sent initially to boarding school at Shawnigan Lake and later to Trinity College School in Port Hope, Ontario, following which their academic careers diverged.

Bruce went to Trinity College at the University of Toronto, while Alan went into business, various pursuits that included stock broking, just in time to experience the market crash in 1929, but ended up at British Columbia Sugar Refinery, eventually becoming vice president and secretary. He was twice married and had three children with his first wife and two with his second. He was an unhappy restless person, witty and delightful most of the time but with a darker side, and died at the age of sixty of liver failure.

Bruce had a much happier life. He had fallen in love, while still an undergraduate at Trinity College, with Jean Campbell of Thorold, Ontario, and they decided to marry despite the fact that Bruce was only nineteen and neither of them had any money. They decided to keep the marriage a secret, but this plan was thwarted when an official of the college, who had gone to examine the register for some unrelated reason, noticed Bruce's signature and felt duty bound to report this because there was a college rule that married men could not "live in." The family, which did not know that Bruce was courting anyone, let alone had married her, was flabbergasted. They had no idea who the girl was, nor did they know anything about her family. He might have ruined his career, but it turned out perfectly, and they were happily married for sixty-five years. He did well at Trinity and articled at his father's law offices in Victoria and Vancouver, following which he was a successful barrister for many years before joining the British Columbia Electric Company as vice president and general counsel. After the provincial government took over the company, he became chairman and president of British Columbia Power Corporation and spearheaded the legal battle against the province to get a better deal for the expropriated shareholders, his conduct in this effort being much praised. He was later appointed to the British Columbia Court of Appeal, where he sat, as had his father, until reaching the mandatory retirement age. Upon his retirement from the bench, he joined the Vancouver law firm of Russell and DuMoulin as a consultant, his advice being much sought, and he occupied the position until his death in 1989. Rocke was of the view that his eldest brother had one of the best brains that he had ever encountered, with an extraordinary memory and an ability to marshal facts that he had never seen equalled.

Primary education for Rocke began in Victoria with two years at St Christopher's School and was followed by four years at St Michael's, where the masters were all English and, with the exception of the headmaster and founder of the school, Kyrle Symons, all uniformly uninspiring to their young pupils. Symons, who had devoted his life to the school, was a superb teacher, and the students revered him – which in those days was analogous to fearing him as well. The school games, not surprisingly, were soccer and cricket. Rocke became head prefect at the school. The principal non-British sport was ice hockey, in which Victoria had a local professional team, the Cougars, which had the temerity to defeat the visiting Montreal Canadiens for the 1925 Stanley Cup, winning the best-of-five series three games to one.[3]

With this thrill fresh in mind, even more excitement was in store for Rocke that year when his parents decided that their mother should take his fifteen-year-old sister, Marian, to France and Switzerland for a year and that the thirteen-year-old Rocke should accompany them. The purpose of the trip always remained a bit of a mystery within the family, and Rocke himself was never quite sure why it occurred. Marian was a gorgeous young teenager and no doubt as unmanageable as today's teens, so it might have been intended to get her out of the environment in which she was then involved. The two elder boys were well ensconced in boarding school at Shawnigan Lake, and Rocke was young enough to be pulled out of his classes without serious damage to his studies. The father was in the process of disengaging from his practice in Victoria, in preparation for a move to Vancouver. Perhaps it was simply time for the Grand Tour and Rocke was a lucky beneficiary.

They took the four-day trip across Canada by train, then had a glimpse of the Chateau Laurier and Rideau Canal before going on to Montreal and sailing on the SS *Melita* for the Continent. On board, they met a family by the name of Ballantyne, from Pasadena, California, and their children, Betty and Billy. Betty was two years older than Rocke and not the slightest bit interested in the smitten adolescent, who then made friends with the younger Billy. After a few days in Paris, the families met again to go to Grenoble, where Rocke and Billy were to attend a local *lycée*.

The *lycée* experience was radically different from what he had been accustomed to in Victoria. The classroom days were nine hours, coupled with heavy loads of homework. There were no sports, either as part of the curriculum or even during recess. The North Americans presented a football to the class, which was thrilled, and they played at recess, dourly observed by the professor. To the shock and dismay of everyone, Billy was suddenly afflicted with a fatal illness (staphylococcal septicemia).

Rocke was then dispatched to Switzerland to attend the École Nouvelle la Chataigneraie in Coppet, just along the shore of Lac Léman from Geneva toward Lausanne. This was a boarding school with a genuine cosmo-politan student body and excellent teaching. It was, Rocke later recalled, typically French – very intense, precise, and particular, while bordering on nit-picking, but good nevertheless for the developing student. He wel-comed it and, even at the age of thirteen, recognized that he needed a lot of such work. They spent the Christmas holidays skiing and skating, including a day in Chamonix, where the first Olympic Winter Games had been held the year before.[4] For Easter, they went to Cannes, where the price he paid for his mornings of tennis was to be dragged in the afternoons to the *dansants* at the great hotels by Marian, where she rev-elled in the attention paid to her still developing beauty by the omnipres-ent gigolos, while the only solace for the uninterested younger brother lay in the superb and ubiquitous patisseries.

Summer of 1926 found the travellers in Britain, with a tour of England and Scotland. England had just recovered from a general strike, and the people were still talking about it, amazed at how well the students had managed to operate the trains and taxis and other essential services. Most seemed to regard the matter – in retrospect and after a settlement that had gone very much in the government's favour – as something of a lark.[5] Rocke was present at the famous (in cricket history) test match between Australia and England, notably the Hobbs-Sutcliffe innings, over which cricket enthusiasts, swaddled in the cocoon of cricket lore, still enthuse. While staying in London, they had the rare experience of visiting a huge estate and getting a taste of a vanishing era. Rocke's father had done some legal work in British Columbia for Sir Robert Kindersley, a director of the Bank of England and of the Hudson's Bay Company, who invited the three to his Surrey estate, sending an enormous Daimler limousine – the corporate jet of its day – to the Howard Hotel in the Strand to fetch them. There were some thirty guests present for a sumptuous lunch, served by liveried footmen and uniformed maids. In the afternoon the guests had the choice of tennis on the new *en tout cas* court surface, cricket (a match pitting family and guests against the household and garden staffs and tenants), golf on the estate's private nine-hole course, or a walk around the estate with some possible shooting. Few estates of this size will have survived the past century's double burdens of upkeep and taxes.

By the time they returned to Canada, his father had completed his professional transition from Victoria to Vancouver, where the family took up residence, but Rocke was nevertheless sent to Brentwood College in Victoria, where he remained for his final three years of high school, becoming head boy in the process. The school was new, developed along the lines of the British public schools. The staff, all English, were not able to engage the students, who remained unchallenged. Sports were all-important and the much-abused English penchant for corporeal punishment was a regular feature of the school. During the summer of his graduation, 1929, Rocke worked in the Hanbury's Mill under the Granville Street bridge in Vancouver, shoveling sawdust for forty cents an hour.

Once Rocke, Marian, and their mother had returned from the European trip, Marian had been sent back east to school, as had her older brothers, but in her case to the private girls school at Compton in Quebec, from which she then returned to Vancouver. She fell in love with a flyer from New York, Samuel Porter Hopkins, and they were married in Vancouver in 1931. While on their honeymoon in Santa Barbara, they attended an air show, where Hopkins was recognized by one of the promoters, who prevailed upon him to perform a few aerial stunts for the amusement of the crowd. To everyone's horror, he crashed into the field in front of the grandstand where Marian was sitting and was instantly killed. Marian was, quite understandably, deeply disturbed for a considerable time, spending a winter in New York with Hopkins' mother and a summer or two in Vancouver. She would never fly thereafter and, indeed, seldom travelled. For any personal contact with her, the family would generally have to visit her.

In the winter of 1932 she went with her mother to Tucson, Arizona, and met some men connected with a dude ranch, the Teepee Lodge, in Wyoming. She became attracted to the idea of life on a dude ranch and resolved to go back to the Teepee Lodge the next summer. Her father did not want her to go alone and dispatched Rocke to accompany her, not something he wanted to do, especially having already organized a summer job for himself, but he was left without a choice in the matter. The summer turned out to be a great deal of fun, during which he rode, played scrub polo, fished, danced, drank corn whiskey (Prohibition was still in effect), and generally enjoyed himself.[6] During the summer, Marian met Allen Fordyce, with whom she fell deeply in love. When the time came to return home, Marian decided to stay, and it was left to Rocke to report to the family on their engagement and decision to get married as soon as possible. Rocke's parents (as his grandparents had been when Bruce and Jean had married without their knowledge) were most upset, never having heard of the intended husband, and feared the worst. A cowboy, as they assumed him to be, could not possibly make a good husband. Marian was, however, determined to proceed – and did. They lived happily together for many years and had three children. Allen was a state senator and operated a huge horse ranch, the Bar-13. Rocke only learned after Marian's death in 1982 that she had died of liver failure, not unlike her brother Alan, who would die three years later.

EAST TO McGILL

The decision had been made to send Rocke to McGill University, and in the fall of 1929 he enrolled in second-year arts. As in many families of English descent, it was quite a normal tradition to send children "away" for their schooling and higher education. The other children had also been sent east for schooling, so it was not completely out of the ordinary that Rocke might be as well. There was an early family sense that he would be special, and he was directed accordingly. British Columbia was seen as too small and too colonial, and there had never been any serious thought that he might attend the University of British Columbia. Rocke himself did not like Victoria and was only slightly more accepting of Vancouver, perceiving both as too small. For a wider view of the world and to create a broader platform, he wanted to get out of British Columbia. Western alienation aside, the family recognized that central Canada was where things "happened." There was then at McGill only a single faculty combining arts and science. Rocke's degree, granted in 1932, would, however, be a bachelor of science in the Faculty of Arts. In those days, students could get into the first year of a normal four-year undergraduate program with a junior matriculation, awarded after grade 11 in Quebec, but one who had a senior matriculation (grade 12 in Quebec and grade 13 in the other provinces) could enter directly into the second year.

However, it was not as though there were no family connections with McGill. On his mother's side of the family, Duncan Rogers was a medical graduate, along with Richard Birdsall Rogers, who played in some of the early McGill football games, became an engineer, and built many of the lift locks in the Peterborough area. On the Robertson side, two of his uncles were also McGill graduates, Herman Melchior Eberts Robertson (a younger brother of his father and a friend of Sir Arthur Currie) and Alexander Septimus Rocke Robertson. All of them were very positive about McGill. Two of his father's cousins had graduated from McGill's medical school, one of whom was Edmond Melchior ("Ted") Eberts, who had grown up in the Winnipeg area and reinforced the sense of the larger stage offered by Montreal and McGill. He would play an important role in the direction of Rocke's studies and was always referred to as "Uncle" Ted. Another decision was that he should become a professional. Business, although not denigrated within the family, was nevertheless not seen as responsive to the calling, high standing, and leadership of someone with his perceived potential. Probably the only two professions given any serious consideration were medicine and law, both of which had significant family precedents. His grandfather and father had been prominent lawyers, and his eldest brother, Bruce, was also a lawyer. Whether due to a sense of the family stock being "lawyered out" or because he did not want to compete with his brother, he opted for medicine.

McGill was a much smaller university than it is today, consisting of some 2,300 students. The principal of the day was First World War hero Sir Arthur Currie, much revered by the entire university community.[7] Rocke met him and was astonished by his extremely retentive memory, one example of which was demonstrated at the principal's reception for freshmen – to which an invitation was extended to all in such terms that it was a virtual command performance that none of the new students even considered not accepting. Waiting to be introduced, they were initially somewhat nervous but became less so as they saw how Currie greeted each student warmly. The only possible connection Rocke might have was that he had been born in Victoria, where Currie had lived for several years prior to the war, although Currie had been away from the city for many years thereafter. Rocke's name was announced in the stentorian voice of the butler.

"Robertson," said Sir Arthur, "where were you born?"

"Victoria, sir," he replied.

"Is your father Herman?"

"No, sir, my father's name is Harold. Herman is my uncle."

"Tell me, how is your aunt Ethel?"

"Very well, thank you, sir."

"All right, Robertson, carry on."[8]

Herman Melchior Eberts Robertson had been a regimental surgeon during the war and later enjoyed a long and distinguished career as a surgeon in Victoria. Aunt Ethel was Ethel Burnham Rogers, who married Harry (George Henry) Barnard. The Barnards were inseparable friends of Rocke's parents in Victoria. She was unable, as the result of a medical accident, to bear children, and the Barnards treated the young Robertsons as though they were also their own children.[9]

Although he may not have fully assessed it at the time, Rocke experienced one element of how Sir Arthur excelled in dealing with people and how his officers and men, while he was in command of the army, and after the war the professors and students admired him for his warmth and his ability to extract their best from them. Memory played a part in this quality and was an instrument that Currie used to establish a bond of recognition wherever possible. Thinking about this later in life, Rocke concluded that the vital element in the relationship was the fact of recognition. How it happened did not really matter, so long as it happened, even if it proved to be a mechanical process, not unlike, he concluded, the playing of a gramophone record in which the grooves are cut and are not readily changed. He got a clue, which later formed part of his more mature assessment of the initial episode, when, a few weeks after the principal's reception, he was walking up the campus driveway and encountered Currie, striding toward him, looking enormous in a fur-collared great coat, swinging his cane. As they passed, Currie waved his cane and roared, "Good morning!" Rocke tipped his hat and hurried on until brought up short by another roar, even louder than the first.

"Robertson!"

Back he trotted.

"Aren't you Robertson?"

"Yes, sir."

"Where were you born?"

"Victoria, sir."

"Is your father Herman?"

"No, sir, my father's name is Harold. Herman is my uncle."

"Tell me, how is your Aunt Ethel?"

"Very well, thank you, sir."
"All right, Robertson, carry on."[10]

Something of the same nature took hold in Robertson, whether in emulation of Currie or on his own initiative, prompting him to generate the same kind of connection through recognition. In addition to extensive diaries and notes, Robertson adopted the practice of keeping notes on cards about colleagues, students, and others, in which he would record facts, names, impressions, and other data. This practice assisted his already retentive memory and allowed him to keep track of the names of spouses, children, birthdays, and other factoids regarding each person, which he could bring to any encounter. The bonds with each were immeasurably strengthened, and they were flattered and impressed that he cared enough to remember them.

Academic life was mixed, with some excellent professors and some who were less appealing to him. Like many McGill students before and after him, he noted that there was little tutoring, not much classroom discussion, and no encouragement of discussion with the professors outside of class. He enjoyed biology, French, the English novel, and organic chemistry. He hated philosophy, the course given by the dean of arts, Ira Allan MacKay, who, he considered, failed miserably in making sense of Locke, Berkley, Hume, and Kant. To be fair, however, the entire fault should perhaps not be entirely laid at the professor's doorstep since Robertson, for his own part, exhibited no indications of any particular brilliance in either of his first two undergraduate years, where his averages were 67 per cent and 61 per cent respectively.[11] Being young and a long way from home for the first time, academic priorities probably did not seriously interfere with having a good time.

Like many of the students of the day, he joined one of the Greek-letter fraternities, in his case the Alpha Delta Phi, which collected many of the sons of well-known, well-heeled, and well-established Montreal families, plus others of suitable social plumage, a category into which Rocke fitted very nicely.[12] Many of these fraternities, between riotous weekend bashes, solemnly positioned themselves as literary societies, and there were regular weekly meetings, at which members would present their essays or speeches, few of which demonstrated any particular merit or revealed budding Pulitzer or Nobel Prize winners. Following each, there would be desultory discussion before more stimulating refreshment was sought.

Rocke's own contribution on one such occasion, dealing with the subject of Helen Keller, was cheerfully rated by the jury of his literary peers (a jury whose uniformly bloodthirsty decisions would have delighted Madame Defarges a century and a third earlier) as the poorest within living memory. However, the fraternity house at 3478 McTavish Street, in which Rocke lived while at McGill – now the site of the building that houses the Students Society of McGill University – was comfortable, and he made many lifelong friends among the presumptive literati.[13] One of his many qualities was that he made friends easily throughout his life and retained these friendships.

His McGill surroundings provided a sheltered and largely conservative social environment that left him generally unaware of many of the important political and societal developments in and around Montreal, as well as at McGill itself. He had no idea of the vocal left-wing voices of his day and even no idea of the Communist activities that were taking place, having heard only a bit about Frank Scott, a fraternity brother somewhat senior to him. Even then, he knew of Scott not as a political figure but primarily as a teacher of constitutional law, spoken of with awe by the law students. He never heard about Leon Edel[14] or Norman Bethune.[15] In retrospect, he rather wished that he had kept his eyes open wider. Left-wing activities at McGill would come back to torment him three decades later.

He played intercollegiate tennis for the McGill varsity team and was a substitute on the football team, allowed, he once observed, on the field only after the team's cause was hopelessly lost – usually shortly after the second half began. Despite his enthusiasm for the Stanley Cup-winning Victoria Cougars and hockey in general, he could skate only well enough to be goalie on class and fraternity teams. He played rugby and reached a college final in boxing (160 lbs). His tennis, however, was considerably more than passable, and he partnered with Laird Watt to win the intercollegiate doubles title in 1934, defeating the dogged Ken Farmer (later to play ice hockey on the Canadian team at the 1936 Olympic Winter Games) and Robert Murray, also of McGill, in five sets. The next two years, following Watt's graduation, Rocke partnered with Murray to win the intercollegiate championships in doubles, earning McGill letters in all three years. They were all good players, with Murray and Watt being invited to try out for the Canadian Davis Cup team, in which they both succeeded.[16] Rocke had a strong service and a good overhead game but was never good enough to defeat either Murray or Watt in singles and carry away the Martin Trophy, awarded for the outstanding singles player at McGill.

His academic program was combined arts and medicine, the latter of which he began in the fall of 1932. The students began at once with anatomy, which occupied most of the first year and a good part of the second. He thought the teaching was fair, with some outstanding exponents, among them Horst Oertel in pathology, a great undergraduate teacher, so effective that his graduates occupied the chairs of several departments of pathology in North America.[17] Doctors Burgess,[18] Scrimger,[19] and Meakins[20] were excellent as well, and he remembered vividly the thrilling and spine-tingling Saturday-morning clinics given by Oertel and Burgess. He could recall so many actual scenes during these episodes that he became convinced that fear (or perhaps any strong emotion) was a great fixative – one was inclined to remember things that were "inputted" when one was frightened. Judging from his marks, he might have had good reason to be fearful in the early years, but sufficient fear had not yet spurred him to great results.[21]

Fear or talent, whatever it may have been, seemed in his two final years to have caused the academic penny to drop, and his performance went through a quantum improvement. He won the Joseph Morley Drake Prize in pathology in 1934–35, his third year. He had failed pathology the previous year and had passed only after writing a supplemental examination. In his graduating year he went to the top of his class, winning the Lieutenant Governor's Silver Medal in Public Health and the Jeanie Forsyth Prize in Surgery to cap off his degree of MDCM (*medicinae doctorem et chirurgiae magistrum*, or doctor of medicine and master of surgery). In the fourth year he got an A in pathology, in surgery, and in obstetrics and gynaecology and a B in public health, in therapeutics, in medicine, and in psychology and psychiatry. In his graduating year he got a B in paediatrics and an A in all the others: bacteriology, pathology, public health, medicine, surgery, and obstetrics and gynaecology. In the volume of *Old McGill for 1936*, the quotation picked by Rocke was from Ralph Waldo Emerson: "Nothing great was ever achieved without enthusiasm." (The full Emerson quotation is: "Enthusiasm is one of the most powerful engines of success. When you do a thing, do it with your might.

Put your whole soul into it. Stamp it with your own personality. Be active, be energetic, be enthusiastic and faithful, and you will accomplish your object. Nothing great was ever achieved without enthusiasm.")

His own academic experiences influenced the way that he later assessed candidates for various positions. He was far less impressed with candidates who had consistently obtained marks of A in every subject throughout their studies. They tended, he maintained, to be eggheads or individuals who did not deal well with reality. He would always seek indications that the candidate had grown through experience and learned from it. He looked at résumés all his life from this perspective and made his hiring decisions accordingly.

University study was followed by a two-year internship at the Montreal General Hospital, an experience that provided him with excellent training. For three months during his first year as an intern he was in charge of the women's section of the tuberculosis sanatorium at Ste Agathe. Other rotations were in medicine under Dr Campbell Howard,[22] surgery under Dr Walter Barlow,[23] and in the Surgical Outpatient Department, attending to casualties of all sorts. As a formative year, it could not have been better. His second year was spent in pathology, which he considered to be a first-class experience, working on postmortems, bacteriology, and surgical pathology, perfect grounding for anything he might elect to do in medicine. Influenced by his "uncle," Dr Edmond ("Ted") Eberts, himself a prominent Montreal surgeon with an appointment on the McGill Faculty of Medicine, he decided to go into surgery.[24] Eberts would prove to be very influential in shaping Rocke's medical education and career path from the time he entered medical school until the outbreak of the Second World War, which occurred while he was studying in England.

LOVE AND MARRIAGE

Not all was hard work and study. Starting in 1932–33, whenever he was able to break free from his duties and studies, Rocke began to go out with Beatrice Roslyn Arnold, and they were soon regarded as a couple. She was always known and referred to within the family and by friends as "Rolly." (I use her full name when I refer to her in this work.) Roslyn was born in Montreal in 1912, daughter of Thomas Arnold and Beatrice Rennie Taylor. John Taylor, father of Beatrice, had a steel-parts business and had lost his wife many years before. He took Thomas Arnold, born in Dundee, Scotland, into the business as a junior. Arnold proved to be a superb salesman, and the business was later renamed Taylor and Arnold. Arnold married the only daughter of John Taylor. Roslyn's name was derived from the Roslyn School (for girls only), which had been founded by Thomas's father, John Porteous Arnold. Thomas Arnold was very interested in sports and was an early member of the Royal Montreal Golf Club, reputed to be the oldest golf club in North America. He was one of three investors who supported the ice hockey club called the Montreal Maroons, which won two Stanley Cups. During the Depression he became the manager of the now-departed Montreal Forum, widely regarded by devout hockey fans as the Vatican of ice hockey. Arnold was well integrated into Montreal society, lived on Ontario Street downtown, and maintained a summer residence, called Arncliff, in Senneville, at the western extreme of the Island of Montreal. During the Second World War he became one of the $1-per-year men recruited by the redoubtable Clarence Decatur Howe to assist in the production of war materials, part of which, in his case, involved moving half-way across the country to Selkirk, Manitoba, where he developed the Manitoba Steel factory in support of the railway industry, which was so vital in the war effort, moving goods and materials to the coasts for shipment overseas.

Roslyn was educated at Trafalgar School in Montreal and at Elmwood School in Ottawa but did not attend university. She was a debutante in the appropriate year during the Montreal Season, and also did unpaid social work. Rocke soon became almost part of the family and spent a great deal of time in Senneville, playing golf and tennis, walking, adding significantly to the grocery bill, and generally bunking-in with the Arnolds, both there and at their Montreal home. The young couple were obviously infatuated with each other and spent a great deal of time together.

There were clearly some ups and downs in the relationship, due perhaps to the length and inconclusiveness of the courtship, judging from some ponderous entries in Rocke's journal, which are, unfortunately, both somewhat cryptic and largely unrevealing of his own feelings. In October 1934 it appears as though some friend of Roslyn got one of their mutual male friends to make a rather "startling disclosure" about Roslyn, which obviously concerned him and gave him "much food for thought" in the future. Presumably, the message was that the relationship should progress toward marriage and at a speed different from the current pace. There must have been some implied ultimatum, but what it may have been was not recorded. He noted rather sophomorically that his "usual method" (whatever that may have been) would, in this case, be very self-ish indeed. There were two alternatives, marriage or a complete spat, the first (temporarily) out of the question and the other a most unpleasant prospect – probably the wisest thing in the long run, but at the moment it seemed too drastic and he was not sure, in any event, that he could stick by it. He would probably find out his own state of mind by doing it and would probably not enjoy the disclosure. It was a most self-conscious dis-closure, awkwardly expressed, and clearly written without much thought before pen touched paper. He decided that he would see her the following day, state the facts, and see what she had to say. His entry the following day noted that he had not had the chance to carry out his plan, and he thought on balance that even if the chance had arisen, he probably would not have done so. The problem, however, as such problems seldom do, did not go away, although it never seemed to come to a head. Still, by the end of October it was clear that something would have to be done. He was squeezed from two sides: by Roslyn's evident desire for some sort of closure and by the demands of his studies and the lack of income that he could anticipate for the next few years. A man in those days was expected to support his wife. He would be regarded as a failure if his wife was forced to work – even if Roslyn had had any such experience. Nor would he have had much appetite for being seen as a "kept man."[25]

One of the flies in the potential matrimonial ointment proved to be none other than Ted Eberts, who had been influential throughout Rocke's involvement in medical school. Eberts had written to Rocke's father on 30 May 1935, just following the year in which Rocke's potential had begun to emerge with his extraordinarily good marks, far better than any he had previously enjoyed. Amid his general enthusiasm and effusive com-ments, he had expressed the hope that Rocke might refrain from mar-rying for the next five or six years! Eberts said he had followed Rocke's work with the greatest interest and pride and felt there was no position to which he might not aspire if from then on and especially after graduation his efforts were properly directed. The "dear boy" had everything – abil-ity and industry, a fine presence, charming manners, and the humil-ity that is a hallmark of greatness. His fourth-year surgical paper, said Eberts, was the best he had ever read, "including a clear and cultured handwriting, which makes a special appeal to the examiner." Here, he went on to express the thought that if Rocke could keep his emotions on ice and "avoid matrimonial complications" for the next five or six years, he could without doubt become a leader in whatever branch of medicine he might ultimately decide to cultivate. Eberts thought he should have two or three years of postgraduate work and a year abroad. Rocke would then be certain of a hospital and teaching appointment, either in Montreal or Toronto, and a distinguished future. He even suggested that Rocke might apply for a Rhodes Scholarship.[26] Eberts advised Robertson that although he had recently resigned from the public service and would shortly relinquish his McGill appointment, he would nevertheless be in constant touch with the hospital and further Rocke's interests in every way. Robertson replied in due course and followed up with the medical aspects and suggestions, but he did not respond to the matrimonial suggestions.[27]

The situation limped along for another year while Rocke finished medical school. He and Roslyn saw each other on every possible occasion, but, he noted, they "had little in the way of gaiety."[28] Reflecting how things "worked" in those days, Roslyn and her mother came out to Vancouver for a visit in the late summer of 1935, no doubt an inspection of sorts, which his parents and their friends and relatives obviously passed with distinction. His examinations finished in May 1936, and by 20 May his mother had arrived in Montreal from Vancouver. Her nickname was "Dainty" – precisely, her family considered, because she was not. She and Rocke discussed the pros and cons of getting engaged. The chief impediment from Rocke's perspective was the fear of Ted Eberts's opposition. This was dealt with, in typical fashion, by Dainty, who summoned Eberts to tea, from which experience he emerged having done a complete about-face, almost to the point of believing that it had always been a good idea for the couple to get married. In the space of a few short days, from 20 to 24 May, the situation had changed from despair to hope. Rocke, relieved of the Ted Eberts albatross, had asked Arnold for and received his permission to marry Roslyn. Roslyn accepted his proposal of marriage, and the engagement was announced on 3 June.

On 24 May, Arnold wrote to Robertson saying how pleased the family was that the two wanted to get married and that they were willing to have this happen, although not without the natural reluctance that would come from seeing their only daughter leave home. They knew it would bring a change in their lives, and while happy that it was Rocke she had chosen, they were in no hurry to see the change occur. By the end of October, however, their feelings had changed somewhat, and both families did not want them to wait too long if ways and means could be found and the marriage did not interfere with Rocke's future, which by now involved going abroad to study. Arnold said that he wanted Roslyn to have some money from him, and this would be $1,800 per year, paid at the rate of $150 per month. He also advised Robertson that she had $10,000 worth of first-class bonds paying 5.5 per cent, a return of $550 per year. Mrs Arnold wanted to give them their apartment for the first year that they were married, and if the couple were to go to Edinburgh or some other European medical centre, he would give them their return tickets. He observed that business conditions were now better, that his own concerns were in black figures and doing well, and that investments were getting back on a dividend-paying basis and increasing in value, all of which was wonderful after what they had gone through with the Depression. Needless to say, he added, it would be his greatest pleasure to increase any allowance to Roslyn when he could, but he thought it best to state definitely what he could do just then.[29]

The marriage took place a year later at 5:00 in the afternoon on 28 June 1937 in the garden at the Arnold home in Senneville, officiated by the Reverend George H. Donald of the Church of St Andrew and St Paul, a well-known Montreal church on Sherbrooke Street West. Thomas Arnold gave away his only daughter in marriage. Her matron of honour was her sister-in-law, Elizabeth Arnold, and Rocke's best man was his fraternity brother George Auld.[30] Rocke noted in his diary, several months later, that the Arnolds had spent months planning for the day and that everything had passed off without a hitch. He had surprised himself by becoming genuinely overcome with emotion from time to time during the afternoon. Roslyn looked perfectly beautiful, and "for the ten thousandth time" he realized how lucky he was to get her. The newly married couple left for Banff and Victoria for their honeymoon. Their new residence together was in the handsome Haddon Hall apartment complex at 2150 Sherbrooke Street West.[31]

STUDY ABROAD

THE CHALLENGE OF FINDING A SURGICAL POSITION

Getting started in a surgical career was not as easy as it might have sounded, even for someone at the top of his class and reasonably well prepared for the purpose during his internship. Positions as surgeons were scarce, especially in the good hospitals, many of which were teaching hospitals connected with medical faculties. Canada was only just beginning to emerge from the lengthy Great Depression that had followed the stock market crash in late 1929 and had continued, with marginal improvement after 1933, until the Second World War. Graduate engineers from McGill in 1935 could get only menial jobs, if any at all. One of them, Robert F. Shaw, who went on to become the president of the Foundation Company of Canada, deputy commissioner general of Expo '67, and a vice principal of McGill, was able to get work only as a night watchman on the Mercier railway bridge. Robertson's fraternity brother Heward Stikeman noted that some of the students they knew committed suicide, faced with the impossibility of getting work following graduation. Stikeman himself, as a qualified lawyer and well connected in Montreal, could eke out a living only by selling insurance, before eventually landing a job in the civil service in February 1939, from which he went on to become the pre-eminent Canadian tax lawyer of his generation. Further credentials, as well as good connections, were required to get any, let alone a worthwhile, position. Who you knew ranked well up there with what you knew. Much thought went into the next stage, by Rocke himself and by his parents, relatives, and supporters. All of them, especially after his splendid final results in medicine, thought he had a bright future and wanted to be sure that he made the right career decisions and that helpful influence could be brought to bear on his behalf. The consensus was that some European exposure would be useful, whether in England or on the

Continent, and there were some extraordinary opportunities for a young surgeon to work with world figures in the discipline.

The big problem with this plan, sound as it seemed, was the growing unrest in Europe, spurred by the activities of Germany and Italy. There was a growing fear that war might be on the horizon, even though it was not yet two decades since the war to end all wars had been terminated. The victors had carved-up Europe, imposing borders and terms of reparations and others on Germany that, in hindsight, made a further war all but inevitable.[1] A year after repudiating the Treaty of Versailles by announcing German rearmament, the National Socialist government of Adolph Hitler had already, in March 1936, occupied the Rhineland with German troops. European politicians protested, but did little more, since everyone knew that no one could possibly be ready for a war until sometime after 1938. Words were all they had, which Hitler knew full well. He played his game of bravado by moving troops here and there, extending claims on behalf of Germany, and threatening to invade if necessary to protect German interests. It was regarded by most of Rocke's advisors as too dangerous to be on the Continent, especially since many of the countries in which one might wish to study surgery at the highest levels were those most affected by the uncertainties. Despite the fact that it was recognized that England was not without risk if any armed conflict were to occur in Europe, Rocke settled on going to Edinburgh with Roslyn and Tam, their first child. They sailed on the Cunard freighter, SS *Antonia*, arriving safely in Greenock, where they were offloaded by lighter on 30 September 1938, and the ship continued to Liverpool to deliver its far more economically rewarding cargo of grain.

Arriving by train the next day in Edinburgh, they encountered anti-Chamberlain demonstrations in the streets. The Scots had no faith in the appeasement approach advocated by the British prime minister, Neville Chamberlain, who had met with both Hitler and Mussolini in Munich on 29 September 1938 and signed the so-called Munich "Peace in our Times" Pact on the following day, reporting this apparent diplomatic triumph to the British public. Rocke's place of work was to be the Edinburgh Royal Infirmary, an institution steeped in medical history. His mentor and patron was Sir John Fraser, Regius Professor of Clinical Surgery at the University of Edinburgh, the last of the master surgeons.[2] There had been early correspondence from Fraser to Ted Eberts ("My Dear Eberts") on 3 October 1938 to report that Rocke had arrived on the

previous Saturday afternoon and was at work in Fraser's ward that morning, where he would observe and attend lectures in preparation for the
Edinburgh fellowship.[3] Because of the European location, he would have
an opportunity for contact with the various teaching systems. The position did not, however, provide him with the possibility of practical surgical work, which he would come to regard as a major shortcoming for
someone interested in becoming a general surgeon. In 1938, undoubtedly
at the invitation of Fraser, he attended the Dinner of the Royal College of
Surgeons of Edinburgh, a formal and protocol-ridden affair in December, at which he was assigned a modestly placed seat and identified on the
seating plan only by surname. Fraser had, like Eberts earlier, recognized
Rocke's teaching potential fairly quickly and had already granted him
some teaching opportunities.

CANADIAN CAREER PLANNERS: THE LOCAL CHESSBOARD

While Rocke was working hard in Edinburgh, his father[4] and "uncle" at
home were almost as busy concerning themselves with his future, especially in the spring of 1939, when his fellowship efforts would, presumably,
come to a successful conclusion. There was a constant exchange of correspondence, each often reporting on letters received from Rocke and from
each other. Writing to Robertson, Eberts had an especially heartwarm-
ing assessment of the son, saying, "I know of no young man ambitious to
go to the top of the ladder in surgery who has Rocke's qualifications, personality, presence, culture and scientific knowledge," and suggested that,
were Rocke to be offered promotion by Fraser in the Edinburgh school,
he might be well advised to accept. Eberts was concerned with the block-
age at the Montreal General Hospital, which had at least a temporary
surfeit of surgeons. On the other hand, the Royal Victoria Hospital had
no first-class person to promote and might consider Rocke, but for such
purpose, it appeared that he would need an English fellowship, not just
the Edinburgh fellowship.

This opened a period of anxious concern on their part, not always
shared by Rocke, that he simply must sit for the English qualification if
he wanted to be certain of a good appointment.[5] Eberts had written to
Fraser to see what Fraser might think about sending Rocke to Budapest,
where he could do public surgery (for a reasonable fee) under the direction of a master. He had also spoken about Rocke to the new principal

of McGill, Lewis William Douglas – who had assumed office, following the untimely death of Sir Arthur Currie, as of 1 January 1938 – "so
that he may not be lost sight of." He speculated darkly, as clinicians do
when contemplating academic administrators, that the time might be
coming when the university would have the final say as to senior hospital
appointments, no doubt grasping but not endorsing the growing importance of academic surgery at teaching hospitals.

In January 1939 Eberts reported to Robertson that he had written to
Sir John Fraser regarding the situation at both the Montreal General and
Royal Victoria Hospitals, adding that Toronto was a possible field "with
infinitely better respects for self maintenance, owing to the homogeneous
English population and the comparatively greater extent and wealth of
its hinterland." He had, with this in mind, consulted Dr Edward Gallie of
Toronto.[6] In the meantime, they both understood, with manly approval,
that Rocke was "working while the light lasts," an essential factor in any
career. Robertson reported to Eberts in February that Roslyn had said,
in her correspondence with them, that because of the deteriorating conditions on the Continent, it might not be advisable for Rocke to go to
Hungary for further experience. The fellowship examinations were fast
approaching, to be sat the following month. News from Toronto, relayed
by Eberts to Robertson in a letter posted 7 March 1939, was not encouraging. The system there was that the Toronto hospitals took in doctors
and trained them for years for the position of chief resident, filling all
vacancies from their own medical school, with the result that the field
was, for all practical purposes, closed to outsiders. Eberts again raised
the desirability of Rocke taking the English fellowship, noting that while
the Edinburgh fellowship had been greatly improved, it still did not have
the same status as the Fellow of the Royal College of Surgeons (FRCS)
(Eng.). Eberts himself had done his fellowship in London, which may
have had some influence on his thinking. This letter crossed with Robertson's letter of 9 March, in which he concurred with Roslyn's conclusion
that under the present conditions it would not be advisable for Rocke to
go to Budapest. There were no indications that Rocke might be offered
anything in Edinburgh, so the possibilities seemed to be an appointment
in some London hospital where he might get some surgery or possibly a
locum tenems. The bottom line, however, seemed to be that he would be
returning to Canada within a year – so where was he to settle?

Roslyn's father, Thomas Arnold, was also part of the Canadian team trying to arrange the best possible situation for Rocke upon his return to Canada. Arnold was about to embark on a trip to England on the *Queen Mary* for the Easter holidays in the latter part of March 1939, after Rocke would have finished his fellowship examinations. Robertson brought him up to date prior to his departure. The possibilities, having eliminated the Budapest option, were the *locum tenems* in England, pursuit of a course of further study in London, especially with a view to getting practical surgical work, or a return to Canada and settlement in Montreal, Toronto, or Vancouver. As for the Canadian options, Robertson said that he would back him in Vancouver and that he thought Rocke could do well there, adding that if Rocke were offered something good in Toronto, it would be well worth considering. The best chance, however, appeared to be in Montreal. Rocke had previously delivered several lectures at the Montreal General Hospital, to the approval of Ted Eberts and other doctors. Robertson thought the authorities at McGill were aware of the fact that in addition to his surgical ability, Rocke was also able to express his ideas as a lecturer, a feature also noted by Sir John Fraser. It was well known that many able men were "poor in exposition." He hoped that Rocke might get a position as a lecturer on the staff of the Montreal General Hospital or at McGill. The salary would be small, but useful, and the position would give him standing as well as permit him to treat his patients in the Montreal General, which would lend him further professional standing.

Other possibilities might be a position as medical officer or assistant medical officer with some insurance company or a "big concern" in Montreal, similar to what Robertson's cousin Harold Eberts, another McGill medical graduate, had done. Such a position would not prevent Rocke from carrying on a general practice. However, the idea of pursuing something at the Montreal General was based only on Eberts' advice and thus seemed little more than a pipe dream. The Royal Victoria was not impossible, and "if it were decided to attempt something along these lines," Charles Martin, McGill's dean of medicine from 1923 to 1936, now retired, could probably be very helpful.[7] Robertson was sure that Martin would do what he could for Rocke, adding the careful touch of a sitting judge, "assuming always that he thought it would be in the interest of the Royal Victoria."

Arnold, interested in the future for both his daughter and Rocke, responded with several thoughts and observations of his own. He was ecstatic about the new transcontinental airmail service;[8] he had received Robertson's letter dated 9 March 1939 and was already replying to it on 11 March. He was grateful for the latest intelligence. He said he had never spoken to Rocke as he would to his own boys because he was reticent about giving advice and felt that Rocke and Roslyn were pretty capable about their affairs. He now felt, however, that he could sit down with him and talk things over, as he had acquired a good deal of information since they had gone overseas. Eberts had read to them the letter Fraser had written about Rocke's abilities as a lecturer, which delighted them, and Eberts was going to show it to Principal Douglas at McGill and to Dr Edward Archibald, former professor of surgery at McGill, chairman of the surgical committee of the university, and chief surgeon at the Royal Victoria Hospital.[9] He mentioned that three weeks earlier Archibald had approached him at their club, pulled him aside, and asked him how the "young people" were getting along. Archibald said that Eberts had shown him Fraser's letter and then went on to say, "now we can't let young men like Robertson get away from us, although we don't want to compete with the General for him." He wanted to see Rocke when he came back, as they wanted him at McGill and the Royal Victoria, and he hoped that he would be in his current position when they did return.

Arnold was, of course, very pleased to hear all of this. He had not related the conversation to Rocke but intended to tell Roslyn, who could then pass on the information. He was sure Montreal was ready for men like Rocke and thought it would be a great help if he could manage to get back while Martin, Eberts, Archibald, and others were still in a position to be helpful. He thought Rocke would be glad to have a chat and talk things over since by the time they arrived in England, Rocke would be freed from his study and at something of a crossroads. He was sure Rocke would be anxious to get to work as soon as possible, as he felt Rocke had called upon his father financially for long enough, but both Arnold and Robertson were sure he would do well when he started. He was sure Rocke would be successful in his examinations, but it was still an anxious time. He then had some tactical advice to pass on, based on his knowledge of the local medical politics. Archibald and Martin were very close, which was helpful, and they were very close with Douglas. Eberts, Archibald, and Douglas were very close. Eberts and Martin were not so close, but this did not matter, so long as one did not mention the one to the other!

While the parental generals planned great things, the foot soldier on the ground was getting ready to face his fellowship examinations. He wrote to his parents on 12 March, describing his preparations for the forthcoming ordeal – "the horrors to come." The previous Monday he had delivered a lecture on the thyroid to the Edinburgh students and was content with the reception it received. The next day he had bade a temporary farewell to Sir John Fraser since he did not want to be present in the ward for the week or so prior to the oral examination, as it would be awkward were he to draw Fraser's ward in the examination. This had left him free to catch up on his bookwork, although despite all his effort he was not sure where he stood. It was very much in the lap of the gods, he said, and something of a toss-up. The examination process was interesting. On 17 March there would be two written examinations, one in the morning on general surgery and one in the afternoon on the chosen specialty – in his case, surgical pathology and operative surgery. The same day, they would get the schedule for the orals, of which there were four, a "clinical" in a ward at the Infirmary and three at the College of Surgeons, in operative surgery, surgical pathology, and general surgery, each lasting between a half-hour and an hour. Sooner or later in such a process, the candidate was sure to be "found out." There were many examiners, and a candidate's chances depended largely on the one before whom he appeared. At the moment, he professed, he was afraid of them all, so it did not much matter whom he drew. He expected he would know the results by 27 March. He had no plans thereafter since all depended on the results, but he had agreed to help Sir John with the making of a film on surgery of the thyroid, which sounded to him like "good sport."

The macro machinations in Canada continued even as the contestant girded his loins for the challenge of the fellowship. Eberts reported to Robertson that he hoped to have a talk with Archibald about prospects at the Royal Victoria Hospital. He knew that Drs Archibald, Bazin (recently retired), and Patch, professor of urology and chairman of the surgical department at the university, were all anxious to put the department on a more "satisfactory" basis. Eberts had in mind that Rocke should in the future be the mainstay of this department. However, he could not help feeling that it would greatly promote Rocke's chances if he were to return with the FRCS (Eng.) and said that he was writing to Rocke in this regard. He was also writing to a retired eminent surgeon, Sampson Handley, formerly chief surgeon at the Middlesex Hospital. Eberts reported himself as doggedly resolved to pursue the subject of Rocke and his future until a satisfactory opening was found. If Rocke returned now to Montreal, Eberts was sure that a place for him would be found on the staff of the Montreal General Hospital, but there was no one there at the moment to whom Eberts should like to entrust his future training, especially in operative surgery. Eberts said he had raised all these matters, in much less detail, in a letter dated 17 March 1939 sent to Rocke, expecting it not to be received until after he had finished sitting for the fellowship, in respect of which he said, "I am sure the result will be as you wish."

Rocke's father passed on the latest intelligence and correspondence to Arnold, then on board the *Queen Mary*, so that he would be current when he met with Rocke in Scotland. Robertson was clearly not entirely comfortable with Eberts's enthusiasm for the idea of the English fellowship and thought Rocke would be "pretty well tired of examinations." Robertson acknowledged that the English degree was more desirable but was not sure the difference would make it worthwhile to stay the additional time in England necessary to secure it. It seemed more important to him that Rocke get back to Montreal while Archibald was still in a position to help him. It did not seem likely that the English would give Rocke much credit for the Scottish credential, and perhaps it would be better to get some practical experience instead of studying for even more examinations. Nor might the McGill authorities be so much more impressed if he were to have the English degree.

Finished with his academic ordeal, but still not knowing whether he had succeeded, Rocke wrote a lengthy letter to his parents on 26 March. He had received no official word of his results, but having previously described the written examinations, he went through the catharsis of recounting the experience of his orals. The first had been in operative surgery and surgical pathology, where he faced four examiners. He thought he had done well in surgery but less well in pathology, although he felt it should have been the other way around. The next was the clinical examination in Sir John Fraser's ward, where he was given a patient and was examined by Fraser, doing not too badly. He felt he had disgraced himself when it came to interpreting the x-rays, although it had not seemed to bother Fraser as much as it did Rocke. He had the "instruments oral" and went verbally through a couple of operations and got through these all right, so up to this point, he felt he had passed everything. The last examination had not, he thought, gone so well, and he felt he had been "downright stupid." He had been nervous about this examination, although he had not been for the others, and could not seem to think along the same lines as the examiners, even though they were "very decent" about the whole thing. This was his main concern, but perhaps, even if he had failed there, he might have done well enough elsewhere to get through overall. He remarked on a mysterious call he had received the night of the last examination – a strange voice – telling him that he had passed. He had no idea who it was and thought it might have been someone's idea of a joke.

Rocke had received Eberts's recent letter regarding the English fellowship and was not only far from persuaded but also strongly opposed to the idea. He did not think its prestige value was any greater than the Edinburgh fellowship, although he acknowledged that he might be wrong in this perception and allowed that it might well be more highly regarded, but if it were, he had not noticed it. He was more certain that its value to him would be very little. In five years he would know a certain amount of surgery, whether or not he took the London examinations. He thought he would do better by applying himself to something more practical for a year. Were he to go to London and spend a year preparing for the fellowship, he would not be any further advanced as regarded his ability to practise surgery than he was at that very moment, having had a year of observation already. It would, in addition, require a full year since there were two distinct stages: primary and final. The primary would focus on anatomy, in the most minute detail, and physiology. He thought he knew enough of these for all practical purposes, but it would nevertheless take a few months to get into shape to write a competitive examination. The next primaries were in July, for which he could not be ready, so he would have to wait until December. If he passed this, and he acknowledged wryly that a small percentage of candidates do pass, he would have to brush up on all the material he had been working on during his time in Edinburgh and write the finals in the spring. Assuming he passed, he would be, a year later, one degree better off but, practically, not a bit further ahead. Added to this combination of uncertainties and no practical advancement in his experience was the matter of expense. He reminded his father, who had been supporting him, that the fellowship had cost £75, apart from living expenses, and that the London fellowship would cost £150 over and above the much higher living expenses that would flow from living in London. He did not think spending all this money simply to advance himself by a doubtful quantity of prestige was at all logical. He also knew that Roslyn was against the idea, a fact that should in itself, he said, be enough to dissuade him.

Not doing something was, of course, well short of a complete answer to how best to occupy himself. This was a harder question, to which his general answer was, "in any other way." As yet, he had no idea what courses were open to him. If he passed the fellowship, he would speak to Fraser to see what advice he might have. The thyroid film was still ahead of them for the immediate future and would require a certain amount of work. He thought he would give serious consideration to a good surgical job in a hospital – anywhere. He might stay on in Edinburgh and work on some problems in the research department and do some work on anatomy and on the wards, very much as he had been doing. The idea of investigative work was not derived from any particular current interest, but in the future he would certainly want to do some such work and this might be a good time to get some grounding. He thought, in fact, that if he could do a reasonable piece of original work and get it published, it would probably do more for his prestige ("curse the word") than would a London fellowship. He did not think this was too likely an outcome – nothing had happened thus far to indicate that he had any bent for research. Or, he mused, he could play golf every day, as he was at the moment. As always seemed to be the case, he added, he could come to no present conclusion. Mussolini was making a speech that evening, the result of which might well, but probably would not, be war.

A cable arrived at the Robertson family home in Victoria the morning of 28 March with the good news that Rocke had been successful in the fellowship examinations. Robertson duly advised Eberts and pressed him again as to the difference between the Scottish and English distinctions. Robertson said he had been told that while in the British Isles the English degree may be considered slightly higher, in America at this time the Scottish degree was considered the better one. He, of course, had no way to judge this and had no doubt that Eberts's view would be correct. He hoped to hear the views of Sampson Handley as well. Eberts was quick to respond, three days later. He was certain that if Rocke could get a start at the Royal Victoria, he would forge ahead steadily and said he would write to Rocke when he heard from Archibald. As to the English fellowship, Eberts was unequivocal, sharing Archibald's views: it was a stiffer examination, and, of course, they demanded the junior fellowship, covering anatomy, physiology, and biochemistry, before one could proceed to the fellowship. Rocke, he felt, had the ability and with some additional coaching could take these qualifications in stride. Archibald admitted that Rocke was a man who should be developed and was very keen about him. Eberts would also miss no opportunity to further Rocke's prospects at the Royal Victoria. He had spoken with McGill's chancellor, Sir Edward Beatty, and two other governors of the university, W.W. Chipman, professor emeritus of gynaecological and obstetrical surgery, and J.W. McConnell, a well-known successful publisher and businessman and a major benefactor of the university. It would have been hard to imagine a more blue-ribbon triumvirate in the Montreal establishment of the day. Eberts had already spoken to the new principal and would renew the attack when occasion offered.

In his letter to Rocke the same day, Eberts was full of advice and counsel. He had had a talk with Archibald, who was going to outline some suggestions after speaking with Dr F.E. McKenty,[10] then surgeon-in-chief at the Royal Victoria, who was returning shortly from vacation. Eberts thought it likely that they would make him a definite offer of a position on the Royal Victoria staff. Archibald's tentative suggestion was that Rocke take up experimental physiology under Dr John Beattie in London, to learn experimental technique, which at the same time would give him very practical training in surgery and, in parallel, prepare him for his junior fellowship (Uncle Ted was nothing if not persistent). Archibald had told Eberts that if Rocke were to secure his English fellowship, it would greatly enhance his prestige at the Royal Victoria. Eberts reminded Rocke that Gallie in Toronto insisted on this for all his senior people. He reminded him as well that Archibald considered the English fellowship by far the more important of the two. Eberts continued by confessing that he had taken it upon himself to say to Archibald that if Rocke were to be given an offer at the Royal Victoria, he thought Rocke might be willing to carry on abroad along the lines suggested by him. Eberts also thought that a few months in Paris and a couple in Sweden to familiarize himself with the various techniques and to improve his French would be useful. He said that he knew this sounded like a big order but that Rocke was destined to play for high stakes and that the groundwork was most important. None of the junior men at the Royal Victoria had any training in experimental work, and this would be insisted upon more and more in anyone destined to head the Department of Surgery. McKenty was said to be resigning in two years, and if Rocke could secure a footing before he stepped down, Eberts thought his promotion would be a certainty.

Rocke's father-in-law, Thomas Arnold, writing to Robertson on 5 April, after the few days that he and his wife had spent with Rocke, Roslyn, and the baby in Edinburgh, appeared to have been much influenced by Rocke's own view of the marginal value of the second fellowship. Plus, he was not a doctor but a businessman who did not know much about life in a teaching hospital and the raging egos and rivalries of surgeons, and no doubt he was hoping that the couple and their grandchild would return to Montreal instead of points west. There was nothing further for Rocke to do in Edinburgh, apart from the thyroid film. Rocke and Roslyn were planning to leave Edinburgh on 1 May and go to London for a month so that Rocke could see some doctors "at work," and Rocke was waiting for word from Eberts's contact, failing which he would get some introductions from Sir John Fraser. Arnold was more persuaded by Rocke's arguments regarding the expense and time required for a marginal increase in prestige. If Archibald, Martin, and Eberts were ready to see him, he should go home, meet with them, tell them of his ambitions and apply for a position.

Arnold thought the young couple might go home during June. His opinion was that Rocke should not delay too long before getting home to meet the influential trio since no young man in Canada had stronger friends than Rocke. Although Martin was no longer active, Martin and Archibald were the closest of friends, and Martin would do anything he could for him, quite apart from Archibald's own interest. Over and above Martin and Archibald, there was Eberts, as keen as he was, and the three of them, Arnold thought, could do anything they wanted, both at the Royal Victoria and at McGill. If they had something to offer Rocke that had a future and wanted him to take another six months, what of it? If it were back in England or in the US, this would not amount to much. Rocke was going back to Montreal a different man from when he left. He had finished an FRCS in Edinburgh in eight months and could (despite Rocke's own estimate) get another in London in one or two. Arnold liked the London scenario – short term – if for nothing more than "show." As far as he could see, some people were "hipped" on the London degree, but he thought they could be persuaded out of it. Arnold believed in striking while the iron was hot, hence his belief that Rocke should go back that summer to meet and discuss with those who could determine his future. It was a somewhat rambling letter, and Arnold did not seem, perhaps not surprisingly, to have a clear idea of what would be involved in getting the London fellowship, but he was nevertheless practical in the sense that he believed, successful salesman that he was, that the parties should meet face to face, to get a better measure of each other.

Rocke himself wrote to his uncle on 8 April, after digesting the advice contained in Eberts's letter of 31 March. He was most grateful for the kindness of Eberts in spending so much time and energy on his behalf. He acknowledged that he had been much perplexed as to what course to follow in the immediate future. The first issue was the political situation, which, besides precluding any thought of studying on the Continent, made him wonder whether or not he was justified in exposing Roslyn and the baby to the "not too hypothetical dangers" of staying on that side of the Atlantic. He thought that this particular difficulty would solve itself one way or the other in the near future. His second concern was a reluctance he had developed during the past year to sit for such an examination as the English fellowship. It had always appeared to him that the primary examination was an impractical approach to a surgical career. The time one would spend memorizing the trivia of anatomy and biochemistry might be far better utilized in making a more direct approach to anatomy and application, together with (as his uncle had suggested) experimental physiology and surgical pathology. This was his own opinion, based on observation, conversation with London fellowship candidates, and his own feelings. He assured Eberts that it was not prompted by a fear of the work involved; rather, his sense of proportion simply rebelled at such an approach.

Rocke acknowledged that his uncle had made it clear that the English fellowship would enhance his chances of an appointment at McGill. If he could not get this appointment without the fellowship, he would have no hesitation to attempt the examinations, but if it were not essential, he believed he could occupy himself in other fields to greater advantage, and it would be with some regret that he would commence anew the memorizing of lists. To recapitulate, he said that he did not "believe in" the English fellowship but, if necessary, that he would make advances toward it and do his level best, although this might not be good enough to get him through without one or two setbacks, which, he acknowledged, was beside the point. His final reluctance concerned money. As his uncle was aware, he was entirely dependent on his father, who had been generous beyond belief. But he knew that his parents' activities, travelling and others, were limited to some extent by the continual out-flow of money to him. He knew his father would back him if he were to go to London for the examinations, but it would still hurt his father to some extent, and he did not feel he was "playing the game" if he did not do what he could to help out. He asked his uncle whether he knew of any scholarship for which he might apply and thought the Royal Victoria Hospital might have one. If he could obtain some help in this manner, he would feel more justified in carrying on. He outlined what little was left to do in Edinburgh and that he would be heading to London shortly to await developments. The experience had been enormously valuable to him. Sir John Fraser had been kindness itself, and he admired him tre-mendously.

There he concluded, having "said his say." He had disparaged, proba-bly unwisely, the English fellowship but had admitted that he was willing to succumb to the system if he had to. His father-in-law would have writ-ten to Eberts suggesting that Rocke come to Montreal to be interviewed by the powers that be. Again, Rocke was not keen to do this unless it was absolutely necessary. He did not believe the time and expense involved would be justified unless there was no alternative. He eagerly awaited his uncle's opinion on this as well as other matters.

Far from their being similarly convinced, the slight opening Rocke had left for the supporters to insist that he proceed seemed to cause them to redouble their efforts in relation to the English fellowship. Eberts wrote to Arnold on 19 April, recounting a conversation he had recently had with Archibald, who in turn relayed a conversation he had had with the Royal Victoria Hospital surgeon-in-chief, McKenty, who was impressed with Rocke and wanted him for the hospital but who insisted that he secure the English fellowship. It was McKenty's intention to make this qualification a sine qua non for enlistment and promotion of the surgical staff at the hospital. Eberts seemed to be of the view that Rocke should make the trip from Europe to meet with McKenty. He thought it should be possible for Rocke to get the name of a first-class coach from Fraser and gave him the name of one of his own friends whom he might contact as well. Eberts followed up with a letter to Rocke, to encourage a visit, if only to put a real person in front of McKenty.

Arnold reported from Scotland to Robertson, saying that Eberts had been hurt by the refusal of the Montreal General Hospital to accept his advice and assessment of Rocke and to persist with their plan to fill all their positions without considering Rocke and was accordingly throwing all of his weight behind Rocke to get a position at the Royal Victoria. As to the English fellowship, he simply observed that had it been known that everyone wanted it, Rocke might have saved himself a year and not done the Edinburgh fellowship. His father waded in with a letter dated 24 April, saying that the public did not realize there was any difference between the two fellowships (if there was) but that within the profession there was a difference, with the English as the hallmark. If the Royal Victoria Hospital were to make him a definite offer conditioned on his taking the English degree, it would be well worth doing so, especially if he could get a scholarship. Rocke should not, in any event, worry about the money because he could attend to that.

The next letter to Rocke came from Eberts, dated 24 April. He had spoken with Archibald and had shown him Rocke's letter, "as I felt that it was a fine piece of English composition." So, apparently, did Archibald. But on to the business: they both agreed with him regarding the primary fellowships, but nothing could be done about it. Archibald felt that Rocke should be able to pass the examination after three months of coaching in London (Rocke's marginal note: "I could not") and that he could then take the final at any time. Archibald had suggested that when the time for the final came, Archibald and Sir John should write to the board, and this he was anxious to do (Rocke's marginal note: "I hope they don't"). Regarding the scholarship, there were several funds, and Archibald thought there might be one of these available for part-time research – but unfortunately only after he had received his fellowship and been appointed to the hospital. The amount mentioned was $750. Again, Archibald had expressed the view that Rocke should come back to see McKenty as soon as possible. The final Archibald suggestion he relayed was that Eberts see Sir Edward Beatty, who was now practically the president of the Royal Victoria Hospital as well as chancellor of the university, and allow him to read Rocke's letter. This was to occur the following day. Archibald hoped that Sir Edward would speak to McKenty and that he, too, would speak to Sir Edward after Eberts had seen him.

The carrot was held out once again. Eberts said that there were three men on the surgical staff of the Royal Victoria, all Canadians, who had taken their FRCS, but Archibald did not think that any of them would prove to be a serious competitor for the senior position in the hospital after Rocke had had surgical training and experience – as Archibald put it, "at the end of a surgical generation," or ten years. Eberts's own view was that if he could win the position of chief surgeon by the time he was forty or forty-two, he would have established a record in the annals of the Royal Victoria Hospital, and he felt this could be done. By then, "of course," he would have acquired a first-class surgical practice. On the whole, the possibilities at the Royal Victoria seemed to him to be, at the present time, the best in Canada for a man of Rocke's calibre. He encouraged Rocke to consider the matter fully and requested that if he decided to accept the advice that Eberts and Archibald had proffered, he let Eberts know when he would arrive in Montreal. On the original of the letter, Rocke wrote that in his letter of reply he had said that he was delighted at the prospects but that he had made "no bones" about the fact that he was against the trip, although he had added that if it were absolutely necessary, he would do it.

Sir John wrote to Eberts on 27 April, clearly as part of the combined effort to promote Rocke's candidacy, noting that Rocke's time with them was drawing to a close (presumably the thyroid film was all but complete). He wished that it had been possible to give him more opportunity for practical work, but Rocke had understood the difficulty and had seen everything they had been able to show him, and he had taken some part in the teaching. As to the teaching, Sir John said that Rocke had shown quite outstanding ability as a teacher. He had the faculty of putting things attractively and clearly, and students had many times expressed their appreciation of his lectures and demonstrations. As to the future, Fraser felt that it would be unwise for Rocke to go to the Continent at this time. Germany, Vienna, and Italy were virtually closed books for the moment, and although he might go to France or Belgium or Holland or the Scandinavian countries, there was at present such a sense of insecurity in all these places that he had thought it best to advise him to spend his time in London. He had given Rocke letters of introduction "to a number of men in that city" and was sure that his time would be spent profitably and well. He closed with the somber observation, "We live in difficult times and the strain of this uncertainty is beginning to be manifest in many ways."

The cumulative effect of all these pressures proved too much for Rocke, who finally and reluctantly agreed that he would study for the English fellowship despite his own serious reservations regarding its marginal utility to him. The young family moved to London, and he commenced the dreary part of studying for the preliminary examinations, with little enthusiasm but considerable determination to do the work necessary to be certain that he passed. He was unable to begin the work soon enough to attempt the July session but was aiming for December, although he thought the whole process might well take a year and a half. The best news of the summer was a letter dated 21 July, addressed to Harold R. Robertson, Esq., FRCS Ed., advising him that at a meeting of the Royal College of Surgeons that day, he had been elected an ordinary Fellow.[11] In mid-August he wrote his parents to say that he and Roslyn were thinking of a brief vacation and closed with the thought that when he was finished he did not know what he would do – by then he should be thinking about learning how to do something, for he would be able to deliver a lecture on any subject but would be of "as much use from a practical point of view as a sick headache." It was a strange system of education that had arisen, but, going back and forth on the question, he had to admit he was enjoying it. The tedium of solitary study was broken during the summer with dissections in the Anatomy Department of the Middlesex Hospital Medical School under professor John Tait, whom Rocke found to be an extraordinarily able teacher. He had been offered a teaching assistantship, effective 1 September, and was looking forward to commencing it immediately upon his return from vacation.

They left for their holiday on 21 August. The European situation continued to deteriorate, and if things were to blow up, Rocke planned to take Roslyn and the baby to Woking and go into London to see Professor Tait for some advice as to what he should do. He was still convinced that there would not be any war and could not believe that Hitler would be such a fool. The only reason he could see for it was that Hitler might have to fight to maintain his personal prestige. The pact with Russia had been a bombshell, but he rather naively imagined that when it all shook down, it would not be as much of a blow for them or such a blessing for the Germans as it appeared at first. The British ambassador was constantly flying back and forth to the Continent bearing messages that everyone hoped would ease the situation, and the media were filled with what

Hitler was doing, although whatever he was doing, it was always menacing. Rocke had seen nothing visceral to suggest a crisis until he had been walking in the village street in Beer, Devonshire, where they were staying and had seen a notice regarding distribution of gas masks. They often looked out across the Channel toward France, wondering what the future would bring.

They returned from holiday on 31 August to find London throbbing with activity. The British fleet had been mobilized, which, for Britain, was tantamount to war. The rail services had been expropriated to enable, if necessary, all the children and their mothers to be evacuated from the city. Everyone seemed to think that the moment war was declared, Germany would send her bombers to London. Sandbags were being placed in front of ground-floor windows, and people were creating space in their basements to store food and generally prepare for the worst. Rocke reported for the commencement of his teaching assignment at 9:00 AM sharp on Friday, 1 September; the students were in place and they set to work immediately. Not fifteen minutes later, Professor Tait arrived to say that the Germans had invaded Poland and that Britain would be declaring war immediately. Plans had been made to move the medical school to Bristol, and the Anatomy Department would start working there the following Tuesday. Tait said that all the other demonstrators were in the Territorial Army and would not be able to move with him to Bristol. Rocke was his only hope – would he stay with him?

Much as he would have liked to support him, Rocke did not accept the offer. Not only did he not want to spend the war doing anatomy, but, much more important, he was by no means certain that he and Roslyn would want to stay in England if there was a war. She and the baby would certainly want to get home to Canada provided that the risk, once the war was under way, was not too great. So he said "no," adding that under the circumstances he should probably resign. Tait agreed that he supposed Rocke should. He resigned from what had been for him a "plumb" job after holding it for about a quarter of an hour. Years later he mused that he had always hesitated when filling out his curriculum vitae as to whether he should include his appointment to the Anatomy Department of the Middlesex Hospital Medical School, where it would look good, even though fifteen minutes was not much of a tenure.

Rocke applied forthwith to the British Army Medical Corps, after which they left London the same day in a huge rented Daimler, lucky to get a conveyance of any kind, with the trains all taken up with mothers and children and no busses or taxis allowed to leave London. They stayed with Rocke's cousin Noel Harris (née Rogers) at Worplesdon Hill in Surrey, where they lived safely and quietly for a month. Rocke dug in the vegetable garden, travelled frequently to London to see whether the Corps would not like to have him, and devoured the news voraciously, all the while wondering whether they should stick it out in England or make a break for home. They, like everyone else, wondered how long the war was going to last. Rumours abounded, including one that there was already a revolution starting in Germany and that Hitler would soon be toppled. Back and forth they went on the matter, saying it would be a shame to abandon the plans for a year of study in London unless it was really necessary. On the other hand, it would be equally shameful to remain in a country that might be overcome by the enemy, or at least be heavily damaged and partially starved, if they could escape then. It was not easy for the twenty-seven-year-old Rocke to make a decision about a return across the Atlantic, which had been made more difficult with the sinking of the *Athenia* a few days after the war had begun. Despite his open invitation, the parents did not proffer any advice on the question. The dilemma was shared by everyone, as he discovered when he asked his bank manager for advice, only to find that the bank manager had a wife and children in England and was wondering what to do with them – did Rocke have any suggestions for him?

A decision, however, had to be made, and one day, while walking together, with the baby in the pram, Rocke and Roslyn came rather suddenly to a conclusion. They would return to Canada as soon as possible. They wondered whether they could get accommodation on any vessel sailing west, having heard that they were all booked for months ahead. Rocke was, accordingly, very surprised when he went to the Canadian Pacific Railway (CPR) offices in London the next day and learned that they could book a passage on a ship leaving from Liverpool in two days. They packed hurriedly, made their farewells, and arrived in Liverpool in time to board the *Duchess of Richmond*, which left port the same night, making its way around the north coast of Ireland and across the North Atlantic. Early the next morning, he went up on deck and saw their destroyer escort disappearing over the horizon. Another passenger ship, the *Samaria*, travelled close to them for several days, but otherwise they were alone and saw no submarines. The voyage home, apart from a vicious October gale, was uneventful. They landed in Quebec on 14 October 1939.

All the carefully contrived plans for Rocke's future career had been rendered moot as a result of a European conflict that would endure for the next five years.

WAR AND BATTLEFIELD SURGERY

Safe in Montreal, they settled initially into an apartment in Chequers Court on Sherbrooke Street West, and Rocke went to see about enlisting in the Royal Canadian Army Medical Corps but was told that he was on the list for the No. 1 Canadian General Hospital (CGH) and that he should wait until the unit was mobilized – an event expected, they said, to take place any day soon. He finally had a chance to meet with the retired dean of medicine at McGill Dr Charles F. Martin, a wise man, who told him to believe nothing that he was told about happenings in the army. Martin told him to proceed as though there were no war. When No. 1 CGH was actually mobilized, he could then drop what he was doing and join it. It would be most unwise, Martin said, for him to sit back and wait for something to happen, and this advice proved to be absolutely correct. He applied to join the staff of the Montreal General Hospital and, with the help of Dr Fraser B. Gurd, was appointed to minor posts in the indoor and outdoor services of both the central and western divisions of the hospital. This gave him plenty to do and he even got some practical operating experience, of which he was in great need, having had so little of it up to then. He carried on in this way until May 1940, when the unit was finally organized. He was commissioned as a lieutenant in the Royal Canadian Army Medical Corps and had to drop everything to become, as he observed, a soldier of sorts.

He thought training for the army in Montreal – which included physical training, military law, first aid, and assorted other matters – was something of a farce, but it was nevertheless all quite business-like and, if one looked ahead, quite exciting. The unit was bound for overseas fairly shortly, and the arrival of Ian, the second of his four children, occurred fortuitously a mere three weeks before the unit left by train for Halifax on 14 July 1940. The unit boarded its ship, the *Duchess of York*, immediately but then waited for nine days before sailing. The men had the extraordinary opportunity of watching the gathering and assembly of convoys in Bedford Basin and their sneaking out of port each night. Their own turn finally came, and the 1,623 men in uniform on board joined a large convoy, protected by a battleship and two destroyers, and were safely delivered in Glasgow a few days later.

Although the crossing had been uneventful, they were greeted by an air raid on their arrival, but there was no damage. They were then put on a train for Aldershot. No one at Aldershot had expected them, and it took some time to find quarters, but they eventually settled into the Badajos Barracks, where they remained for two and a half months. There was some more training in the mornings, with marching, physical training, revolver practice (for the officers), map reading, and similar activities. The revolver practice was a mixed bag, he wrote, "Personally, I'm scared to death of the things, but so far we have not been given any ammunition so all is well." Full parade drill with all equipment prompted the observation that "We look more like overloaded Christmas trees than anything else." The rest of the day was essentially free, and they played tennis, went beagling, or simply loafed around, the latter soon becoming an activity, he wrote, at which they became exceedingly competent. Around them the Battle of Britain raged. They were south of London and could often see enemy planes and the occasional aerial dogfight. He was among the lucky ones who got leave to go up to London to work at various jobs. Robertson went to the Royal College of Surgeons of England in August 1940 to help professor John Beattie with some experiments and basic physiological studies related to shock from hemorrhage. Lodged at London House, an establishment on Mecklenburgh Square founded by Commonwealth families (especially Canadian) near the British Museum, one night in early September after dinner, the Canadians witnessed the first massive air raid on the city, which targeted the East London docks. He maintained a vivid memory of the huge fires, a steady horrible glow with flares here and there as more bombs were dropped. There was a steady hum of aircraft and the static crackle of anti-aircraft shells. That evening presaged an almost continuous series of night bombings of London and other strategic targets.[1]

Robertson was promoted to captain in September 1940. In October 1940 the unit finally found a hospital in which to work, at Marston Green, on the outskirts of Birmingham, well away from any other unit of the Canadian army. The hospital had been built as an emergency medical services unit for both civilian and military casualties and was perfectly good, although they had very few patients. The raid on Coventry on 15 November 1940 was unique. British cryptographers had managed to break the codes used by the German forces. They knew that an air raid was planned for that day and that the target was Coventry. They also knew that if a massive evacuation of the city were to occur in advance of the raid, the Germans would undoubtedly conclude that the British had advance knowledge of the attack, perhaps because their codes had been compromised and should be changed. The strategic decision made under Winston Churchill was to let the raid occur without warning the inhabitants of the city, a harsh price but one, given the desperate circumstances during the Battle of Britain, when the fate of the country was at stake, that its leaders were compelled to pay. Robertson and other members of the unit were close enough to witness the raid, knowing nothing of the strategic background, and went the next day to help with the medical care of the survivors. They took in 140 patients from Birmingham hospitals, which were being cleared to make space for raids expected to follow the 15 November raid. Robertson did not add much to his modest surgical experience to date, dealing primarily with fractures.

On 11 January 1941 they had a visit from Professor Howard Florey, who was then working at the Medical Research Council on experiments related to shock of all types. Florey introduced Robertson to the exciting potential of a new antibiotic, called penicillin, which he was developing. Robertson would later have the opportunity to evaluate it in relation to war wounds.[2] In March he visited the Army Blood Transfusion Service in Bristol, where he learned that the experience of Norman Bethune during the Spanish Civil war was being applied in the current war. Field transfusion units were being added to shorten the time between injury and blood transfusion. This meeting exposed Robertson to the world leaders in blood transfusion at the time. He and Dr Jack Gerrie, who would become director of plastic surgery on his return to McGill and the Montreal General Hospital, met with Sir Harold Gillies, an internationally recognized plastic surgeon specializing in the reconstructive surgical consequences of war injuries. During the week of 7 April 1941, following another raid on Coventry, Robertson had his first exposure to gas gangrene, which made an indelible impression on him – "as horrible a business as I have ever seen."

There were not too many air raid casualties, and the only time they had sufficient work was when a large number of children were transferred from the Birmingham Children's Hospital to keep them out of harm's way from air raids following the November 1940 bombings. However, the experience did serve as an introduction to army administration and to the leadership required to organize and manage a general hospital surgical unit. He worked closely with nursing colleagues to build and establish functional operating rooms but was continually frustrated by the army bureaucracy and inactivity.[3] One common result of having too little to do was that trouble brewed, especially among the officers, some of whom decided that the commanding officer was not doing his job properly and should be replaced, which they made known to senior officers in the Canadian military headquarters. A small group of the officers, among them Robertson, while not enamoured of the commanding officer, felt that he was an honest, hard-working, and well-intentioned officer and that there was no cause to remove him from his post. As time went on, the schism in the officers' mess became more and more apparent and increasingly unpleasant. Eventually, a board of enquiry was appointed. Its hearings, held in private, were tense and searching. The findings favoured the commanding officer, who had done no wrong. His supporters were elated, but despite the board's findings, the officer's reputation within the unit had been seriously damaged and he could no longer command it well. After a decent interval, he was posted to another unit and, not long after that, was sent home.

Robertson spent his wedding anniversary on 28 June 1941 operating on a compound fracture of the femur ("good amusement") and dined with Phil Hill, Bill Turnbull, Cam Gardner, and Palmer Howard, recording in his diary that "The wedding anniversary was noted by the conspicuous absence of the bride which was most unfortunate." On his birthday the same year, 4 August, he commented, "I was operating all day hacking and slashing with complete abandon. Being a sentimentalist, I left the hospital earlier than usual and returned home to write to my spouse, pups and parents, all of whom have played some part in my birth, subsequent existence and perpetuation." He also noted, perhaps not with equal sadness, that "whiskey was extremely hard to come by on this warring island." The preparation and waiting continued. The Americans were not yet in the war despite the covert assistance given to the English, and no one was remotely ready to move toward the Continent, where, if victory was to be achieved, the fight would eventually have to be taken. Apart from the operations of the British navy at sea and the army in North Africa, it would be almost three years before Operation Overlord could be planned, staffed, and executed, with only the Sicilian and Italian campaigns in between.

After a year in Marston Green, in the fall of 1941, the unit was moved closer to the action, in Horsham, Sussex. It was a newer hospital in which care was delivered in twelve associated huts, having a total of 600 beds. They had better quarters, more advanced surgical capabilities, and much more work to do, and they were located closer to London and to friends in other Canadian units, all of which led to a boost in morale. Robertson got some real experience in the treatment of injuries – most of which arose from motorcycle accidents – leading him to speculate that riding a motorcycle was considerably more dangerous than being a military pilot. He attended a lecture from Sir Reginald Watson-Jones, who wrote the classic textbook in orthopaedic surgery and who provided considerable assistance and wisdom in support of the units' fracture management program. Robertson could not fail to learn from this exposure and came away with a greatly expanded sense of fracture management at Horsham. "It's great fun when they turn out well and awful to see the mistakes limping away, but most instructive in either case." He met professor José Trueta, a Barcelona surgeon and a world renowned leader in wound care and debridement (the removal of damaged tissue or foreign objects from a wound), on two occasions, once at Oxford on 29 November 1940 and again at Marston Green on 1 March 1941. These concepts of wound debridement were immediately applied within the unit at Horsham and subsequently when they were operating under real battlefield conditions.

The Royal Army Medical Corps had developed considerable experience with field surgical units during the fighting in the Western Desert in 1941–43, but the Royal Canadian Army Medical Corps did not form any such units until well into 1942. Two units were established initially. Major Frank Mills[4] was given command of No. 1 Cdn Field Surgical Unit (FSU) and Robertson, also promoted to major, command of No. 2. The units consisted of two officers (a commanding officer, who was a major and surgeon, and a captain, who was second in command and an anaesthetist), a corporal, and eight other ranks (two orderlies, two operating room assistants, three drivers, and a batman). The units had three vehicles: a special surgical van with a generator, drawers for instruments, racks for tables and other equipment, and cupboards for miscellaneous equipment; a large truck for tents, personal equipment, and stores; and an eight hundredweight vehicle for personnel. The idea for the field surgical units was to get as close as possible to the action and operate in tents or buildings equipped out of the units' vehicles.

The activities of the units' members consisted largely of training themselves, mainly with respect to the use of the equipment they would be taking with them. They would clear out one of the operating theatres in the hospital and set up their own tables, anaesthetic machines, and instruments. After a few practice runs they performed some real, albeit minor, operations to test the sufficiency of their set-up. The next step, which was designed to bring them closer to what would be the "real thing," involved choosing a field at some distance from the hospital and then setting up the tent and operating tables, spreading the instruments, getting the sterilizers operational, and going through the motions of performing operations. Once they had become reasonably competent in these drills, they would take patients from the hospital and perform minor operations under genuine field conditions. The patients (Robertson called them "victims") were always fully informed about what they planned to do and entered into the spirit of the exercise with cautious enthusiasm. As luck would have it, nothing went wrong and no patient suffered more than he would have if the operation had been performed in the hospital. Even so, looking back at the situation some fifty years after the fact, he shuddered at the thought. In today's litigious society, one can only imagine the anticipatory saliva of plaintiffs' lawyers.

Robertson's unit received some of the casualties from the disastrous venture at Dieppe in August 1942, and the occasion produced at least one amusing story, here told in much the same language as recorded by Robertson. Among the batch of wounded in the Dieppe raid who were sent to their hospital at Horsham was a young lad with a wound in his foot – not very severe, just enough to keep him in bed for a few days. Robertson was making his rounds on the third day that the man was in his ward, when the patient asked him whether he could speak to him alone. The nurses withdrew, the curtains were drawn around the bed, and Robertson was shown the reason for the secretiveness. The patient had a full-blown case of gonorrhea. As Robertson gazed on the unmistakable signs of the disease, his mind began to flash back. He knew that for two or three weeks before the raid the troops had been cooped up in barracks enclosed by barbed wire and that none of them had been able to get out. He knew as well that since the soldier had returned to England, he had been in a bed in his ward. So he asked him how on earth he had gotten this?

The lad replied that when they landed on the shore at Dieppe, he went up the beach and into the town, shooting away. Suddenly, he heard a whistle and looked up. There in an upstairs window was a pretty girl, beckoning to him. So he thought, "what the hell," and went in. Later on, he heard more whistles – different ones – and he knew that they were supposed to retreat, so he jumped up, put on his clothes, grabbed his rifle, and ran down the street and across the beach. He had nearly reached the boat, but just at the last minute, "that's when I got this bloody wound in my foot!"

The more military aspects of the units' training were derived from involvement in various exercises, the most important of which, involving the whole First Canadian Army, occurred in March 1943 and was code-named "Spartan." During the week in which they participated, they moved about the south and west of England following their division. They set up their equipment in many different places and performed mock operations on mock casualties that were brought to them by field ambulances. The weather was awful, being cold and wet, but they learned a good deal about finding their way in the dark, getting out of the mud, scrounging for food, and finding shelter, all of which were essential to survival in actual war. When not out on their training exercises, they worked in the hospital. Time passed quickly, rumours of invasion flew all around them, and having (they thought) trained themselves adequately, they grew restless.

They waited for the call to action.

WAR SURGERY: THE SICILIAN AND ITALIAN CAMPAIGNS

Eventually, the call to action came. Despite knowing it would come, they were completely surprised. On 20 May 1943 Robertson received a call from London. The assistant director of medical services (ADMS) of the First Canadian Division wanted to make sure they were all set. Robertson assured him that they were ready for anything – was something about to happen? "Do you mean to tell me that you have heard nothing?" he was asked. "Not a thing," replied Robertson. "In that case," he was ordered, "you had better get up to London at once." When he arrived at the Staff Headquarters in St James's Square, he was surprised to see his friend, Frank Mills, commanding officer of the No. 1 Cdn Field Surgical Unit (FSU) on the steps of the building, who had received essentially the same phone call. They went together into the office of the ADMS and were again asked by the incredulous officer, "Do you mean to tell me that you have not had any instructions about a move?" They both said, "yes sir." "Well," said the ADMS, "I'll tell you now that you are to be ready at 0800 hours tomorrow to leave for an overseas expedition." He was unable to tell them where they would be going, just that they should pack all their equipment in crates that weighed no more than eighty pounds and that they would not be able to take their vehicles with them.

Apparently the 51st Highland Division had originally been designated for the mission, but in response to pleading by the Canadian authorities, they had been replaced by the First Canadian Division. In the resulting confusion, the Canadian planners had forgotten to bid for space on the ships for the field surgical units. The two doctors pointed out the obvious – they simply had to have their vehicles and could not rely on others to move their equipment. Apart from this, the most important vehicle of all was the large surgical van with the built-in generator, without which they would be unable to operate. The only concession they could wring from the ADMS was that they could keep their vehicles until the last moment, in the hope that someone might relent, but that, no matter what, they had to pack all their equipment and be ready to move at 0800 hours the next day.

Robertson rushed back to the hospital, where he commandeered the unit's two carpenters and all the crating materials that could be found. The entire unit worked all night, and by 0600 hours all the gear had been packed and stored in the vehicles. Robertson told the men to get what sleep they could, but to expect a call before long, and went to bed himself with an ear cocked for the call. It did not come that morning and did not come at all during the entire day. When it did come, the unit was ordered to move at once to a nearby Canadian hospital, where they were to receive further orders. Limited as his army experience may have been, it was enough to make him wary, and he was not surprised to find, when he reported to the commanding officer of the hospital, that no one expected them. They settled in nonetheless and were soon joined by Frank Mills and his unit, and they all waited six days before getting another signal ordering them to proceed at once to Bothwell, near Glasgow, where they were to report to an English casualty clearing station. Sensing, at last, that they were nearing a convoy that would take them somewhere, they hurriedly complied with the order. Upon arrival they were, by now, no longer surprised that the commanding officer of the casualty clearing station had not the slightest inkling that they would be arriving. Space was found and they spent fifteen days with the unit. Much of the time was spent trying to find a place in the convoy for their vehicles, and they were eventually able to make a deal: if they were to bring the empty surgical van to a certain dock at a given time, it would be filled with anti-malarial equipment. When it had reached its destination and had been emptied of its contents, they could then claim it. They were unable, however, to get anyone to take on their other vehicles.

Almost four weeks after the indication that they would be leaving the following morning, they finally embarked on their ship, the MS *Batory*. They had thirteen days of frustrating practice landings in Scotland, most cancelled due to bad weather, before they set sail in convoy, still having no idea of their destination. The issue of tropical drill, mosquito netting, and anti-malarial gear pointed to the eastern Mediterranean, Burma, or Africa, but this could easily have been part of a diversion or misdirection aimed at the enemy. They had no idea where they were going, and the excitement was intense. Only after being at sea for several days were they informed. All of the officers were called to a meeting in the main lounge of the ship, where the commanding officer told them they were headed for Sicily. The officers commanding the various units were then given their general and specific instructions. The general instructions consisted of detailed maps of Sicily and aerial photographs of the landing sites and of the important landmarks in the surrounding countryside. The specific instructions dealt with every move the unit was to make upon landing. These were simple enough: having been landed on one of the beaches, they were to make their way to a certain point on a road about three miles inland, where they were to attach themselves to a British field dressing unit. There, they were to await orders. Robertson and his second-in-command, John Leishman, pored over the maps and photographs for hours, to the point that they felt they had mastered them thoroughly. They had been told to memorize and then to destroy all of the material they had received. This done, they settled down to enjoy the rest of the trip, which to their pleasant surprise, was uneventful. They heard that a submarine had sunk a ship in one of the other convoys but saw no signs themselves of any German ships or planes.

The passage through the Straits of Gibraltar in the middle of the night was, for those who had been living with black-outs, little short of thrilling, with all of the bright lights ablaze. The night before the landing on Sicily was very exciting, with convoys converging on the island from several points in Britain, Alexandria, and the United States, the latter country now fully involved in the war following the surprise attack by the Japanese on Pearl Harbor on 7 December 1941.[5] There were hundreds of vessels of all sizes, battleships, cruisers, monitors, destroyers and other warships, landing craft, motorboats, ocean liners, freighters, and tankers. It was, for the young Robertson, a marvelous sight, and he recognized and admired this remarkable feat of organization on such a grand scale, even though there were many smaller organizational failures at ground level. There was some concern about whether it might be too rough to land, but Admiral Cunningham assured them the waves would subside enough to allow for a safe landing early the following morning.

The assault troops started their landing at 0245 hours and met with very little resistance, with the result that there were practically no casualties at first. The noncombatants were confined to their quarters and instructed not to emerge until they received orders to do so, but they were nevertheless required to be ready to move on a moment's notice. This meant that they were fully dressed with all their personal equipment (gas masks, water canteens, revolvers) hanging off them. They were eager to hear how things were going, but no one paid the least attention to them as they sat on their bunks, sweating profusely, wishing that their turn would soon come. All they could do was listen to the clatter of boots on the decks above and the roar of the barrage laid down by the monitors and other heavy naval craft.

Mid-morning arrived. They wondered if they had been forgotten. Robertson decided to disobey the order to remain below decks and sent one of his men to reconnoiter. He came back with the disturbing news that most of the troops had left the ship and that the FSU unit did not seem to fall within anyone's disembarkation plans. They were clearly going to have to make their own way ashore. They all went topside to be met with a most impressive and confusing sight. Many of the vessels they had seen the previous evening had anchored off the coast near Pachino. The monitors had settled on the bottom and were firing at a village barely visible in the distance. Landing craft were scurrying between the ships and the shore, transporting troops and supplies. They were the only unit left on their own ship, and it was only with great difficulty that they persuaded a young lieutenant to come alongside and take them ashore.

As they neared the beach, Robertson asked him which one it was, as the land ahead of him bore not the slightest resemblance to the photographs he had so assiduously memorized, but thought that if he knew which of the three landing beaches they would be on, he could find his way by map to the rendezvous. The lieutenant said he had no idea to which beach they were headed and, frankly, did not much care. His instructions were to put people ashore as quickly as possible; his passengers could bloody well find their own way once he had landed them. They were landed some one hundred feet from shore and waded in through water up to their armpits. Thus baptized, he said later, and not a little confused, they at last reached the territory of the enemy.

He left his men to wring out their clothing while he made a short tour to see if he could determine where they were. The first sight to impress him was about five hundred Italian soldiers lined up with their mess tins at the ready, waiting to be fed. They were the first prisoners of war, who had simply given up when the first Allied troops appeared on the beaches. They were not war-like folk and had obviously had enough of the Germans who had overrun their country for several years. All they wanted to do was to get back to their ordinary lives. It may have taken some of the edge of triumph off the Allied landing on the European continent, but it certainly saved lives on both sides of the conflict. After some exploration, he managed to find a recognizable landmark, and it was easy thereafter to find his way. More difficult was finding the field dressing station that was to be their temporary host. The plan had been for the unit to establish itself somewhere on a stretch of road about one mile in length between two recognizable points. He marched his by now dry but tired and hungry unit to one end of the stretch, settled them there and then walked up and down the stretch of road until dark, without finding the field dressing station or finding anyone who had ever heard of a field dressing station. The real meaning of micro military planning began to strike home when Robertson and his unit discovered that the medical unit with which they were to make contact had not landed at Pachino but, through some misunderstanding, had been taken off to Malta.

They had a rather lonely night on the ground, made worse by a substantial enemy air raid met by a furious barrage from the ships anchored in the bay. As they lay, uncomfortably exposed, on the ground, they thought they might be more at risk from fragments from their own anti-aircraft shells than from the enemy bombs. When dawn finally arrived, Robertson and Leishman set out to find First Division headquarters, which proved to be a more difficult task than they had expected. None of the units they encountered had the slightest idea where headquarters was. The fighting units were moving north at a fast pace in accordance with the main battle plan, and headquarters was, no doubt, fully occupied in maintaining contact with them. Finally, they found headquarters and were ordered back to the beach area to help the Canadian 9th Field Ambulance, old friends. The Field Ambulance had no equipment and nothing for them to do, but they told them where they might be useful. The No. 1 Canadian Field Dressing Station was set up nearby with a British field surgical unit whose members had landed with some instruments in their packs and had been operating all night. Perhaps Robertson's group could relieve them. Delighted at the prospect of being able at last to help someone, they gathered their men, commandeered a jeep, and set off to find the British, who were not far off and who greeted them warmly. They were pleased that the Canadians could give them a break. Robertson's unit set up quickly and did five cases.

That same evening they moved inland to another location, and the following day, still with the No. 1 FDS, they moved farther inland to a location called Bompalazzo. As the troops drove north into the heart of Sicily, Rocke's unit and the other Canadian medical units followed them closely, setting up in tents and schoolhouses and even wine cellars to deal with the flow of seriously wounded Canadian soldiers, as well as some German casualties and civilians.

The major problem, however, was that they still had no equipment. They finally located their vehicles, but for some time they had to borrow instruments and supplies from the field dressing station, which was not set up to treat major wounds. Each day they would return to the beach to see if they could find some of their own equipment, which, it appeared, had been rather generously distributed among the ships in their convoy and was scattered in dribs and drabs along about a mile of beach. Gradually, they built up their stock of basic materials, much of which came from recovery of their own crates and some of which was either borrowed from other units or captured.

On two occasions during the Sicilian campaign, Robertson was given permission by the ADMS to enter an abandoned hospital and to take away anything he needed. It was an eerie feeling to walk into an absolutely empty hospital. In one case, there was a large unexploded bomb on the floor of the main entrance hallway. The beds in the ward were all dishevelled and in some were the bodies of patients who had been unable to escape when the bombardment started. The doors of the cupboards were open and clothes scattered on the floor, everything pointing to a frantic exodus. In the operating theatre, however, everything was spotlessly clean, ready for the next day's slate of cases. He had the difficult task of choosing the instruments he needed – and only those he needed – although he was sorely tempted to open his knapsack and fill it with everything it could hold. He did find that he had come away with a few instruments that he could not possibly use in a field surgical unit, but the combination of weeks of deprivation and the thought that the unexploded bomb in the lobby might go off at any moment may have accounted for extras.

It was not until the Sicilian campaign was half over that they figured they were fully equipped, although the lack of equipment did not prevent them from being surgically active. They soon adapted themselves to the extraordinary conditions, which were quite unlike anything they had experienced in their training exercises. It was summer, with its heat and dust, and dysentery was with them throughout the campaign. Although the air temperature in the shade was not excessively high – perhaps 90 degrees Fahrenheit – in the surgical tents, with the sun beating down on the canvas, with no draught and the sterilizers in full operation, it was at least 120 degrees. They operated without gowns, stripped to the waist. Orderlies used magazines (one of the many contributions of *Maclean's* magazine to the Canadian war effort) as makeshift fans to keep the operators cool and to keep the flies from landing on the exposed wounds. Normally working alongside No. 1 Field Surgical Unit, they first decided to work twelve-hour shifts to provide twenty-four hour coverage. On the first day, they tossed a coin to see who would get the night shift and who the day. Robertson won the toss and chose to operate at night, which proved to have been a grave error because although it was easier to work at night, it was practically impossible to sleep during the day because of the heat. Later in the campaign they decided to work twenty-four-hour shifts, which proved to be more satisfactory.

One of the real menaces throughout the campaign was the flies. The unit was well supplied with an insect repellent called Flit and fly swatters, and the men were constantly at work to keep down the creatures, but if they let down for a moment, they would be deluged. One example near the end of the campaign involved a young British soldier with an abdominal wound affecting the stomach and colon. The wound was severe, but the patient was in good condition and had an excellent chance to survive. At the time, they were using a large school building in Agira. A day or two after the operation, they got word that they were to move south to a rest area and that all the Allied troops were to leave Agira. By this time all Robertson's patients were fit to be moved except the one with the abdominal wound. They had strict instructions not to move patients with abdominal wounds for at least a week after their operations, based on experience in the desert war, where many had died or developed serious complications as a result of being moved too soon. He would have to hold the young soldier with him until he was ready to stand the trip to the base. On the third postoperative day, he saw the long thin line of the Allied tanks, artillery, infantry, medical units, and service corps filing out of Agira.

He looked forward to a few days of rest and quiet, with only one patient who needed little care, as he was coming along very well. He had kept three men with him, with plenty of food, drinks, medicine, drugs, and Flit, and felt quite secure. The first sign of trouble was that as soon as the troops were out of sight, the people of Agira began to swarm into the school looking for loot of any sort. The mayor's promise to keep civilians out of the "hospital" was unenforceable, and they had no way to stem the tide. Along with the civilians came flies – millions of them. There were now only four in the unit working to keep the flies at bay, whether by swatting or Flitting, far too few to do any good. The effect on all of them was remarkable – they loathed the flies and were depressed by the constant swarms around them.

Their patient, normally a tough, rather impassive individual, was the most affected. Even though he was protected by mosquito netting and very few flies managed to get to him, he was deeply disturbed by the huge collection of flies on the outside of the netting. He begged Robertson to take him to a hospital down the line where the flies would be controlled. Robertson told him that it would be dangerous for him to be moved and that he would have to wait for another three or four days. The patient became more agitated, and with each hour Robertson's own resolve weakened, until he finally decided that it would be more harmful to the patient to keep him there against his will than to move him. Preparation for the move was extremely careful, but by sundown they were ready, with a naso-gastric suction in place and an intravenous running, and gently hoisted the patient into the van. They drove at a snail's pace through the relative cool of the night and delivered their charge to a British hospital early the next morning. He seemed unaffected by the trip, although Robertson still felt guilty. He feared that something would go wrong that could have been avoided if he had had the strength to keep him in Agira for another three or four days. The flies had defeated him and he feared that he would come to regret his failure. For months he searched every mail delivery for a letter from the patient, who had promised to let him know how he fared. He had not thought the man would break the promise and so had come to the conclusion that he must have died. But in December, four months after Robertson had left him at the British hospital, a letter arrived saying that he was fully recovered and that he had thought he should wait until he was ready to rejoin his unit before writing.

In the rest camp they had an opportunity to reflect on their first weeks in action. In the course of thirty-six days they had operated in six places: in a barn near the Pachino beach, in tents set up in olive groves, in school houses, in the dining room of a private house, and in a wine cellar. They had performed countless operations with a mortality rate of approximately 18 per cent. Nearly all of the men had been seriously wounded; chest and abdominal wounds, compound fractures of the extremities, and burns were the commonest injuries. They had been faced with extraordinarily difficult problems that would have taxed the abilities of fully experienced war surgeons, and they were not well trained for the job. Robertson had had some experience with motorcycle injuries but had seen only two or three gunshot wounds of the extremities, and he had never dealt with an open abdominal or chest wound. This sort of injury did not often occur in civilian life. There were many times, especially in the early days of the campaign, when he desperately wished that he had someone to guide him, an experienced surgical consultant. By the end of the campaign, they were becoming accustomed to the difficult conditions and had learned to avoid some of the traps that lay in wait for the beginner. The rest camp was not completely restful. Malaria had become a serious problem, and all medical hands were called upon to help take care of the victims, some of whom were desperately ill.[6] But for the weary surgeons, it was nevertheless a relief from the war-wounded, and they slept well and ate better than they could have imagined while out in the field. They had the luxury of their first piece of bread since prior to landing at Pachino.

Probably the most remarkable episode for them was a visit from the commander-in-chief of the British Eighth Army, to which the Canadian forces in Sicily belonged. When the announcement was made that General Bernard Montgomery would come to inspect the brigade, the troops were thoroughly annoyed. They wanted to rest. They did not want to polish their boots and be ready for inspection. Why did the general not just leave them alone? On the day of the visit the men, disgruntled as only soldiers can be, formed three sides of a square on a nearby field. They expected to have to wait a few minutes – inspecting officers were always late – but after an hour of standing in line in the blazing sun, they began to get restless. Some of the men could be heard to curse the general and all his probably unmarried ancestors. All of them grumbled about being late for lunch; it was already lunchtime and he had still not arrived.

It had got to the point that the officers were wondering how much longer the men would hold their ranks when a cloud of dust appeared in the distance, raised by Montgomery's little open car. As it approached, he stood up and waved to the men. The car came to a stop in the middle of the three-sided square. Montgomery called out to the men to break their ranks and gather around him. He did not want to inspect them, just to have a few words with them. He said he was sorry he was late, but he had had so many people to see that day. Then he turned to his adjutant and said, "Tell me, are these Canadians from the east or the west of Canada?" The adjutant replied, "both." Montgomery turned to the troops and shouted a question, "Which is better – the east or the west?" The men, now beginning to think that the general was not all bad, responded with deafening shouts. Montgomery then explained that it did not really matter where in Canada they came from, as all Canadians were magnificent fighters, and said he would not dream of undertaking the attack on Italy if he did not have the Canadians with him. He continued on in the same vein.

The effect on the men was miraculous – in the space of ten minutes he had won them over completely. It never occurred to them that he had probably said the same thing to every group he had met that day. All that mattered was that he had said it to them. As they walked away from the field to get their much-delayed lunch, the men were jubilant, hooting, laughing, and slapping each other on the back. Robertson thought at the time, and the thought persisted some fifty years later, that Montgomery's performance was the best example of crowd-swaying he had ever seen.

The rest period lasted about two weeks. By the end of August they set off north to station themselves near the shores of the Strait of Messina, where all the Allied armies were gathering for the attack on Italy. Their instructions were to stand ready as soon as the attack barrage started but to await orders before moving. For the second time they were forgotten. The invading forces started to move at about 0230 hours, under cover of a massive artillery barrage. The men sat up, fully dressed, and watched the spectacular fireworks from their vantage site. Expecting to be called at any moment, they gulped down a hurried breakfast, later a hurried lunch, and in due course a hurried supper, but still no one called them. Finally, Robertson sent one of his men down to the beach to find out what was happening. He returned with the report that there seemed to be great confusion, with various units jockeying for places on the transport craft and no one in apparent command. They concluded that they were obviously going to have to make their own way, or they would be stranded on the shore forever. Down they went to the beach and ranged about until they found a craft with its gates open. They simply drove their vehicles aboard and were soon underway, on a beautiful evening with clear skies and calm waters. There had been no air activity to speak of during the day, so they settled in for a peaceful crossing.

When they finally beached at Reggio di Calabria it was nearly midnight. Fearing that the enemy might launch an air raid, Robertson was anxious to get the unit ashore. His vehicle had been hoisted to the top deck, and after they touched down he could hear the portal open and the sounds of two or three vehicles leaving. Then there was silence. Sensing something was wrong, he sent his corporal down to find out what was happening. He came back to say that Robertson would not believe it, but the naval lieutenant said that someone had stolen a mirror from the washroom, and the captain had ordered that no one was to leave the ship until the mirror was returned. Robertson made his way to the portal and confronted the lieutenant, who confirmed the corporal's report. He asked what efforts had been made to find the mirror. None had been made. He then asked who was the senior army officer aboard. The lieutenant did not know. After a quick survey, it turned out that it was Robertson; a colonel had been on board the first vehicle to leave, and now Robertson was, presumably, the senior representative of the army. He got all the army officers together and had them break into pairs and go to each vehicle on the ship and tell the occupants to surrender the mirror – no questions would be asked and no disciplinary action taken if they simply gave it up. A few minutes later they all met. No one had surrendered the mirror. He then went to see the commander of the ship, who said of course he knew why Robertson was coming to see him. The commander said he had just given the order to allow the troops to disembark with their vehicles; he hoped Robertson would understand his reason for taking such an extraordinary action – basically interrupting the invasion of Europe because a mirror was missing – but sailors were a superstitious lot and regarded the loss of a mirror as a sign of bad luck to come, just as they did the breaking of one. He had needed to be seen to have done everything in his power as commander to retrieve the mirror because if he did not find it, his ship would forever be regarded as an unlucky one.

The mirror crisis behind them and ashore in Italy, within a matter of hours they were established in a large modern school building in Reggio di Calabria, the finest city they had yet seen and practically abandoned by its inhabitants. The invading troops, including Canadians, could not resist the temptation to loot – not the first time in history that armies had ever resorted to such practices. The doors to shops were pried open, and the looters entered and seized anything that came to hand. Customary or not, Robertson found it an unpleasant business, relieved somewhat by the sight of some Canadians who had broken into a hat shop and come away with a great deal of headwear. They had donned and paraded around in gentlemen's top-hats and broad-brimmed ladies' garden party bonnets, draped over a tank and waving to the bemused onlookers like members of the royal family. The stay in Reggio di Calabria was short, and there were few casualties in the early part of the campaign; the Italians surrendered four days after the Allied troops landed, and the Germans withdrew farther north to establish defensive positions.

Thus began the laborious but inexorable process of pushing the Germans out of Italy. The Allied troops were never far behind, and the FSU moved frequently so that it could be as close to the front as possible. Between the landing on 3 September and mid-December, they had changed the unit's location eight times: from Reggio to Potenza to Motta

Montecorvino to Volturara to Riccia to Campobasso to Civitanova to Rocca San Giovanni and finally to St Vito Chientino, just south of Ortona, where they stayed for several months.

As they moved north, autumn gave way to a miserable winter with rain and persistent cold winds. The roads, not particularly good to begin with, crumbled under the heavy military traffic, while the dirt roads and paths were deep in mud. The fighting grew more desperate as time went on, and the casualties increased accordingly. This particular phase of the campaign ended with the battle for Ortona in December, at which time the surgical unit was settled in a school building in St Vito. The operating theatre was in a large room, big enough to house all the unit's equipment as well as a large stove that fuelled the sterilizer and protected the men from the extreme cold and dampness. They were not alone, sharing the building with No. 1 FSU, No. 1 Field Transfusion Unit, and a field dressing station, which carried out the resuscitation. The upper floor was used as the ward accommodation.

Robertson came away from his experience with a deep appreciation of the extraordinary work of the regimental stretcher bearers and the field ambulance men. The combination of their effort and the proximity of the FSU meant that even during the most difficult period of the campaign, the fight for Ortona, fully two-thirds of the casualties reached them within six hours of being wounded. As anyone familiar with the treatment of trauma knows and as Robertson and his colleagues learned first-hand, the shorter the delay between being wounded and receiving treatment, the better the chances for recovery. Given the difficulties to be overcome by the bearers, including the active fighting going on all around them, the deep mud, and the poor visibility, it was a magnificent effort. Despite this, the terrible conditions affected the wounded considerably since the cold, the wet, and the mud combined to deepen the shock caused by the wounds and doubtless were factors in the development of gas gangrene in a number of cases. As during the Sicilian campaign, Nos 1 and 2 FSU combined to provide twenty-four-hour service. Not having the oppressive heat to deal with, they experimented with eight- and twelve-hour shifts, but settled once again on twenty-four-hour rotations, which proved efficient and not unduly tiring.

He also came away with a particular understanding of the role of nurses in the recovery of patients. He recounted this in a speech that he gave almost thirty years later at a graduation ceremony for nurses.[7]

He was discussing health care in general and the education of doctors and nurses, including the combination of theoretical and practical work, and expressed some concern that perhaps there was, at present, a bit too much emphasis on the theoretical. Here is the example of what he learned about the value of good nursing during the war:

> Let us recall that technology is the nurse's servant; that she may use it well or badly and her effectiveness will vary accordingly – to some extent. But her guide, her motivating force, the thing that determines whether she is to be a superb, a good, a mediocre or a poor nurse, is something innate – not taught. It is a natural quality, probably the one that has led her into nursing in the first place. I cannot find a name for this quality so, for want of a word, I shall illustrate my meaning by a story.
>
> The scene is laid in a Field Surgical Unit in Italy during the Second World War some 28 years ago. The unit was established near the front and was about 50 miles ahead of the nearest hospital. There had been a lot of action at the front and there were a good many casualties. The weather was bad and the trip to the hospital by ambulance over the atrocious roads would test the stamina of anyone; it was more than a severely wounded man could stand. Thus we had to hold on to some of our bad cases much longer than we would have liked, and after a few days we had a ward (actually a schoolroom) full of seriously ill patients who had been with us for some time and whom we simply couldn't move. We had some paraplegics, some chest and abdominal cases, some very real problems, and we had no nurses. The men in the unit, all trained "on the job," did their work magnificently; they nursed as best they could, as well as any men could, I judge, but as the days wore on the patients became more and more unhappy. One saw unrelieved restlessness or discomfort here, a developing bedsore there; in short one saw things happen that shouldn't happen, and that we couldn't stop. Just when our spirits were at their lowest ebb we got word that two English nurses were being sent forward to help us out. As soon as the patients heard the news they perked up, and I have to allow that it wasn't the prospect of better nursing that inspired them at first.
>
> At long last the nurses arrived to be at once meticulously inspected by even the sickest man, and a wave of disappointment

spread over the ward, for, to put it in the softest way, these two were
not the kind of nurses that soldiers dreamt about. They were, as an
English officer put it diplomatically, singularly poorly endowed, or
so it seemed for the first two minutes or so as they nervously and
bashfully entered the ward, covered as it were, with confusion at
having to face the inevitable test of male scrutiny which they knew
they were unlikely to pass. But if they failed the first part of this
test, that was their only miss. From the moment they had their
sleeves rolled up and started to work, it was clear that something
was happening in the ward that hadn't happened before – that
couldn't have happened before because there hadn't been anyone
who had the gift that these women had, of being really able to
nurse, to comfort, to reassure, to encourage, to do all those things
that nurses can do, and can do best while simply taking care of the
patient's creature comforts.

I've called this a gift, and so it is, this ability to nurse, but it
is one that must, in order to be fully effective, be developed by
experience. This pair of nurses that I came to admire so greatly
as they showed us up for the oafs that we were as far as nursing
was concerned, had gained their experience in a British hospital
a good many years before the war. I venture to say that they had
practically no so-called scientific training. A touch of anatomy and
physiology, perhaps, a fairly extensive practical course in decorum
probably, but no real science as curriculum people like to think of
it. I doubt that they knew what a red blood cell was, but they knew
whether a patient's colour was good or bad; they knew nothing
about fluid shifts or membranes, but they knew at a glance whether
a patient needed water and they knew how to get him to take
it. They probably wouldn't know anything about an electro-
cardiogram machine but they deduced a lot from feeling a patient's
pulse; they had probably never heard of Applied Psychology but
they could outperform most psychologists, I have no doubt. It was
great to see them moving down the ward in their first swing to
see what needed to be done. A look and a word or two with each
patient and they decided how to handle that boy from there on.
In this their judgment was virtually infallible. In short, they had
it. They knew their job. Once at work they exuded confidence in
their own ability to make people feel better, and the men felt it and

responded, and the results were wonderful to behold. The men relaxed. They started to sleep a bit – to eat a little – to recover.

It was a great experience for all of us to see this quality that I have been trying to describe at work in such a dramatic fashion and in so concentrated a form. Such an extraordinary opportunity seldom arises. I hope it never does again. But of course in every ward, in every hospital, one can see the same sorts of things, for the conditions that call for help are found everywhere in civilian life and the urge to respond to the cry for help is universal and awaits development in every woman. My plea, so far as nursing education is concerned, is that this quality be not submerged by theory but that, on the contrary, it be nourished by practice at every step.

The volume and urgency of cases in a wartime environment required a particular organization, and the observant Robertson carried back much of this experience for postwar application, discussed later. The casualties were brought on stretchers into the Field Dressing Station, where they were assessed. Those who had relatively minor wounds and were in good condition were transferred as soon as possible to ambulances, which took them to casualty clearing stations or hospital units in the rear. The seriously wounded were kept in the Field Dressing Station, resuscitated, and eventually operated on by one of the field surgical units, following which they were retained in one of the wards until they were judged fit to stand the trip back to the hospital. The stay with the FSU could last from twelve hours to ten days, the longest "guests" being generally the abdominal cases. In the period of 179 days while Robertson was in Italy with No. 2 FSU, the units dealt with hundreds of cases, with an overall mortality rate of 15 per cent. The largest single group was the abdominal cases – there were fifty-one – which had a mortality rate of 35 per cent. Chest wounds were common, as were compound fractures of the extremities. They dealt with very few head wounds, since the patients with such wounds travelled well and there were good neurosurgical units in the rear area.

Only once during the two campaigns were they shelled directly by enemy artillery, when the target was the building they occupied – "a most disturbing business," he noted later, in the stiff-upper-lip fashion of the day. The advance positioning of field surgical units, usually within five miles of the fighting front, often resulted in them sitting between the major artillery units of the combatants, as was the case during their stay in St Vito, when the projectiles flew overhead in both directions during barrages that often lasted for hours at a time. Although they never considered themselves in any particular danger, many of the patients were deeply upset by the noise and the memories of having been on the receiving end of this deadly fire. One enemy plane dove down on St Vito and fired some cannon shots from low altitude in their direction, one of which passed through the second-story room in which Robertson was sleeping, through the roof of the cab of the surgical van parked outside (where three of the men were sitting), and through the windshield, before burying itself in the ground, but no one was hurt and it proved to be a one-of-a-kind attack. They noted, with some black amusement, that the shell had gone right through the red cross painted on top of the surgical van, supposedly to protect it from enemy action. The Allied forces had command of the air, and the German 88 millimetre guns generally left the medical establishments alone.

After nine months in the FSU, Robertson was brought back to a base hospital (No. 14 Canadian General Hospital) at Caserta, just to the northeast of Naples, where he remained working on chest cases under Dr Sandy MacIntosh for three months, until he was sent back to England. The return convoy consisted of many merchant vessels and a large escort of naval vessels. On the first morning out, he was called to see a young English sailor who had ruptured his appendix a couple of days earlier. It was obvious that he would be ill for some time, but they had only enough intravenous fluids for two or three days. He informed the captain of the vessel, who told Robertson to notify him when they were about to run out of the fluids and he would take action. When the time came, a signal was sent to the admiral, who issued an order. The fleet stopped moving, and a destroyer moved from one vessel to another, picking up cases of intravenous fluids. By the time the exercise was over they had enough to last at least a month. While all this was going on, Robertson lifted the boy so that he could see through the porthole that all the ships were standing still. He was overcome when Robertson explained to him that this was being done for him, and all he could think of to say was "coo lumme!" By the time the ship landed at Liverpool he was improving, and

Robertson had every hope that he would recover. He gave the boy his address and asked him to let him know how he got along, but he never heard from him.

By mid-July 1944 Robertson was back in England, assigned to No. 6 Canadian General Hospital in Farnborough. It was just over a month since the D-Day landings in Normandy. The perception was that the war was going well and that victory was inevitable, although few predicted that it would take close to another year to be achieved. The hospital was very busy treating the casualties shipped back from the Continent by the trainload, often several hundred at a time, and it took a great deal of organization to get them sorted out and assigned to the proper wards for treatment. This experience of streamlining trauma care would also be valuable for Robertson's later career. Many of the patients would have received the same battlefield surgery that Robertson and his unit had been providing during the Italian campaign.[8]

In late September the consultant in surgery for the army, Colonel Joseph Arthur MacFarlane, hinted that it might be possible, should Robertson be so inclined, for him to be sent back to Canada.[9] Having been away from Roslyn and the two boys for well over four years, this was a decision that took no time to make. In October, along with 10,000 others, he sailed on the *Queen Mary* bound for New York. By then the German U-Boat threats had diminished considerably and the transatlantic voyage was uneventful. The only excitement was that Bing Crosby was aboard, returning from entertaining the troops in France and Holland, although they were unsuccessful in persuading him to entertain those on board. Landed in New York, Robertson took the train to Montreal to be greeted by Roslyn and the two boys. The elder, Tam, now six and a half years old, was a bit wary of what he perceived to be a faintly menacing stranger, while Ian, at four and a half years, was, he recalled, "merely perpetual motion."

Next ahead was the decision of what to do.

It was a different Robertson who returned from the war. Even though he regarded his surgical training as "patchy and incomplete," there is little doubt that the huge amount of surgery thrust upon him, and under very primitive conditions, had expanded his experience and provided him with far more confidence than the untrained junior who had set off in 1940. The military experience had also helped him to focus on surgical and administrative priorities. These related to trauma and to the development of civilian systems based on the military, underscoring the vital principle that whatever the system might be, it must, as had been drummed into the military surgeons, minimize the time between wounding and definitive care. The leaders he had met while in the military had greatly influenced him. Sir Howard Florey was involved in shock-related research, but the even more important introduction of penicillin was impressed upon him when he had the chance to test it in several clinical cases and noted the dramatic effects on gas gangrene victims. From Trueta, he had learned the important addition of debridement to wound management in the military setting. Although he did not yet know how important they would be, the relationships he established with colleagues in a wartime environment would last for the rest of his life, and these colleagues would continually support each other professionally and otherwise.[10] Beyond this, he had had extraordinary contacts with Canadian and international medical leaders. Wilder Penfield, then neurosurgeon-in-chief at the Montreal Neurological Institute, had spoken with him about many things, including trauma and trauma systems, but also about the almost certain advent of a universal medicare system in Canada. All of the others were to play some future role in Robertson's career.

POSTWAR: VANCOUVER AND
EXPANDING HORIZONS

The principal dilemma was whether or not to stay in Montreal. Shortly after his return, Robertson reported to Ottawa and Brigadier Warner, who offered him his choice of chief of surgery at the Queen Mary Veterans Hospital in Montreal or at the Vancouver Military Hospital. Montreal was clearly the better position from an academic perspective, especially since there was not even a medical faculty at the University of British Columbia (UBC), but the downside was that there were several Montreal surgeons senior to Robertson who were still overseas and who would be returning within the foreseeable future. He thought they would resent him for having usurped their positions and that the situation would become most uncomfortable, so, after some soul-searching, in November 1944, Lieutenant Colonel Robertson accepted the appointment as surgeon-in-chief at the Vancouver Military Hospital. The family packed its worldly goods in crates and set off by train for Vancouver.[1]

The Vancouver Military Hospital had only recently opened as a temporary facility, located at the Shaughnessy Veterans Hospital, designed to care for the many casualties expected to arrive from the European and Pacific theatres. Robertson took over at once upon his arrival in November as chief of surgery. Shaughnessy Veterans Hospital had been in existence since the First World War and in the early 1940s had moved to splendid new quarters, along with its surviving veterans and a growing number of more recent ones. The surgeon-in-chief at Shaughnessy was Dr A.B. Schinbein, who had held the post since shortly after the end of the First World War. Robertson found him to be a superb surgeon, sound in both judgment and technique. He half expected the rugged individualist, usually blunt and often crusty, intensely proud of his status as the leading surgeon in the province, to be resentful of the intrusion represented by his arrival, but he found him, somewhat to his surprise, to be kind and helpful.

Schinbein carried on as chief of surgery for a year or so and encouraged Robertson to join him in his work at Shaughnessy. Schinbein himself came often to the Vancouver Military Hospital to consult on difficult problems, and in the process Robertson learned an immense amount from him. He recognized that he had an enormous amount to learn since his surgical training had been patchy and incomplete. The only practical surgery he had had, over and above his academic training, had been in the army, so; while he had plenty of experience dealing with wounds, his civilian practice had been limited to a few months of rather poorly supervised work in 1939–40, while he was waiting to be mobilized. Added to this was his relative lack of exposure in matters of administration. It was true that he had good training in army administration and that his time in the field surgical unit had given him a valuable introduction to the rough-and-tumble of administrative survival in the field. However, he still had much to learn about the more subtle, but no less hazardous, jungle of the administration of a clinical service in a nonmilitary hospital. After Schinbein's retirement in 1945, Robertson became chief of surgery at the Shaughnessy as well.

Fortunately, there was much to be done, and learning was done on the job. There was a steady flow of sick and injured patients from the training establishments in the region, as well as sporadic shipments of wounded from overseas. The necessary services had to be organized and supplied with both staff and interns.[2] To attract good interns, however, it was necessary to be able to teach them, which involved developing a course of lectures. For those who aspired to the level of fellowships in surgical specialties, the hospital had to provide facilities for anatomical dissection. The hospital also had to arrange for an amendment to the provincial Anatomy Act to permit undertakers to release subjects for the purpose of dissection. Once these basic functions were organized, the staff moved on to developing a small research unit in connection with the department of pathology, where they started some projects – investigating venous thrombosis, the preparation of arterial grafts, the effects of splenectomy, and the ever-troubling problem of hospital infection. The latter project was headed up by the hospital pathologist, Dr J.C. Colbeck, who devised ingenious methods to follow contaminants through the hospital, a project of deep interest to the surgical service.

EARLY EXPOSURE TO THE ROYAL COLLEGE

In June 1945 Robertson received the certification in general surgery from the Royal College of Physicians and Surgeons of Canada. His certification was based on his interrupted training program in general surgery as a result of wartime activity.[3] The Royal College had emerged by way of the Canadian Medical Association over the course of the early and mid-1920s, as medical specialization was becoming increasingly prevalent, but no formal structure had emerged for dealing with the granting of credentials and licences for the specialists. The further need for coordination of advanced postgraduate training in all medical and surgical disciplines had added to the impetus to create a body responsible for such activities. The Royal College, spearheaded by a group of physicians from Regina, who were assisted by colleagues in Montreal and Toronto, began its activities in June 1929, charged with the principal task of certifying the professional competence of new specialists. It is not a licensing body as such but monitors the level of all medical specialty training in Canada.

On 14 November 1946 Robertson was awarded a fellowship by the Royal College, *ad eundem gradum*, entitling him to the distinction of the postnominal Fellow of the Royal College of Surgeons (FRCS) (Canada) to go along with his Edinburgh fellowship earned before the war. At the time, as had been the case when he studied in Edinburgh, there was a difference between having a certification and being a Fellow, both decisions falling within the competence of the Royal College. His established prominence within surgical circles in Vancouver and his recognized leadership abilities led to early election to the Council of the Royal College in 1951, at the age of thirty-nine, followed by re-election to a second four-year term in 1955. From the beginning, he was on several important committees, including, from 1951, as a corresponding member of the Committee on Credentials of the Surgical Division. He was an examiner for the Fellowship in Surgery from 1953 to 1955, on the Committee for the Approval of Hospitals in December 1955, and for several years a member of the Committee for Annual Awards. A combination of wisdom, personal charm, and leadership skills advanced him to the Executive Committee, first as a member-at-large from 1953 to 1955 and later as vice president from 1955 to 1957. He served as the Royal College's representative to the American College of Surgeons' Board of Governors from 1952 to 1955, a position that opened the door to the entire leadership in US surgery and lifelong associations with leading surgeons throughout the United States.

One area in particular that showed his leadership and ability to tackle difficult problems in a tactful manner was the Certification Program, which had led to a double standard within the Royal College, that of certification and that of full fellowship. The first was perceived as the technical or professional qualification and the latter as something of a "club" whose entry criteria were mysteries known only to the initiated. The issue had been controversial for many years. The council had attempted to address the matter in 1939, putting forth the view that any new certificants should be admitted to the Royal College at once and as a matter of course. The opposing view was that certification should be at a lower level and that there should be no automatic relationship with the Royal College itself. Fellowship should be awarded only at some later date after review by a credentialing group of the Royal College. In 1953 Robertson moved that the council form a committee to study the Certification Program. Since no good deed seems to go unpunished, he was appointed as the chairman of the Robertson Committee that was to study the problem and to make recommendations, which reported to the council in 1955. The committee supported the maintenance of the two standards but made important recommendations to the effect that the training requirements for certification be made the same as those for fellowship. The council finally adopted the recommendations in 1959, and the first graduates of the Certificate and Fellowship Program were produced by 1965.

In the meantime, in 1957, a second committee, chaired by Dr E.H. Botterell, and of which Robertson was a key member, recommended that the certification examination be discontinued and that certificants be brought in as full members of the Royal College. The recommendation was rejected by the council, apparently on the basis that it would have required an amendment of the statute incorporating the Royal College. The solution was to establish a single examining board for both certification and fellowship, which had the practical effect of ending the double standard. Robertson thus played a critical role in the resolution of a thorny and divisive issue, the solution to which produced a considerably larger and stronger Royal College.[4] Throughout his career Robertson would be a strong advocate for the concept that specialty training should ultimately fall under the aegis of a university program and that there be a more extensive screening program that would involve local evaluations, and this eventually led to the in-training evaluation report system that was developed and perfected in the 1970s. He also emphasized the need to evaluate trainees and programs on their quality rather than simply on the length of time involved. This was a recurrent theme for Robertson throughout his medical life and one for which he advocated wherever he was involved, particularly in the teaching hospitals.

HOME AND FAMILY

Robertson purchased a home in the fashionable Shaughnessy area in Vancouver at 1361 Minto Crescent, just off Granville Street between 32nd and 33rd Avenues. It cost $17,500, which probably meant that he had some help from the families since his military salary and hospital stipends would not have supported an expenditure of this magnitude. Tam and Ian were already part of the family scene, and to this prewar contingent were added Bea in 1946 and Stuart in 1947. All four children would go on in due course to rewarding careers, but only one of his grandchildren would follow him in medicine.

The two elder boys attended Athlone School in Vancouver and did their high school as boarders at Shawnigan Lake School on Vancouver Island. Tam then attended and graduated from the University of British Columbia. He went on to work for the investment dealer firm of A.E. Ames & Co., first in Montreal and then in Paris, before moving to Ottawa to join the federal Department of Finance, where he became responsible for treasury bill auctions and later for the Farm Credit Corporation. He contracted Parkinson's disease and was particularly debilitated by it, dying from its complications in early 2007. Ian studied at McGill University after doing two years at the University of British Columbia and followed this by attending Harvard University, where he did exceptionally well in the master of business administration (MBA) program. He became associated with Maurice Strong and was involved in the early days of the Canadian International Development Agency. Bea attended Miss Edgar's and Miss Cramp's School in Montreal and then had a "finishing" year at a Swiss school, there being no apparent interest in the family that she pursue a university education. She worked at the Royal Victoria Hospital for a group of doctors and then, as a mother, moved to Ottawa with her husband Joel Freeman, a McGill medical graduate. When their three children were older, she worked at the Royal College in an administrative position and is an administrative assistant at the Neuroscience Research Institute at the University of Ottawa's medical faculty. Cynthia, one of her three children, is the only medical doctor directly descendant from Robertson, a graduate of the medical school at the University of Western Ontario. Stuart is a lawyer in Toronto, where he specializes in media law and has been characterized as the dean of the media law Bar of Canada.

THE UNIVERSITY OF BRITISH COLUMBIA MEDICAL FACULTY

By early 1950 Robertson had become chief of surgery at the Vancouver General Hospital, and although he continued as chief at Shaughnessy as well, he spent less time there than previously. He developed a small private practice, using Dr Schinbein's quarters in the local Medico-Dental building on West Georgia Street, where he got some additional, if not very lucrative, experience. A medical faculty at the University of British Columbia was definitely in the works. It was a time of physical expansion and increase in status for the university, and for the latter purpose in particular, it was all but obligatory that it have a faculty of medicine. The formal steps to create it were taken in 1949, with the appointment of Myron Weaver from Minnesota as the first dean of medicine. Pressure was added to the situation by the announcement of the university president – somewhat the reverse of the "if you build it, they will come" syndrome – that students would be admitted to the faculty in September 1950. Establishing any new faculty, let alone a faculty of medicine, is an enormous task: staff had to be appointed, premises found for the preclinical years, arrangements made with teaching hospitals, and teaching, office, and research facilities designed and built within the Vancouver General Hospital and elsewhere. Weaver worked well and effectively. Robertson was appointed professor of surgery in February 1950, one of the earliest of the professorial appointments in the new faculty and the first in surgery.

Getting ready for the teaching work, Robertson went on a tour of some of the prominent medical schools in North America, which produced a mixed bag of results and as many bad experiences as good. Nearby was the University of Washington, which had a recently established faculty that Robertson thought might generate some useful tips, but having spent the day with the university's professors of medicine and surgery, he concluded that although they were very friendly, they were not very helpful. One thing was clear, however, and that was a lack of interest in undergraduate teaching, a feature not by any means restricted to the University of Washington, as it seemed to be a common denominator in most of the medical faculties, where the preoccupation appeared to be with research. At Minnesota, the source of the UBC dean of medicine, he met with Dr Owen Wagensteen, one of the giants in American surgery, who was also very hospitable but obsessed with an anticancer program, believing that if the surgeon were aggressive enough, he could get rid of the patient's cancer, in many cases, an approach that led him into the most drastic operations and reoperations, which seemed more like butchery than surgery to Robertson, who was glad to see this craze disappear a few years later. In New York he encountered more butchery in some hospitals and some good work in others but not much that would be of use back home.

In Baltimore he found the most exciting developments that he was to encounter. It was the era of the "blue baby" operations, a procedure devised by Alfred Blalock and a superb example of how breakthroughs can occur as the result of interdisciplinary exchanges. The whole idea for the procedure came out of a lunch discussion in the hospital cafeteria with Helen Taussig, a pediatric cardiologist, about failed research enterprises. Blalock had been describing how he had been unsuccessful in producing pulmonary hypertension in dogs by anastomosing (surgically connecting adjacent blood vessels) the subclavian artery to the pulmonary artery. The anastomosis had worked well, but the animals' raised pulmonary blood pressure had not had the expected effect on the pulmonary vasculature. Taussig expressed amazement that it was possible to anastomose a systemic artery to the pulmonary artery. If this were technically feasible, she reasoned, it would be worth trying the procedure with infants suffering from congenital pulmonic stenosis (abnormal narrowing of the artery). Blalock agreed to try. The results were better than anyone had dared hope, and it opened up a whole new vista in surgery. As for Ohio State University and the University of Michigan, they were hospitable but yielded nothing of particular interest. At the University of Toronto he reconnected with Dr MacFarlane, who had been the senior consultant overseas during the war and whom he had come to know quite well and to admire. The general bottom line, however, remained the same – no one was much concerned about the undergraduate and everyone wanted to display their research prowess, often by rolling out a battery of machines or electronic devices to show what wonders they could perform. Some of the surgery that he saw was magnificent; some was disgusting. In the end, he learned very little that he could put into practice as a budding professor of surgery in a new faculty of medicine.

The teaching that resulted at the University of British Columbia was very conservative. Harold Copp had gone on the faculty's behalf to Case Western Reserve at Cleveland to learn about its new and revolutionary program of integrated teaching but had come away none too impressed, so they all settled down to reproduce their McGill and University of Toronto models. Looking back many years later, Robertson felt they had probably missed a great opportunity to improve on the past since they were not hampered by any particular traditions, having an entirely clean slate before them. They rationalized that the methods they had grown up with had been the result of generations of trial and error and that to break away from them would almost certainly lead to failure. In any event, they were under the gun to be ready for the September arrival of the first entering class of the faculty. They still had formal lectures, which Robertson thought was probably a mistake. Students only responded to brilliant lecturers, who were few and far between. Robertson did not view himself as in this class of formal lecturer – he felt that he did not spend nearly enough time trying to make his lectures interesting and did not use the illustrative material readily available in the wards and research laboratories. He was much better at bedside teaching and enjoyed moving about the ward with the students discussing the cases with them. So, too, he enjoyed what they called the "side room clinics," in which they would bring in cases from the ward for discussion in the greatest detail. He thought that he was good at this and that the students seemed to both enjoy and benefit from the sessions. Indeed, he abandoned formal lectures altogether when he came to McGill.

Construction of a medical school building commenced in 1950 at the Vancouver General Hospital, joining the hospital at several levels. The surgical and medical staff offices, teaching rooms, research laboratories, and lecture theatres all adjoined the hospital. The most important links were those binding the teaching facilities with the wards that housed the teaching beds, a close-knit arrangement that suited the school's purposes well for several years. It took somewhat more time to set up and staff the animal quarters, operating theatres, and the various laboratories, but before long there were quite respectable activities in both medicine and surgery under way. At Shaughnessy Hospital there were three main surgical research projects. One dealt with the issue of hospital infection since there was a virtually worldwide epidemic of staphylococcal infections, particularly in hospitals. The hospital pathologist, Christopher Colbeck, was especially interested in the problem and worked with the surgical staff to investigate how the infection was spread and how to control it. The work was well recognized and led to several publications in prominent journals and textbooks. Robertson himself did research work on the reaction of the venous endothelium to blood clot, trauma, and other factors, which also produced several published articles, but not much attention was paid to the work beyond some mention in literature on thrombosis and tissue repair. Once the laboratories were opened at the Vancouver General Hospital, he moved the project to the new location. Allan McKenzie worked on the development of aortic grafting, then widely employed in the United Kingdom and the United States, spending much time experimenting with ways to prepare and store human and artificial grafts, which involved a lot of work on dogs.

At the British Columbia Research Council[5] on the grounds of the Vancouver General Hospital, they began the preliminary work on open-heart surgery. A team of Ross Robertson (a thoracic surgeon unrelated to Rocke Robertson), Peter Allen, William Trapp, and Philip Ashmore learned to use the heart-lung machine in the laboratory. Using dogs, they went through the complete ritual of open-heart operations, opening the heart of the anaesthetized dog, performing some sort of operation (such as making a hole in the interventricular septum and then repairing it), closing the heart and the chest and bringing the dog out of anaesthesia. They would then nurse the animal as carefully as they would a human subject. The question was when they would be allowed to operate on humans. This was a decision for Robertson to take, unlike the current policies of bringing such matters before an ethics committee, and his word on the matter, as surgeon-in-chief, was law – provided that what he ordered turned out to be right. Having no precedent upon which to rely, Robertson decided that if the team could produce a 75 per cent survival rate in a sizeable number of operations on dogs, they could move on to treat humans. Mere weeks later, the team arrived at his office to say that eighteen of the last twenty-four dogs operated upon had survived. Robertson gave his permission to proceed, and within days the first operation was carried out in the hospital. To everyone's great relief, it went well and the patient survived. In short order thereafter, open-heart surgery became almost a routine procedure.

Development of the surgical teaching services at the Vancouver General Hospital was, in Robertson's opinion, surprisingly easily achieved, with all of the subdivisions (orthopaedics, urology, neurosurgery, plastic surgery, thoracic, and ear, nose, and throat) fitting quite smoothly together. In each, there was some teaching of the undergraduates to accomplish, to which was added the graduate training program they had developed for each service. There were two general surgical services, one of which was headed up by Robertson and the other by Dr T.R. Sarjeant. All the "public" general surgical cases were admitted to these services, and any beds not used by them were filled by patients of the teaching staff of each service. These "private" patients were used for teaching in the same way as the "public" patients. Storm clouds rose on the horizon shortly after they had put the plans for the general-surgery teaching ward into effect. The superintendent of nurses announced that she was bitterly opposed to mixing male and female patients as the plans had contemplated. There was bound to be trouble, she predicted. The doctors, who were determined to have two mixed general-surgical services, pointed out that they already had similar arrangements in the private and semi-private wards, with males and females in adjacent single, two-bed, and four-bed rooms. This had no impact on the official nursing opinion; public ward patients were, somehow, different. Robertson recalled that, as this argument reached its height, he was horrified to learn that one of the male patients from Dr Sarjeant's service had made his way down the corridor during the night and got into the bed of one of the female patients. This could have been a serious set-back. A debating point fell into his hands when he learned, later that day, that on the very same night an intern had made his way into the nurses' quarters and had been surprised in the bed of one of the usually closely guarded trainees. The expected uproar regarding the patient never came – understandably enough – and the issue of the mixed surgical wards disappeared.

Progress in development of the faculty was slowed in the early years as a result of illnesses suffered by Dean Weaver, who was forced to take long periods of sick leave on two occasions. Each time, Robertson was drafted to substitute for him, which gave him valuable administrative experience but reduced the time available for surgery. During his administrative episodes, in addition to managing the day-to-day affairs of the faculty,

Robertson set himself the objective of completing the plans for the pre-clinical department building. There had been some temporary huts that the dean had worked desperately hard to make ready for the students, but it was clear that proper quarters were required. There were indications to the effect that if plans could be prepared in time, there would be money available for construction. Plans could be completed, however, only if the chairmen of the various departments could reach agreement as to the allocation of space. This led to many heated discussions and near-agreements, always foiled at the last minute when one of the disputants would balk at the necessary compromise. In the end, they missed the opportunity, and Robertson acknowledged it as a failure in his first experience of administrative bargaining.

Robertson made his own contributions to the body of academic medical literature. The traditional measure of an academic career is an individual's curriculum vitae. Robertson's c.v. was personally typed and grossly underestimated his productivity in the academic arenas of clinic work, education, and surgical research. This was in modest contradistinction to many of today's academic c.v.s, which record in mind-numbing detail practically every conference, phone call, interview, and student encounter. In Robertson's case, there is little mention of his monumental role in surgical administration or delivery of health care. His first published paper occurred in conjunction with Fraser B. Gurd and appeared in the *Canadian Medical Association Journal* in 1943, the result of work done in the Department of Surgery at the Montreal General Hospital prior to his military experience.[6] It relates to the interesting topic of fluid and electrolyte balance in the surgical patient and addresses important developments in the replacement of body fluid in the context of operations as well as the inability of patients to take sufficient water and electrolytes by mouth. It is based on several cases of bowel obstruction involving the loss of large volumes of body fluids and the need for replacement by the intravenous route. It discusses methods of assessment of volume loss and appropriate replacement of both water and essential electrolytes. This work clearly was the stimulus for Robertson's life-long interest in pre- and postoperative care of the critically ill patient.

The first written record of Robertson's military experience came in a publication in 1945 in the bulletin of the Vancouver Medical Association. It is entitled "Activities of a Field Surgical Unit" and describes the changes that were necessary in the medical-service system related to the dramatic transformation in the style of warfare. Mobile field surgical units were developed, and while they were first used in the Spanish Civil War, Robertson gives credit for their emergence to a British surgeon, D.W. Jolly, who published a book describing such a unit, including its medical composition and an outline of the equipment required.[7] Robertson describes the first Canadian surgical units formed late in 1942 and sent with the First Canadian Division to Sicily in July 1943. These units could set up in almost any location and were strategically located with the military line of attack, where they functioned in tandem with a field transfusion unit – first developed by Bethune in the Spanish Civil War – and a field dressing station. The three components were grouped together and described as an advanced surgical centre (ASC). The sole purpose was to provide a surgical facility near the front line for patients, whose chance of recovery would be jeopardized by a longer delay. The location of the ASC was balanced to be close to the front lines yet far enough away to be out of the range of field artillery. Robertson noted that this plan resulted in an average interval between wounding and admission of approximately five hours, down from averages during the First World War of twelve to eighteen hours. During the Sicilian campaign, which lasted only thirty-one days, the two Canadian field surgical units set up their location in seven different areas and prompted the following comment by Robertson:

Perhaps one of the most interesting features of this field surgery is the constant changing of location. In peace time or in a base hospital in war time, one is brought up to operate in a proper operating theatre and one becomes accustomed to and somewhat dependent upon its fixtures and conveniences. In the field it is different. There are no fixtures and the conveniences are sometimes very scarce. This is not to deny that field surgery is pleasant – for it is undoubtedly enjoyed by all those who take part – nor is it to say that it is not efficient – for it often is. But it does mean that a certain amount of ingenuity is required to produce satisfactory surgical conditions on all occasions.[8]

The results are of clinical interest, and Robertson describes several hundred cases where operations were performed on seriously wounded men evacuated from the divisional front. These included a broad array of injuries, including those to the abdominal wall and the underlying viscera, to the chest, and to the lower and upper extremities, all of which were the major components of this experience. Serious head injuries and facial maxillary wounds were usually sent on to specialty teams in the rear if the patient's general condition allowed for the travel. The recorded rate of mortality in this group was 15 per cent of the operations but was probably slightly higher, as several patients were operated on more than once. There were also a large group of patients admitted to the ASC who died prior to any surgical procedure.

This experience led Robertson to think about better systems for injured civilians. He accumulated an enormous repertoire on the history of trauma systems. He often stated that Napoleon's surgeon, Larrey, was most important in emphasizing the role that the surgeon should play in organizing all aspects of care to the injured patient. He credits him with developing the first "trauma system." Larrey worked to improve sanitation, procurement of food and supplies for the sick and wounded, and training of medical personnel, while emphasizing the importance of rapid evacuation of the wounded from the battlefield. Robertson also underlined the importance of a system, known as Emergency Medical Services, that evolved in Britain under the direction of the Ministry of Health, designed to deal with mass civilian casualties as well as victims of the military conflict. The British organized all civilian hospitals and civilian physicians into the British Emergency Medical Service. This system established guidelines for the organization of trauma centres, their locations, corridors for prehospital transport, and triage, as well as mobile surgical teams that could be deployed close to the areas of casualties. Trauma centres were classified, based on their resources, for the first time in history.[9]

Robertson frequently spoke of how useless were the immobile medical units used in the First World War in the face of the rapid pace (notwithstanding the many set-piece trench warfare battles during the war) of troop movements. This gave birth in the United States military to the auxiliary units, composed of special surgical teams that travelled to the front lines in order to treat wounded soldiers. The Canadian field surgical units had adapted this model. During his preparation phase at Marston Green, Robertson had had the privilege of hearing a lecture by José Trueta, the great Spanish surgeon, who clearly had a major influence on his own thinking. He often quoted Trueta's dictum: "Surgical aid to casualties in the front line is impeded by many factors and has to be adapted to varying conditions, but the main basis of success is to have the wounded patient on the operating table at the earliest possible moment." This principle was the motivating factor for Robertson, upon return to civilian medicine, to develop a trauma system for care of the injured civilian. Robertson always considered, like Larrey, that the coordinator or conductor of the trauma orchestra should be a general surgeon, who would work collaboratively with surgical specialists in a designated trauma centre (which he termed a "Level I trauma hospital," as described by Henry Hamilton Bailey). His guiding principle, drummed into him by Truetta and the war experience, remained that the single most important variable in trauma care was reduction of the time between injury and definitive surgical care. There had to be a prehospital program of field and air ambulances, along with a rehabilitation program, which he had seen work effectively in Marston Green and Horsham. He also believed that a university teaching hospital was the best location for a Level I centre because it could provide the added features of education and research, which would continue to improve trauma care. There is no question that Robertson's major contribution to the field of surgery was in changing the trauma system in civilian hospitals to provide a high level of care in the shortest possible interval from injury to definitive care.

His next publication was derived from his wartime experience and was published in the *Canadian Medical Association Journal* in 1946.[10] He frequently referred to this work in his diaries and chastised himself for the delay in its publication. It related to a patient who suffered a serious crushing injury and the resulting complications. The paper was written in collaboration with William Mathews, who was one of Robertson's close military associates at Marston Green and Horsham. Mathews was later to become pathologist-in-chief at the Montreal General Hospital, and he was one of the many military comrades with whom Robertson maintained an extremely close personal friendship and professional relationship.

The next series of publications were published during his tenure at the University of British Columbia while working at the Shaughnessy Veterans Hospital and the Vancouver General Hospital. They all focus on three major topics – venous thrombo-embolism, wound and hospital-acquired staphylococcal infections, and pre- and postoperative care of surgical patients, with a special emphasis on care of patients with intestinal obstructions and early elements of surgical nutrition. All of the papers on venous thrombo-embolism basically address the various mechanisms for injury of the endothelial layer of the vein, whether by pressure, chemical irritation, or surgical manipulation. They examine the basic hypothesis as to whether a pre-existing blood clot can initiate an inflammatory change in the lining of the blood vessel, which thereafter perpetuates the process of thrombosis in a vein. These studies were all based on Robertson's impressions, during his military experience, of the consequences of massive pulmonary embolism. He also considered this to be a major problem upon his return to civilian medical care, where in-hospital pulmonary embolism produced a significant number of unexpected deaths in postsurgical patients, which was reflected in his attempt to take a clinical problem to the laboratory first and then change clinical care.[11]

Perhaps his major area of interest while in Vancouver was the whole problem of wound infection, again derived from his interest in the care of wounds during his years in England, Sicily, and Italy. His collaboration with J.C. Colbeck and W.H. Sutherland led to many publications on aspects of hospital infection. This interest in the infected wound itself became centred on mechanisms leading to the spread of hospital-acquired staphylococcal infections. He looked at mechanisms that were related to the wound and those related to the infected patient, such as the number of patients who carried staphylococcal organisms in their nasopharynx prior to surgical procedures. He also examined mechanisms where this infection spread among the hospital population – both patients and staff – and the hospital environment.

His contributions in this area were leading-edge and resulted in invitations to speak on the subject at the American Surgical Association, which is the premiere surgical organization in North America, and also to give the highly prestigious Moynihan Lecture. The keynote lecture on "Wound Infection" was delivered at the Royal College of Surgeons of England on 6 May 1958 and reflected the work done with Dr J.C. Colbeck and Dr W.H. Sutherland in both the Department of Surgery and the Department of Pathology at the University of British Columbia.[12] His approach to a complex and major hospital problem, which came to light in the postwar years and perhaps related to the overuse of antibiotics, focused on mechanisms of infection control. These included the establishment of an isolation ward where infected patients were concentrated in a special area of the hospital. It addressed, in addition, several infection-control measures, such as special care of the environment and methods for laundering blankets, pillows, and mattresses. He also outlined a schema for the spread of hospital-based infections from patient to patient, from patient to staff, and then from a hospital personnel to another group of patients. The recommendations were very significant and played a role in hospital infection-control techniques in both the United Kingdom and North America. One of the first things that Robertson would do when arriving at the Montreal General Hospital in 1959 would be to establish an isolation ward and an infection-control program. His classification of wound infections from the Moynihan Lecture was classic and was a leading work for many years. It is probably the topic that resulted in Robertson's invitations to become visiting professor at several North American medical schools during his tenure at the University of British Columbia.

The third area of Robertson's publications from Vancouver focuses on pre- and postoperative care, particularly in the management of bowel obstruction, and this is undoubtedly related to the stimulation he received from Fraser B. Gurd during his early days as a surgical staff member at the Montreal General Hospital. It was also the beginning of his major interest in surgical nutrition, which was one of the subjects he wanted to pursue when he established the University Surgical Clinic shortly after his 1959 arrival in Montreal. His recruit, Dr Gustavo Bounous, headed up a team that made monumental discoveries in the area of surgical nutrition, including the development of an elemental diet that resulted in the feeding of predigested material to the nutritionally depleted surgical patient via the normal intestinal track. While this work was led by Fraser N. Gurd and Gustavo Bounous, the foundation for all of the studies was clearly laid by establishing it as a primary focus of the McGill University Surgical Clinic.

Robertson's basic interest in surgical research can be discerned in a book chapter that he wrote on the relationship between Edward Archibald and Norman Bethune, centred on the "new medical science."[13] Robertson discusses the situation in the Department of Surgery at the time when Norman Bethune returned to McGill in 1928. Bethune worked with Edward Archibald, who was at the forefront of establishing new efforts in surgical research within the McGill Department of Surgery. Robertson notes the difficulties experienced by a clinician in the university context, which involved adding research activities to an already overburdened career. He credits Jonathan Campbell Meakins for establishing the University Medical Clinic at the Royal Victoria Hospital in 1925 and Archibald for making similar efforts shortly thereafter in the Department of Surgery, and Archibald had recruited Norman Bethune to be a leader in the area of thoracic surgery. Robertson summarized the situation thus created:

> There were facilities albeit primitive, for surgical experimentation and the hospital was fully equipped to enable its staff to treat and to follow the course of patients under study. There was unquestionably an atmosphere of intense eagerness and enthusiasm. McGill again was abreast to the times. It had entered the era of the so called new medical science which was characterized mainly in the present context by the systematic study of various categories of disease by bringing together the clinical and the basic scientists to study the causes, the course and the factors that influence the course of diseases.

This concept was undoubtedly foremost in Robertson's mind when he established his research efforts at the University of British Columbia in the area of venous thrombo-embolism, hospital-acquired infections, and nutritional support of the surgical patient. They were also the driving force in Robertson's rapid moves at the Montreal General Hospital to reintroduce "a new medical science" to a hospital that was predominantly clinical based.

These calls on his time and his administrative flair were to set a pattern that would keep him from being able to maximize his skills as an operating surgeon. The better he got at running the services, the Department of Surgery, and the Faculty of Medicine in Vancouver and later in Montreal, the more he was called upon to increase his commitment in this direction. Every meeting, every conference, every visit, every lecture, every paper took him out of the operating room. Surgeons have to be supremely confident in their decisions, their actions, and their techniques, and the only way that this confidence can be acquired is by constant work and repetition. They have to get to the point of their intervention as quickly as possible, perform the operation, and close the incision with the minimum time for the patient under anesthesia and a minimum of operative shock. Robertson paid a surgical price for his extraordinary abilities as a conceiver, organizer, and administrator. It was the same story when he moved to Montreal. In the year prior to his appointment as principal of McGill, he was able to perform only about sixty operations at the Montreal General Hospital, perhaps 10 per cent of the operating load of a fully-engaged general surgeon. There was no doubt that he was a fine surgeon in his own right but also little doubt that he never reached the degree of operating skill that would have been commensurate with his expectations of himself. In many of his journals, correspondence, and conversations, there is a constant theme of not having done enough surgical work. The unstated message was that he knew that lack of constant practice diminished the skill and proficiency he could bring to a particular case. His personal loss in this regard, however, was far more than offset by the benefits that his other skills provided to generations of surgeons, physicians, and patients and to the advancement of medicine and surgery. There would be no book written about Robertson as an operating surgeon, with a stainless steel scalpel in his hand. The Robertson with a mental scalpel is a much different proposition.

THE BENEFITS OF NETWORKING

Although it would be many years before the term "networking" became a term of art, Robertson had an unerring instinct and ability to develop a broad range of contacts, associations, and friendships that made him even more effective in his work. His networking had begun with the extended Robertson family, expanded during his student years at McGill University, been enhanced during his time in the military, and been honed once he returned to Canada. While the vast majority of those in the postwar generation have little, if any, experience with the military, one should never discount the powerful associations and friendships that were developed in the crucible of war and how durable they remained throughout the lives of those concerned. To this experience was added the development at the University of British Columbia of a new faculty of medicine, which always attracts leading scholars and physicians, and later his appointment to the prestigious Faculty of Medicine at McGill University. And on top of all the experience and opportunities, he had an engaging, articulate, intelligent, and ambitious mind wrapped in an attractive and friendly personality – people recognized him as someone destined for prominence.

In the early years of the new faculty at the University of British Columbia, there were several outstanding visitors. Robertson, like many physicians, had a very retentive memory and thus had clear recollections of them even years after many of the visits. Sir Geoffrey Keynes was noted for his work in such different fields as blood transfusion, cancer (on which he had extraordinary views that would turn out, thirty years later, to have been correct), and surgery of the thymus gland. When he had visited the University of British Columbia in 1956, his main interest outside his medical involvement had been to find a book that was reputed to have once belonged to the mystical poet William Blake. Robertson and Keynes remained friends for years, and it was Keynes, sharing an interest in books with Robertson, who had encouraged Robertson to persist with expanding his collection of dictionaries, which, over time, came to be one of the largest, if not the largest, private collections of dictionaries in the world. Robertson would later donate the collection to the University of British Columbia and publish, with one of his grandchildren, a monograph describing the collection. Sir James Learmouth, professor of surgery at Edinburgh University, was best known at the time for his attentions to King George VI, upon whom he had performed a lumbar sympathectomy in Buckingham Palace several years earlier. Although his visit to the university was successful in all other respects, he refused to give any interviews to the media, which caused the university some mild embarrassment. The background to the refusal was his disgust with the press following his intervention with the king, when they followed and hounded him for days before and after the operation and used any and all means to get photographs of anyone or anything connected with the case. Sir James resolved never again to have dealings with the media. Robert Milnes-Walker, professor of surgery at Bristol University, was well known internationally for his interest in management of the bleeding in cirrhotics but had such a wide breadth of surgical knowledge and experience that all the advice he gave to them during his stay was especially valuable.[14]

There were nonsurgical visitors of importance as well, including Sir Howard Florey, one of the collaborators in the production of penicillin. Robertson remembered his visit during the war to No. 1 Canadian General Hospital at Marston Green, when Florey had given a thrilling account of the results of the first clinical trials of penicillin, which had been extraordinary and otherwise unachievable. By the time of his postwar visit, Florey could share the difficulties he and his colleagues had faced while trying to get the pharmaceutical companies to undertake commercial production of penicillin. The batches used for the clinical trials had been produced in the Oxford laboratory. Despite the urgent appeals of Florey and his colleagues, the British companies refused to move forward. They were already fully committed, indeed overcommitted, to meeting the needs of a country at war and could not take on anything more. Florey looked elsewhere. He filled his briefcase with penicillin cultures and set out for the United States, where, once again, he was unsuccessful. None of the large companies he approached were willing to accommodate him. On the verge of concluding that he had exhausted all the possibilities, he happened upon a relatively small company by the name of Pfizer that agreed to take on the considerable task of producing penicillin commercially. It was chilling to them all, even well after the war, to think how close Florey had come to giving up and how many additional lives would have been lost had he failed.

There were, in addition, many American visitors, of whom Robertson considered the most prominent to be Richard Cattell, surgeon at the Lahey Clinic, who stayed for several days, giving lectures, making ward rounds, and enthralling staff and students alike with accounts of his surgical adventures. Perhaps the greatest of these had been in 1953 when Anthony Eden, foreign secretary in the British government, had undergone a cholecystectomy (removal of the gall bladder) in a London nursing home, during the course of which the common bile duct had been damaged. Eden had a biliary fistula and was incapacitated. It appeared that there was no surgeon in Britain with experience in the repair of the common bile duct. The typically British explanation seemed to be that such damage so rarely occurred in Britain, where only fully qualified surgeons were allowed to operate, that no one knew how to fix a type of damage that should never have occurred in the first place! As luck would have it, Cattell had extensive experience in common duct repair and was in Europe at the time. He was invited to see Eden and advised him that he should have an operation. There followed an interview with Prime Minister Winston Churchill, who asked whether Cattell would perform the operation in England – there was a matter of national pride at stake. Cattell replied that he would operate only in his own theatre, with his own team, instruments, x-ray facilities, and so forth. There, he could expect a good result, but he could not be at ease in any other place. Churchill countered that he was prepared to duplicate Cattell's theatre, down to the last sponge. Cattell could bring over his own nurses and orderlies, his operating table, his instruments, indeed anything at all that he might require. Even knowing how sensitive the situation was, Cattell was firm. He knew that Churchill would do everything he could to help, but he also knew that he could do his best work only in his own shop, so he would have to say "no." At this point, Cattell recounted, Churchill, without blinking an eye, launched into a discussion of world affairs, occasionally engaging Cattell in conversation, but for the most part it was a fascinating monologue. Abruptly, Churchill stopped, turned to face Cattell, and said, "Once more, Dr. Cattell, will you do this operation in London?" "No, sir," he replied, and the interview ended. In the end, the operation took place in Boston and was successful. Eden outlived Cattell.

In February 1956 Robertson was invited by another wartime friend, Francis D. Moore, to be the surgeon-in-chief *pro tempore* at the Peter Bent Brigham Hospital in Boston, one of the teaching hospitals associated with Harvard University, and visiting lecturer at Harvard University.[15] This was a major recognition; Robertson was only the second Canadian ever to have received the appointment. Although a completely honorary position, he would be nominally responsible for the entire surgical service of the hospital for a week. His duties included giving a public lecture as well as attending the regular clinico-pathological conference and the x-ray conference, teaching the medical students, and working with the resident staff. This was an extremely prestigious appointment and Robertson worked hard to prepare, knowing that he would be pitted against some of the most respected surgeons on the continent and the brightest of the Harvard students. He was filled with the usual doubts as to whether he could hold his own in such circumstances. The week, when it came, seemed to go by in a flash. The Robertsons stayed with the Moores, with whom they became lifelong friends, although Robertson himself stayed at the hospital for two nights "on call," and they met many interesting people, both medically and socially.

He came away with several new ideas that could be applied at the Vancouver hospitals and in the medical faculty and witnessed a number of new surgical and other techniques, including a kidney transplant, assisted in some operations, was requested to make diagnoses, and conducted ward rounds. Robertson's public lecture ("Observations on Venous Thrombosis")[16] was, as he observed, "politely received," and he felt he did quite well at the two conferences, emerging relatively unscathed from the good-natured traps set for him by some of the practitioners. He found the Harvard students, with whom he made several ward rounds, to be impressive, noticeably superior to the students at the University of British Columbia, and much better in biochemistry and physiology, although relatively weaker in pathology, physical signs, and anatomy. This meant that when he got backed into some highly scientific corners, he could work his way out by introducing some anatomical or histological question or by demonstrating a physical sign that they had not yet encountered. He had an amusing discussion with the chief orthopaedic surgeon, who took him mildly to task about the number of cases that were being referred to Boston for consultation and who thought that Robertson should "tighten things up." As the discussion continued, it turned out that all the patients were coming from Winnipeg and that the doctor had thought this was where British Columbia was. All in all, it was a delightful experience, and the remarks of the colleagues and students were particularly generous. Later, in 1965, Robertson and Moore would receive honorary doctorates from the University of Glasgow at the same Convocation.[17]

A similar occasion arose in 1958, this time in Great Britain, when Robertson was invited to take over the professorial unit as temporary director from Sir James Paterson Ross, one of the most famous of British surgeons,[18] at Saint Bartholomew's Hospital in London.[19] This, too, was an enormously prestigious honour, and as Robertson looked at the pictures hung in Sir James's office, he considered himself to be "the smallest fry by far" to have held the position.[20] He was the first Canadian to receive such an appointment. Adding to the general honour of the appointment, he was named a Perpetual Student of Barts, a special distinction that had been conferred only upon the previous holders of the temporary professorship, plus the Dukes of Windsor and Gloucester. The two weeks were not unlike what he had done in Boston. He met with the students and staff, did some teaching, reviewed the research projects, and gave a public lecture (the Moynihan Lecture) at the Royal College of Surgeons of England. There were, he concluded, significant differences between the two medical schools. The English students were much younger and more carefree than their American counterparts, who were much more earnest and struggling to excel. The research at Barts was much simpler than at the Brigham, and there was obviously much less money available for research, so while the staff members did their best with what they had, the results at this stage were unimpressive, certainly not at the level of the splendid clinical performance and unique history of the institution. The pity seemed to be that although there was excellent research being done and published in both England and Scotland during the late 1950s, very little came from Barts.

Robertson's own teaching was later recognized by the University of British Columbia when it established the H. Rocke Robertson Award in 1982, presented annually since 1983 for outstanding clinical teaching. A large plaque, with a picture of Robertson, hangs on the wall at the office of the UBC Department of Surgery at the Vancouver General Hospital, and the winners' names are engraved on it.

By 1958, after fourteen years in Vancouver, Robertson was a well-established surgeon, with a reputation that had spread throughout Canada and the United States as well as to Great Britain. He was known to have been instrumental in the development of a new faculty of medicine, had been recognized as a leading academic, was the initial professor of surgery at the University of British Columbia, was known as a capable and forward-looking professional, and was obviously entering into the peak years of his surgical career.

MONTREAL GENERAL HOSPITAL

It is difficult to piece together the precise sequence of events that began to unfold in 1958. This much, however, is clear. McGill University and its two principal teaching hospitals, the Montreal General Hospital and the Royal Victoria Hospital, had invited a special committee of external academic surgeons to undertake a comprehensive survey of the Department of Surgery with a view to determining how it was functioning "in regard to the care of the sick, the teaching of students and the conduct of research."[1] The chairman of the committee was Professor Robert Milnes-Walker, an eminent English surgeon from the University of Bristol, and the other members were Dr Frederick G. Kergin, a professor of surgery and renowned surgical educator at the University of Toronto, and Dr Francis D. Moore from Harvard University Medical School and the Peter Bent Brigham Hospital.

In June 1958 the committee, after meeting with the medical staffs of the Department of Surgery and other departments, as well as with university officials, reported with regret on an observed tendency for staff surgeons to lose interest in original work as they became more active in practice. More significantly, the committee noted, "both inside the Department ... and outside it, that there was a lack of guidance and direction at the summit." The committee was particularly critical of the Royal Victoria Hospital but recommended that neither of the current surgeons-in-chief at either hospital be reappointed and that "every effort should be made to attract academic surgeons of the highest caliber."[2] The report, which the committee thought should have been kept confidential except for a summary of the recommendations, caused an uproar, especially at the Royal Victoria Hospital. A confidential supplementary report was issued in December 1958.

Central to the recommendations of the committee was its assessment of the modern concept of surgery. Today's surgeon was no longer merely a person who operated. Modern physiology, biochemistry, and physics had all had their impact, and a department of surgery that was to be in the vanguard of progress must be permeated by such influences. The committee concluded that surgery was changing its outlook at the present time more rapidly than any other branch of medicine and that unless a medical school was right up-to-date in its teaching, it would fall by the wayside. Surgical progress was such that the student must be imbued with the spirit of advancement and change so as to continue to be receptive to changes throughout a professional life. In surgery, just as in medicine, there were many problems that affected not only the treatment of individual patients but also the outlook of treatment in a wider sense; these problems could be solved only in a laboratory. It might be necessary in many such investigations to bring the patient into the laboratory or even to provide a small ward that would act as such an investigation laboratory within the hospital itself.

With respect to the position of surgeon-in-chief, the committee had two comments:

> In any department, the concept of surgical advance and surgical scholarship is the product of the stimulus of the head of the department, and we consider that if this atmosphere is going to pervade the department it must be inspired from the top. We are not aware of any department of surgery where major progress has been made as a delegated responsibility while the head occupied himself solely with clinical practice and thinking ...
>
> The whole of our recommendations will stand or fall on the selection of new surgeons-in-chief at the two hospitals. We gave careful consideration to the possibility of appointing present members of the staff to these posts, but came to the conclusion that no present member fulfilled all the requirements that we envisage, and that there would be advantages in appointing men who had shown their ability elsewhere. We believe, as one of those whom we interviewed expressed it, that the University and Hospitals should go out into the world and find the best men and make the posts sufficiently attractive to bring these men to Montreal. They should look for men under fifty years of age who have already shown

their ability as academic surgeons, who will fit in well with their
colleagues and who have had some experience of research. They
must be able to provide that dynamic spirit which can stimulate in
others the need for progressive research. We believe that there are
such men available who would be attracted by the facilities which
Montreal can offer to do this work and who are less interested
in material rewards. The appointment of two such men would,
we believe, bring McGill University right back to the forefront of
surgical progress.[3]

In Montreal, Fraser N. Gurd (one of those considered by the special
committee for the post but not recommended)[4] believed that Robertson,
with whom he had interned during the summer of 1938, was the best
candidate: "I had already come to the conclusion that Dr. H. Rocke Robertson of Vancouver would be the best choice for surgeon-in-chief. As
founding chairman of the Department of Surgery at the University of
British Columbia and acting dean of the medical school, he had gained
the experience so sorely needed at McGill. His personality and charm
would assure the full support of all concerned. The only question was,
would he leave Vancouver?"[5] Interestingly, Milnes-Walker, as chairman of the committee, had written privately to McGill's principal, Cyril
James, on 17 June 1958, prior to the completion of the committee's formal
report, specifically mentioning Robertson as the one name on which all
the members of the committee were agreed for surgeon-in-chief at the
Montreal General Hospital.[6] Milnes-Walker had been one of the distinguished visitors at the University of British Columbia's medical faculty
a few years earlier and had met Robertson at this time. Francis Moore
had arranged for Roberston to be the surgeon-in-chief *pro tempore* at the
hospital in February 1956, so there could be little doubt that he would
have been favourably disposed to Robertson's appointment. Kergin, in
a Canadian academic surgical environment, would undoubtedly have
known Robertson as a fellow academic. Given the major deficiencies
in the development of surgery in both hospitals and the challenge that
would face the next surgeons-in-chief, as well as the desire to better
integrate the hospitals' surgical departments with the academic mission of the university, it was a massive vote of confidence in the abilities
and potential of Robertson on the part of this blue-ribbon committee
of experts. Milnes-Walker also told James that Robertson had spent a

day with him in Bristol approximately two weeks prior to the date of his letter, before leaving for a month on the Continent in early June.

Robertson's diary for 30 May 1958 records that, in the course of a brief tour he and Roslyn were taking through south-western England, during the period of his stint at Saint Bartholomew's Hospital in London, he visited Bristol, where he met Milnes-Walker at the Bristol Royal Infirmary and spent the day with him. While Milnes-Walker was busy, he talked with Dr Miller, a lab expert, and with Joe Peacock, who had spent some time at Michigan and who was interested in Raymond's disease. He lunched at the hospital, watched Milnes-Walker do a case at the children's hospital, and then drove with him to see the Clifton suspension bridge that had been built in 1864. He recorded the story of a frantic young woman who had attempted to commit suicide by jumping off the bridge (it was a favourite suicide spot) not long after it was built, only to be saved from death by the parachute effect of her petticoats. She lived to be 100 years old and recounted this experience on her hundredth birthday on a program aired by the British Broadcasting Corporation. They then drove out to the Milnes-Walker's place, southwest of Bristol, a large house in open country on about ten acres of land with a view of the Mendip hills. They toured a bit, seeing Roman lead mine ruins and a forbidding Cheddar gorge, ate at a pub near Cheddar, and then returned to where they had stayed the night before. Robertson noted that they liked the Milne-Walkers very much. No mention was made in the diary of any discussion regarding his future nor of Milne-Walker's chairmanship of the special committee to advise McGill University.[7]

Milnes-Walker reported to James that he was was not certain that Robertson could be attracted back to Montreal from Vancouver, but he had not felt himself to be in a position to make anything but general comments on the possibilities to him. He went so far as to suggest that James consider waylaying Robertson in Montreal on his way back from Europe to discuss the matter with him. There is no indication in the records that any such meeting between James and Robertson occurred, and it is highly unlikely that it would have.

The first piece of correspondence regarding the matter was a letter from the dean of medicine, Lloyd Stevenson, dated 28 July 1958, within a month after the special committee issued its report, in which Stevenson expressed himself as delighted to hear a "rumour" that Robertson might be interested in coming to Montreal. Robertson's own notes of any first encounter place the contact in the fall of 1958, which is clearly wrong. His recollection was that he had been called out of a case conference at the Shaughnessy Hospital to take a telephone call from an old war friend, James Shannon, an orthopaedic surgeon at the Montreal General Hospital.[8] Shannon said that he and David Wanklyn, vice president of the Montreal General Hospital, would like to come out to Vancouver to see him but did not explain the purpose of the proposed visit.[9] Robertson wrote that he returned to the conference wondering, perhaps briefly, what it was all about, but it should not have taken (and probably did not) a nanosecond to make the fairly obvious guess. Robertson was very much aware, in the small world of academic surgery, that McGill and its teaching hospitals had been actively looking into some reorganization of their departments of surgery, especially since the contents of the report had found their way into the public, and he knew perfectly well the capacities of the two who wanted to meet with him. Nor is it clear how much about McGill's intentions Milnes-Walker may have hinted at or let slip during his encounter with Robertson during the spring.

Shannon and Wanklyn were coming to Vancouver to say, in person, that they wanted Robertson to become surgeon-in-chief at the Montreal General Hospital and chairman of the Department of Surgery at McGill University. They had, they said, McGill's full blessing to approach him on their joint behalf. In keeping with the way that such matters work in practice, they had no formal offer to make. It is bad business to make offers that may be turned down; word gets around. They were paving the way – as enthusiastically as possible and relying on their friendships – for discussions that would lead to a formal offer that would be known, before it was formally made, to be acceptable. Besides, there was some personal history involved in this particular matter.

FIRST BOUNCE

This was not the first approach that had been made to Robertson on behalf of the Montreal General Hospital and McGill University. The background to the original offer arose from the fact that at the academic level, by the mid-1940s, McGill had more or less concluded that it needed to move in the direction of having a full-time professorship in the Department of Surgery.[10] The professorship issue was not without its complications. The concept was for each of McGill's main teaching hospitals, the

Royal Victoria and the Montreal General, to have a full-time professor of surgery, who would in turn also be surgeon-in-chief of his hospital. In addition, there would be a full-time assistant professor in each of the two hospitals, who would be the director of surgical research. The Royal Victoria Hospital embraced the concept immediately. In January 1946 the Montreal General Hospital's medical board considered whether the hospital should move in the same direction. The attending surgeons supported the idea of a surgeon-in-chief but with significantly limited authority. Even more strictures were to be imposed on the assistant professor, including a prohibition against any private practice. McGill rejected this idea and, in its response describing why it would not accept the proposal put forward by the Montreal General, made the political mistake of holding up the practice of the Royal Victoria Hospital as the desirable yardstick – a huge tactical error, given the often bitter rivalry between the two institutions. This led to posturing, opposition for the sake of opposition, and bellicose statements by the Montreal General surgeons to the effect that teaching was one thing and internal hospital affairs quite another. McGill might influence the former but should stay entirely out of the latter.

When order was at last achieved, the Montreal General agreed to follow the same policy as the Royal Victoria, and a selection committee was appointed by the university Senate to identify candidates for the two positions. The first surgeon-in-chief position at the Montreal General Hospital was to be offered to Fraser Baillie Gurd and the assistant pro-fessorship to Robertson.[11] The offer to Robertson was much favoured by Gurd, who had hoped Robertson could be persuaded to return to Mon-treal and perhaps to succeed him as surgeon-in-chief. Evidently, Robert-son was aware of these machinations and may well have been willing to consider the possible appointment, but Gurd, writing to his son Fraser Newman Gurd, then studying in Philadelphia, expressed the fear that the filibustering tactics on the part of the attending surgeons at the Montreal General had been such that it would be impossible to get Robertson to fill the post of assistant professor: "He has evidently become fed up with waiting for definite information and has, I believe, purchased a house in Vancouver with the intention of staying there permanently."[12] By the end of June 1946 the committee had made its recommendations, which were accepted by the medical board of the hospital and sent to McGill for action. Inexplicably, McGill did not act on the matter for some eight

months, and it was not until March 1947 that the joint appointment of
Gurd as professor of surgery and surgeon-in-chief was confirmed and
the offer extended to Robertson. By then, Gurd was of the view (although
he hoped he was wrong) that Robertson was now comfortably ensconced
in Vancouver, had a large practice, and might well refuse the appointment.

Cyril James had written to Robertson at the Shaughnessy General
Hospital on 26 February 1947:

Dear Dr. Robertson,

A good deal of water has passed under the bridges since I had the
pleasure of talking over with you at my house the proposed reorganization of Surgery at McGill University and the Montreal General
Hospital.

Since that time a Selection Committee has been set up, consisting of representatives from both the Hospital and the University,
and after very careful consideration of the whole problem that
Committee has recommended that Dr. Fraser Gurd be appointed
as First Professor of Surgery. The Committee also wishes to recommend to the Board of Management of the Montreal General
Hospital and the Board of Governors of McGill University that you
should be appointed as the first full-time Assistant Professor of
Surgery and I have been asked to ascertain whether you would be
willing to allow me to present your name to the governing bodies
of the two institutions. Such a nomination is, as you will know
from your experience, almost the same thing as an appointment
but I would not wish to go through the formalities until I have
heard from you.

I am attaching a copy of the general agreement between the
Hospital and the University in this matter, since it defines the
major elements in the plan and you may wish to refresh your mind
on our discussions.

May I add an expression of my own personal hope that you will
find it possible to return to Montreal and accept this appointment
which would become effective at the earliest date at which you
were able to come into residence. You are already a friend of David
MacKenzie who would be your colleague in the experimental sur-

gical laboratories, and I can assure you that all of the members of
the Department of Surgery would give you a very warm welcome.

With renewed good wishes, I remain ...

Robertson characterized the offer as one of a semi-full-time post at
the hospital, which had many attractive features, especially since he was
devoted to the Montreal General Hospital and would have liked to rejoin
it. The salary, however, was very small, and to live reasonably well he
would have had to supplement the salary by income derived from private
practice conducted from offices elsewhere in the city. At the same time,
there was a growing possibility that the University of British Columbia
(UBC) would establish a medical school, where he thought he stood a
fair chance of getting an appointment, and he was enjoying his work in
Vancouver. Robertson's letter of response, dated 11 March 1947, uncharacteristically blunt in matters of this nature, made it clear that McGill's
delay in reaching a decision had not gone unnoticed.

Dear Dr. James:

I am certainly greatly honoured by the recommendation of The
Selection Committee that I be nominated to The Board of Management of the Montreal General Hospital and The Board of Governors of the [sic] McGill University as full-time Assistant Professor
of Surgery as explained in your letter of February 26th, 1947.

I clearly recall our discussion on this subject in March of 1946.
At that time I had not made any permanent commitments in British Columbia. Upon my return from Montreal I waited for some
considerable time for word from you. A point was reached where,
for personal and economic reasons, I had to make a final decision
as to where I would live. I, therefore, wrote to Dr. Gurd on the 17th
of April 1946 and asked him if he could give me any information
concerning the progress of the discussed plans. His reply on the
20th of April left me without any assurance that an early decision
would be made. I, therefore, replied on the 29th of April indicating
that I had decided to remain in Vancouver. The whole question is
now re-opened by your letter. On further serious consideration, I
have been forced to conclude that I must stand by my original decision to stay here.

I fully realize the import of this decision and can only say that the choice has been a most difficult one and has been made after most careful thought. In doing so I am relinquishing an opportunity which at one time was my ambition and one which I would have seized eagerly had it presented itself at an earlier date.

Yours most sincerely ...

James was left with nowhere to go and gave no explanation for the delay when he replied to Robertson on 24 March 1947:

Dear Dr. Robertson,

Naturally, I find the contents of your letter of March 11th very disappointing indeed, since you were the unanimous first choice of the Selection Committee for the Assistant Professorship of Surgery. I am especially sorry that we have lost you by such a narrow margin of time; but as a matter of fact I was not in a position to write to you about this matter until last month. I know that my colleagues on the Committee will fully share my own disappointment, but I can realize that the impossibility of our letting you know the McGill decision sooner put you in a very difficult position in Vancouver.

May I wish you the brilliant success that I feel confident awaits you in your future career, and with best personal wishes always, I remain,

Cordially yours ...

As McGill's principal, James was in perpetual recruitment mode. One never knew whether this particular wheel might come full circle again. He had to remain on better terms with Robertson than Robertson with him.

In the meantime there were exciting developments relating to the physical plant of the Montreal General Hospital. It had become increasingly clear that the hospital was overcrowded and had to move. The central division, then located at 66 Dorchester Street East (now René Lévesque Boulevard), and the western division, which had amalgamated with the Montreal General Hospital on 1 January 1924 and was located where the Montreal Children's Hospital is today, could not cope with the demands on them. A new hospital was required. The location of the new hospital was to be farther west, following the demographic patterns of the growing city. The preferred location was a property on Pine Avenue at Côte-des-Neiges owned by the estate of Judge Alexander Cross, which the hospital's Board of Governors had agreed was the only available and suitable site for construction of a new hospital.[13] The purchase of the property was not completed until 1948, and financial campaigns to raise the funds for construction began immediately thereafter.[14] The new hospital opened its doors in 1955.

SECOND BOUNCE

The stars and the planets may have been lined up by 1958 and some preliminary indications been given that Robertson might be receptive to the right offer, but this did not make his move to Montreal by any means automatic. The opening of the possibility led to several days and weeks of weighing the pros and cons of coming to Montreal. The family had had nearly fifteen good years in Vancouver. The two elder children were well established at the University of British Columbia, and the younger two, aged eleven and twelve, were getting along well in school. None of them would be set back by such a move. Robertson's parents would be sad to lose them from Vancouver, while Roslyn's would be correspondingly delighted to have the family back in Montreal. The couple had relatives and friends in roughly comparable numbers in each place.

Professionally, there was much to be gained for Robertson from a move to the Montreal General Hospital and McGill, which were far in advance of the University of British Columbia and the Vancouver General Hospital in the eyes of the world, although Robertson, in situ, could be forgiven for thinking (possibly even correctly) that the actual difference was perhaps not that great. After all, he had been involved in building both of the latter to their current levels of surgical achievement. Both he and Roslyn were enthusiastic and apprehensive about the prospect: she was excited but, at the same time, hated to leave a world in which she had been happy and secure; Robertson was strongly influenced by the possibility of professional enhancement, having no doubt concluded that he had likely gone as far as he could go in Vancouver. Montreal would be a promotion and bring a new challenge.

There were details to be explored. Dean Lloyd Stevenson had first to raise the concept of the "ceiling" that would apply if Robertson were to come to McGill as what was termed a "geographical full time" appointment.[15] The salary ceiling was a mechanism designed to encourage full-time research and teaching by establishing a maximum amount that the individual could earn, principally from fees generated in private practice. Anything earned above this maximum would not accrue to the individual but to the department, so any personal financial incentive to do a significant amount of outside work was deliberately removed. Stevenson was anxious to know, provided that the salary and total income package was satisfactory, whether Robertson had no objection in principle to the establishment of a reasonable ceiling. Robertson promptly replied, on 1 August, that he was not yet convinced, finding the pros and cons hard to weigh, saying only for the moment that the prospect of returning to Montreal was decidedly attractive in many respects. He had, however, no difficulty with the concept of ceilings and would gladly accomodate himself to the McGill pattern. Nevertheless, he would be keen to maintain his present standard of living, but he assumed that this would present no great problem. More important, he would want assurance of a budget and working space sufficient to maintain a staff of clinical and laboratory assistants such as he then had at the University of British Columbia. From the informal discussions that he had had and from Stevenson's letter, he gathered that Stevenson had thoughts along the same lines, so he was looking forward to hearing more.

Stevenson replied on 4 August that he hoped they could come to a mutually satisfactory agreement and that full discussion would be required. Much of this would best be done in Montreal, on the spot, where Robertson could see what was planned. There were visits for meetings with the university side, the hospital side, and members of the various departments during the late summer and fall, culminating in a letter from James, on behalf of McGill, and from W.W. Ogilvie, on behalf of the hospital, dated 24 November 1958. Robertson did not send his reply until 5 December, in which he said that while he had a sincere interest in the position, he would, before making a final decision, first have to discuss the matter with the University of British Columbia's administration. He also sought clarification on several points that had been discussed but either were not included in the offer letter or were unclear, some of which related to his own remuneration and some to the budgets for salaries of other full-time geographical appointees, laboratory space, clerical staff, and moving expenses. Most important for him, however, was a commitment to providing the facilities and space necessary to make major progress in research, plus the ability to attract good people. It is very likely that the governors of the hospital had not thought that it would be such an expensive proposition to get a surgeon-in-chief whom they might have assumed would be an easy catch – after all, it was the Montreal General Hospital. They were put in a position of having to raise considerable funds to meet the requests put to them by Robertson, but to their credit, they undertook to do so, with the result that McGill and the hospital replied on 10 December, accepting all the points raised by Robertson.

There was some risk involved for both McGill University and the Montreal General Hospital as well, which may well have been one of the reasons they were willing to negotiate at such levels with Robertson. They were in possession of a damning report from the special committee regarding the state of surgery at the hospitals and the university, which would eventually have an adverse impact on the development of both the Faculty of Medicine and the hospitals. Robertson, although someone who might well, given his McGill connection, be interested in the position, could not be regarded as a "sure thing." He was heavily involved as chief of surgery at the Vancouver General Hospital and had been actively involved in starting and running the new Faculty of Medicine at the University of British Columbia. He was well respected, had written definitive papers on medical subjects, had attracted the attention of national and international medical organizations and faculties, had been invited to give the Moynihan Lecture, and had been visiting professor and lecturer on many occasions. If McGill and the Montreal General Hospital tried to recruit him and failed, it would be a crushing blow to their prestige.

Later that month, now presented with an offer that was clearly much more attractive than the one made a decade earlier, he came east for final consideration. He had lunch at the University Club in Montreal with Cyril James, William Ogilvie, and Lloyd Stevenson. They reached a verbal agreement: Robertson would accept their offer. He would start to work at the Montreal General Hospital and take up his teaching responsibilities effective 1 July 1959. In retrospect, it was all but unimaginable that Robertson would have refused to accept the appointment, particularly since they had responded favourably to all of his concerns regarding the scope of the academic mission were he to accept. McGill had the foremost medical faculty in the country, and the Montreal General Hospital, as one of its teaching hospitals, was well known on the medical landscape as a leading teaching hospital. Added to this was the fact that the original plan, which had included the 1947 offer to Robertson, had not produced the outcomes sought by both McGill and the Montreal General Hospital (as well as by the Royal Victoria Hospital), shortfalls clearly identified by the special committee. This was to be "take two," with even greater expectations than on the previous occasion and an urgent need for someone who could come in, take over, and lead by example in an environment that had more than its share of type-A personalities. It was an opportunity that no ambitious academic surgeon could possibly resist.

By now an inveterate collector of books, Robertson celebrated the decision by going to the Mansfield Bookshop, then next door to the University Club, where he made a lucky find. The proprietor pulled out from beneath his desk a battered, but complete, copy of the first edition of Malthus's *Essay on Population*. It had been brought into the shop by a Mr Babbage, who said that it had belonged to his grandfather, Charles Babbage, a well-known mathematician in the nineteenth century whose work was considered by some to have been the mathematical origins of the modern computer. Robertson later had the book repaired by John Grey of Cambridge, and for many years it was one of his proudest possessions. Balancing off the Malthus, he also bought a copy of D.H. Lawrence's *Lady Chatterley's Lover* and spent the return trip between them.[16]

On 24 December 1958 Robertson wrote to Ogilvie and James to say that he had had a chance to discuss the situation with the president of the University of British Columbia and that he was now in a position to accept the invitation to come to McGill and to the Montreal General Hospital. He did so, he said, with the full appreciation of the honour they had bestowed on him by extending the invitation and in the most earnest hope that he might justify their confidence.[17]

The official announcement was made on 8 January 1959. Fraser Gurd wrote immediately to Robertson, saying:

The announcement of your appointment here was made public today, and I would like to tell you at once how delighted I am that you have accepted.

During the day, since the news came out, I have been thinking what Dad [Fraser B. Gurd] would have thought of the curious turn of fortune's wheel which should bring you back to the Montreal General at such an important juncture in its history. It took only a minute to conclude that he would have been immensely pleased and immensely proud.

You will be heartened to know, I am sure, of the upsurge of spirit and enthusiasm apparent among all ranks here today. The period of doubt as to your decision was demoralizing but is now a thing of the past. No one could get off to a better start than you will, in terms of goodwill and sincere support.

MOVING EAST

Anyone who has changed cities after a decade and a half of residence and a lifetime of association with relatives and friends in one city knows what a hectic strain is connected with such a move. At home, the children were considered first and arrangements made that would be the least disruptive for them. Tam, the eldest, would remain in Vancouver and complete his degree at UBC. Ian would move with the family and complete his final two years of undergraduate study at McGill. Bea would be enrolled in the private Miss Edgar's and Miss Cramp's School for girls, and Stuart was to attend Lower Canada College, a well-known private school for boys. Finding a new house was next. During his December visit, to conclude the arrangements regarding his joint appointments, Robertson had been horrified by Montreal prices and, perhaps so influenced, had not much liked any of the houses shown to him. To no one's surprise, Roslyn did considerably better when she came back east in February, finding just the right house – one that Robertson had previously condemned as hopelessly ugly when it had been shown to him – and they made arrangements to buy it. The Vancouver house was easily sold at a price he thought remarkably high: it had been bought in 1945 for $17,500 and was sold in 1959 for $40,000. He learned in 1989 that the same house was listed for sale at $1.4 million! There was a predictable round of parties and dinners, and he was profoundly touched by the mementoes and gifts presented by colleagues, students, interns, residents, and hospital trustees. The most outstanding gift was a full set of the *Oxford English*

Dictionary, an inspired choice for someone with an obvious and declared interest in the history of the English language and dictionaries.

Professionally, during the first half of 1959, although Robertson was still physically in Vancouver and undoubtedly discharged his responsibilities at the two hospitals and at UBC with his customary abilities, his active and inquiring mind was already partly in Montreal, planning for what he would accomplish upon the formal commencement of his duties.[18] The Montreal General Hospital had existed in Montreal since 1 May 1819 (only two years after the founding of the Bank of Montreal) in various forms and locations, but the new hospital, halfway up Mount Royal and bounded by Côte-des-Neiges to the west, Cedar Avenue to the north, and Pine Avenue to the south and east, referred to at the time as the "new" Montreal General Hospital, had been opened only four years prior to Robertson's arrival in Montreal. Having had no part in the inevitable compromises and trade-offs inherent in any project of the magnitude of a general hospital, he was not bound by any such arrangements and, as an experienced medical practitioner and academic, immediately began planning for improvements to the physical plant. Part of the wooing exercise had been to show off the new state-of-the-art hospital, so he already had a good idea of what was there, how it had been set up, and to some degree, how it functioned. He knew from experience, if not instinct, that if architectural "surgery" was called for, it would be best to get it done early, during the honeymoon period that would follow his arrival. With this in mind, he did not wait until he got to Montreal to start the analysis and planning.

Little thought had been given (reflecting the hospital attitude to research identified by the special committee) to providing space for full-time staff and research. Nor, inexplicably, had thought apparently been given to the need for postoperative recovery rooms or intensive care units. Sitting in Vancouver in the early months of 1959, he spent hours sketching plans of animal quarters, animal operating rooms, research laboratories, offices, an intensive care unit, and an infection unit. Fraser Gurd was particularly helpful with respect to the planning of the research laboratories, and they were in constant communication. In Montreal the architect supplied information about potentially available space, measurements, and comments on the sketches Robertson sent to him. By the time he arrived in Montreal, the planning was well advanced. It did not take long to work out the details, and the hospital's Board of Management set aside a generous amount for the changes.

Robertson was also thinking about the academic portion of his joint positions. There had been discussions with Lloyd Stevenson, the dean of medicine, during the lead-up to McGill's offer, and Stevenson wrote in early January, bringing him up to date on the parallel process at the Royal Victoria Hospital and providing him with the current teaching schedules and lectures for surgical physiology and surgical pathology (both coming under experimental surgery) and for the undergraduate program. Stevenson sought Robertson's advice on making better use of the surgical staff at the Montreal Children's Hospital in the course of undergraduate teaching and on adding a separate segment to the program in pediatric surgery.[19] As far as the dean was concerned, the whole new curriculum was an experiment that was to be the subject of searching criticism as they proceeded. As to the hospital, he passed on the observation that Robertson's plan to establish a traumatic and reparative surgery unit, obviously discussed during the earlier visits to Montreal, was likely to go well.

A NEW BROOM

Upon his arrival, and after a short experience with the existing facilities, he set out to enlarge an out-patient department that was, in his view, grossly inadequate. Drawing up the floor plans for it was easy, but resistance developed from the nursing staff, which had been largely responsible for the original design and did not welcome the drastic changes Robertson proposed. The nurses did not believe that opening up the whole area and doing away with the small cubicles would improve its efficiency. Eventually, they capitulated – they could read an organization chart as well as patients' charts – but Robertson never believed they were persuaded that the changes were helpful.

The radiologists, however, with the additional gravitas attaching to full members of the medical profession, mounted a stronger resistance. Robertson wanted to establish an x-ray unit in a room contiguous with the out-patient department so that patients requiring x-rays would merely have to be wheeled into this room, instead of having to be conveyed to an elevator and taken up to the fifth floor, where the main radiology department was located. In Robertson's plan, the films would be sent up to the x-ray department in a pneumatic tube, where they would be developed and read, and then the report and the films would be returned, also by tube. In the meantime, the patient – who under the existing circumstances had to sit or lie, often for hours, in a draughty corridor without a nurse in attendance – would be put back to bed in the out-patient department to await the results in relative comfort under the surveillance of the nursing staff. The radiologist-in-chief argued that the satellite x-ray units were wasteful and dangerous and that he could not countenance their establishment. He and Robertson had one or two "fairly brisk arguments," and the radiologists eventually came around, swayed, Robertson thought, by hospital "public opinion."[20]

Robertson had turned his personal attention to the problem of infection in surgical wounds immediately upon his arrival at the hospital. The problem of infection had increased dramatically in the 1950s, when a number of antibiotic-resistant strains of bacteria (such as *staphylococcus aureus*) began to appear. The problem, which had been a preoccupation of Robertson since his days in the army, was one that he had pursued in Vancouver and about which he had had many discussions during his visit to Harvard University and its teaching hospitals in 1956, as well as at many other hospitals. Robertson instituted a number of reforms, including new operating room arrangements, preparation techniques for patients being operated upon, and much stricter rules for postoperative dressings. An infection committee was established, an infection control nurse appointed, and more accurate records maintained. Combined with these changes, there was a major study of hospital infection, which was unfortunately abandoned when Robertson left in 1962. When he visited the Montreal General Hospital on 8 August 1969, he noted in his diary that he had been rather disappointed with the Intensive Care Unit, perhaps because he had been shown an awful case of a man whose aortic valve had become infected and whose legs were dead. Throughout his round of ward and intensive care visits, he had got the very definite impression that people had stopped worrying about infection and that all of his "preaching" had gone for naught.

A traumatic and reparative unit was established under Frederick M. Woolhouse. This had been a particular interest of Robertson, again going back to his experience as a surgeon during the war, and one that he had identified as a priority in his earliest discussions with the hospital and McGill. They also began to gear up for work in the field of cardiac surgery. The Women's Auxiliary (a formidable and effective force in support of the Montreal General Hospital) had presented the hospital with a heart-lung machine some months before Robertson had arrived on the scene, but the surgeons had no idea how to run it. Once the lab was established, they learned how to use it and began to simulate operations, getting ready for the real thing. Institutional rivalries then entered the picture. Robertson received a visit from his counterpart at the Royal Victoria Hospital, Donald Webster, who informed him that the Royal Victoria's view was that it would be "unwise" for the Montreal General Hospital to take on cardiac surgery.[21] To do so, Robertson was advised, would be to disrupt the then current arrangement, by which the full load of such surgery was comfortably handled by the Royal Victoria and the Montreal Children's Hospitals.

It is not difficult to imagine the impact that such a suggestion would have had on the ambitious Robertson, who had already gained some experience with such operations in Vancouver. He told Webster that the Montreal General Hospital intended to proceed, noting that for them to stay out of the cardiac field would be to assign themselves to a secondary role, because cardiac and major vascular surgery were going to be – indeed, already were – in the vanguard of surgical progress. Webster thereupon retired from the fray, but the Royal Victoria, not inclined to give up, sent in its most persuasive negotiator, Dr Ronald Christie, physician-in-chief, to press Robertson to reconsider his position.[22] Determined not to be seduced by Christie's charm, Robertson once again refused to relent. The final volley in this skirmish took the form of a letter from the medical board of the Royal Victoria Hospital stating that members of the board were unanimous in "deploring" his decision to commence heart surgery at the Montreal General. Robertson undoubtedly replied in some formal manner, but the real reply was the performance of the first open-heart operation at the Montreal General shortly thereafter, on 30 June 1960.[23] Fortunately, nothing went wrong. Anthony Dobell, a surgeon on the staffs of both the Royal Victoria and the Montreal Children's Hospitals, helped to solve some of the transitional angst when he joined the Montreal General staff (no doubt, speculated Robertson, to the dismay of the Royal Victoria) and operated for several years at all three hospitals. Such surgery continued at the hospital for decades and seems to have survived a more recent putsch within the Quebec health care system, where a bureaucratically invented concept of "complementarity" was invoked as a purported basis for attempting to locate all cardiac surgery in yet another hospital, which would have diminished the ability of McGill and its teaching hospitals to attract the best students, researchers, and clinicians and, furthermore, have eliminated the creative tensions that arise from having competing institutions in a city the size of Montreal.

Chemotherapy was making its presence felt in the treatment of certain malignant diseases, and this field was taken up by several of the doctors, including Lawrence Garth Hampson, Simeon James Martin, John D. Palmer, and Harry J. Scott. Dr Ian W.D. Henderson was recruited from Harvard as a full-time assistant surgeon and brought with him a knowledge of chemotherapy for cancer patients. Teaching in the wards was reorganized to reach second- as well as third- and fourth-year medical students. The University Surgical Clinic was opened in 1960, and a regular feature if its activities included attracting residents who would stay on for a program leading to a master of science degree in experimental surgery, many of whom went on to careers as surgeon-scholars. Continued improvement in the handling of emergencies led to the Montreal General Hospital being recognized as an outstanding model for the organization of hospital emergency departments.

RESEARCH MISSION

Far more difficult than alterations to the bricks and mortar was creating the paradigm shift in the direction of basic research within the Department of Surgery that had been a central tenet of the special committee report that had led to Robertson's recruitment. There had never been much original research done in the surgical department of the Montreal General Hospital. Whatever ardour that might have flickered in staff members had been effectively dampened by the complete lack of laboratory space. Failure to include such space when the new facility had been planned simply reflected that despite the structural changes effected in the late 1940s with the appointment of a surgeon-in-chief, surgical research had never developed as a priority. Generations of surgeons had passed through the department, teaching conscientiously, but without any commitment to or serious thought of doing personal basic research. Those who were inclined to do so were constantly under pressure to do surgical work in order to earn their livings and wanted to make certain there was no perception, on the part of referring doctors, that they were "unavailable" for surgical work, which, as a practical matter, would have led to such doctors no longer referring cases to them.

Most of the surgical research in the department had been, essentially, a family affair. Dr Fraser B. Gurd had made a major effort to get work started in the Donner Building on the McGill grounds opposite the Royal Victoria Hospital near the intersection of Pine Avenue and McGregor (now Doctor Penfield) Avenue, and his son, Fraser N. Gurd, had carried out a number of good studies there at great expense of time and effort. When all was said and done, the fact of the matter remained that at the time Robertson joined the hospital, Gurd was the only hospital staff member with significant research experience, so they needed to start virtually from scratch. Robertson felt that it was vital to get work going in the new laboratories; it would be most unsatisfactory if they were still vacant for long.

Robertson had negotiated for two "geographical" full-time posts in the department and, by agreement between them, offered the first to Gurd, who would be provided with a secretary and would have an office in the hospital in the surgical clinic to be constructed on the ninth floor of the hospital. This would come with a promotion to senior surgeon, giving him charge of a surgical service, and appointment as associate director, under Robertson, of the University Surgical Clinic. Over and above being relieved of the expenses for an office and secretary, Gurd would get a salary of $10,000 (with benefits) and be entitled to retain income from private patients, with a ceiling of a further $15,000 per year, all of which was enough to allow him to take the position without any significant loss of net income.

Robertson had brought William Mersereau with him from Vancouver. In fact, part of his negotiations with McGill and the hospital had specifically involved Mersereau, including his salary and moving expenses. A competent laboratory man, he soon settled in to the new hospital environment and continued work on a long-term vein endothelium project that had occupied him for years, filling one of the research facilities. Fraser Gurd occupied another, and there they stood for some time until they learned of a Taiwanese researcher, Mei Chi Lo, who was doing some work on zinc, which appeared, possibly, to have some effect on cancer of the prostate. They installed him in one of the labs, where he worked with great industry, but without getting the results he had hoped. The medical network produced another lead when an American friend of Robertson, Harris Schumacher, called to say that there was a young Italian who had been helping one of his colleagues but whose allowable time in the United States was about to expire.[24] He wondered whether Robertson might have some use for the man, Gustavo Bounous, and assured Robertson that he would not regret taking him on, should he decide to do so. Robertson jumped at the chance, and Bounous proved to be a superb worker, an original thinker, and a magnificent technician who stayed for many years. The search went on for a laboratory director, someone with extensive general experience in laboratory work, whose job it would be to initiate and help set up studies and to generally supervise the work in the lab. The first selection, John W. Trank, a physiologist from the University of Minnesota, seemed to fit the bill, but Robertson felt that he spent most of his time tinkering with his own intricate machinery and never seemed to enter into the life of the laboratory at large. He would leave for another important position after a year or so.[25]

Despite a cautious start, there were several interesting research projects underway within a short time and more on the drawing boards as Robertson worked to encourage members of the surgical department to take some initiative in projects within their own specialties and to move beyond simply doing competent surgery by assigning to each staff surgeon a particular area of interest. Alan Thompson, later to become surgeon-in-chief at the hospital, made many interesting findings arising from a study on pancreatitis that was carried on with the help of Bounous and others. Bruce Williams studied burns in rats and proved to be one of the best of the clinician-researchers in the hospital over a lengthy period, publishing many useful papers. Laird Wilson, a busy orthopaedic surgeon, did some research in bone healing. Pat Cronin, a cardiologist, was given lab space while they had it to spare in order to study the effects of interference with coronary circulation. Fleming McConnell published a paper on the effects of some of the radio-opaque substances used in radiography on the venous endothelium (which were dramatic – the venous endothelium of the rat's vena cava was badly damaged), but no one seemed to pay much attention to it. The original venous endothelium project on which Robertson and Mersereau had been working, while perhaps not exciting except to those immediately involved, nevertheless produced interesting results. Notably, they were able to demonstrate the degree of pressure necessary to damage the endothelium and also to follow the process of thrombus formation or healing in a denuded vessel. Robertson was pleased to see a significant reference to this work in a text entitled *Tissue Repair*, published more than ten years after their own main publication on the subject.[26]

Harold Elliott's retirement had left the hospital without a neurosurgeon, and Robertson set about recruiting Joseph Stratford, who was then heading up the neurosurgical department at the University of Saskatchewan.[27] It was a particularly elegant courtship, one that began in early March 1962 and was completed by the end of April, including plans and commitments for expanded and exclusive facilities in the hospital for neurosurgical patients, appointment to the medical faculty with the potential for promotion to full professorship, a residency training program in neurosurgery in conjunction with the Montreal Neurological Institute, operating room access and procedures, a starting date of 1 August 1962, and a range of other details. It took McGill until the end of August to confirm the academic appointment, but Robertson had assured Stratford that it would all work out as they had agreed, and Stratford resigned from his Saskatoon positions and moved east on the strength of Robertson's assurances. At one of the early encounters, Stratford had been invited to dinner at Robertson's home at 661 Clarke Avenue and there met Lloyd MacLean, from Minnesota, who, unbeknownst to Stratford, was being recruited by Robertson at the same time to become chief of surgery at the Royal Victoria Hospital.

Stratford was not the only surgeon to be recruited and come to the Montreal General on the strength of Robertson's verbal assurances. David S. Mulder was a student in the Faculty of Arts and Science at the University of Saskatchewan when he was offered early admission into the Faculty of Medicine's class of 1962, the second full class in the faculty. With his medical doctorate in hand, Mulder had accepted a residency (after the customary year of internship) at Toronto's Sunnybrook Hospital. Robertson knew the head of surgery at the University of Saskatchewan, Eric Nanson, as well as Joe Stratford, and met Mulder at the graduation ceremony, where Mulder was the class valedictorian and Robertson the main speaker. Robertson said that Nanson had told him Mulder was "O.K." and that he wondered why Mulder wasn't coming to the Montreal General Hospital? Mulder replied that he had not applied there. Robertson said that if Mulder would accept his handshake, there would be a job for him at the Montreal General Hospital on 1 July 1963. He should show up, find Mrs McMurray, and this would be all there was to it. Mulder recalls his father being worried about moving his wife and the first of their children all the way to Montreal when he did not even have a scrap of paper to confirm the existence of a job.[28] He took the plunge, however, and sure enough, on 1 July, Mrs McMurray was fully prepared, even to the extent of having his name badge all ready to wear. Working with Fraser Gurd, he obtained a master of science degree in surgery in 1964. Mulder went on to become a leading general surgeon and eventually surgeon-in-chief at the Montreal General Hospital for the remarkable period of twenty-one years, from 1977 to 1998.

Professorial rounds were conducted each week, at which the interns and residents were called upon to defend their treatments of the patients for whom they were responsible. Robertson was a believer in the Socratic method, very much along the lines of the Osler tradition. He would first ask to see the patient for a hands-on examination and then look at the x-rays, where he often found things that had not been noticed by the radiologists. He was an outstanding diagnostician, with impeccable anatomical knowledge, and could take apart a diagnosis and treatment in an instant. He proved to be an exceptional teacher, one who never criticized the doctors involved but, by suggesting a course for consideration, opened their eyes to what might be possible if they learned to be equally observant. He could do three or four cases in this manner in the course of an hour. After rounds, even after it was known that he would be leaving his position at the Montreal General Hospital, Miss McCairn (who had been with the medical corps in Sicily) would serve tea and biscuits in the office, and they would talk of other things than surgery. Mulder recalls that he and Rea Brown, also recruited by Robertson as a general surgeon, were doing an experimental heart valve operation on a dog one day and learned that Robertson would be looking in on them. They wanted to be sure to impress him and not get anything wrong and, in their excitement at the prospect of his visit, put a clamp on an artery instead of a vein, which resulted, to their huge embarrassment, in a virtual explosion of blood, just as Robertson arrived.[29] Brown, undoubtedly in part due to Robertson's influence and interest in the field, became the leader of the trauma unit. Others recruited into the Department of Surgery by Robertson included Mike Laplante, Harvey Brown, John Hinchey, Norman Poole, and Bryce Weir.

The establishment of the University Surgical Clinic at the Montreal General Hospital revolutionalized its Department of Surgery and continues to be an important factor in academic activities within the department. The University Surgical Clinic, established by Robertson, and the University Medical Clinic, established by Douglas Cameron, have now fused and were the foundations for the establishment of the Montreal General Hospital Research Institute, which is today one of North America's pre-eminent hospital-based research institutes.

Morale throughout the entire Department of Surgery improved remarkably, justifying the conclusion reached by the special committee that had recommended Robertson for the position – leadership started at the top with the example set by the leader. Here was someone with ideas and the organizational ability to implement them as well as the personality to generate the support of those working with and for him. He made them better at their professions, which they could recognize and which only spurred them on to improve themselves even more. It was a superb chemistry. The many organizational changes stood the test of time. The animal and other labs were a great success. Thirty years later they were still functioning well, and there had been practically no changes in their structures, as was the Infection Unit. The Intensive Care Unit that Robertson had designed had proved to be much too small, and after a few years significantly more space was allotted to it. The out-patient department had to be expanded to meet the demand, but the basic principles of the design had been maintained. The new era in surgery sought by the Montreal General Hospital and by McGill University had finally arrived. Its standard bearer was Rocke Robertson.

Observers at the time, and even now, recognize that although the period of time that he spent as surgeon-in-chief at the Montreal General Hospital and as chairman of the Department of Surgery at McGill was relatively short, Robertson's impact on both was quite remarkable. He had jump-started an approach to the new medicine that has remained to this day and that is one of the many reasons why the Faculty of Medicine at McGill remains one of its leading faculties, with a worldwide reputation for generating important progress across a broad range of disciplines.

TRANSITION FROM SURGEON TO PRINCIPAL

MONTREAL GENERAL'S LOSS, McGILL'S GAIN

There were other currents at work that would have an impact on the Montreal General Hospital and McGill's Department of Surgery. In June 1962 Lloyd Stevenson, dean of medicine, advised Robertson that he was on a list of possible candidates to succeed Frank Cyril James as principal and vice chancellor of the university.[1] James had been in the position since 1939, and there was a feeling among members of the Board of Governors (perhaps not one shared by James) that it was time for a change. Under some pressure, particularly from the chancellor, R.E. Powell, James had submitted his resignation, and the search for his replacement was on. That his name might be on the list came as something of a surprise to Robertson. He had never expected such a possibility and, while flattered even to have been considered, was initially unsure whether he would be able to do the job well. His initial discussion with Roslyn led him to think she was none too keen on the idea, which would necessarily involve giving up surgery. All he knew for certain was that until some decision was made (probably by someone else, he speculated), he was certain to be disturbed – perhaps acutely disturbed if someone approached him.[2]

Even before there were any overt steps taken to approach him, however, he began a typically careful consideration of the pros and cons of accepting such a position, should it be offered. On the one hand, he dreaded getting deeply enmeshed in university politics; when serving as acting dean of medicine at the University of British Columbia, he had encountered such politics and had not enjoyed this aspect of the experience. He also felt that he owed something to the Montreal General Hospital. Having been there for only three years, could he decently leave it so soon? On the other hand, there was no doubting the attraction of the prestige of the post of principal of an institution such as McGill University. He was then fifty years old and recognized that he did not have many more years of active surgery ahead of him. In fact, since 1950, when he had joined the staff of the University of British Columbia, he had been doing less and less surgery each year as his administrative load increased. So far as the Montreal General Hospital was concerned, he felt (already considering the possibility that the new post might be offered to him) that he had, arguably, done precisely what he had been commissioned to do – to develop the surgical service for teaching and for research. Once he learned that he was on the list, even though the matter was not pressing and he had plenty of time to decide whether to let his name stand as a possible candidate, he had started to mull things over in his mind.

He was next contacted by Stevenson on 16 July, who asked him, on behalf of the chancellor, whether he would allow his name to stand on the shortlist for principal, which would necessarily involve some interviews and related formalities. Robertson said immediately that he would allow this and, after hanging up the telephone, wondered whether he had not missed a convenient moment to withdraw. If, by chance, he were to be chosen, it would be awkward to refuse, and he was still by no means certain that he wanted or was suitable for the job. He felt inadequate in many respects and thought he would not relish many of the controversies in which he would inevitably become involved. At the same time, however, even the thought of having the opportunity to assume this important job was quite exciting – he could not deny this, even to himself. In any event – whatever his feelings – he was now committed to go further. In some ways, he wrote in his diary, he hoped that someone else might be selected and that he would not be faced with the decision, even though he did not know who else was in the running. This is undoubtedly an overstatement. He knew perfectly well how selection committees operated and how appointments were made and would not have allowed his name to stand were he not willing to say "yes" if the offer came through. Roslyn had no clear cut view either way but expressed no disagreement with his interim decision.

On 20 July he had his first contact with Chancellor Powell, who invited him to his magnificent office at Alcan, of which Powell was the chairman, where they talked for an hour before he took Robertson to lunch at the Mount Royal Club. They talked generally about McGill, reviewing its problems and prospects, and Powell asked what Robertson would do were he to be given a free hand. Robertson said he did not know enough about the problems to outline a policy, which did not seem to displease Powell, who did most of the talking – a proper enough role in the circumstances. Robertson had the impression that they were seriously considering his appointment and that the list had been reduced to three or four candidates. The mundane details of the position included a salary of $35,000, house and furniture, car and chauffeur, expense account – all very exciting, but Robertson was careful not to let himself get too enthusiastic. Powell told him they would talk again. Through July he read histories of McGill and its statutes and discussed the matter with Roslyn. He thought he should tell the Montreal General Hospital administration that the possibility was out there and found, somewhat to his relief, that Powell had already advised David Wanklyn and Kenneth Blackader, so the principal players at the hospital were aware. July faded into August with no news, but on 5 September, Powell called him to say that he would be in touch soon.

"Soon" proved to be 13 September, and Robertson went to Powell's brand-new office in Place Ville Marie, the opening day of the new complex, where Powell discussed with him the possibilities of the principalship. Powell told him he was one of the few survivors of the elimination process and, in general, led Robertson to believe, although Powell did not commit himself in any way, that he might be appointed. He had surprised Robertson by saying that he had the full support of the faculty, especially since he was practically unknown to members of the university staff apart from those in the Faculty of Medicine. Robertson could not imagine how they could express themselves strongly in his favour. The best he might have hoped for would have been a somewhat passive "nothing against" position. It was reassuring to think that, should he be appointed, there would not be too many internal people disgruntled in the process. Robertson, no fool regarding the importance of signals, told Powell that he would accept the position were it to be offered. Relieved at having made his own decision, he went straight home for lunch with Roslyn and, after going over the ground again and again, came away with the impression that she was rather keen on his getting the job – as he was, at least that day.

In early October his friend Dr Alan Mann called to "congratulate" him, having apparently heard some rumour. Robertson had heard nothing. Four days later, Mann had lunch with him to say that the reason for the delay was that, recently, the name of Arnold Heeney had been reintroduced and been strongly backed and that John Deutsch was still a contender. Robertson recognized that he was doubtless trying to prepare himself for a "loss" by not being disturbed by such formidable competition and that he felt some relief at the thought that he might not be chosen. He suspected that were it not for the natural dislike for losing a contest, he would be delighted not to get the job. It would be like playing in a tennis tournament and saying that he would be satisfied to have got into the semi-finals. In the meantime, the uncertainty remained a distraction, and every time he sat down to read or write, thoughts of the possible new job crowded in on him, and things that he could normally do with great ease were piling up around him.

Powell called him a few days later to say that the Senate advisory committee, chaired by Stanley Frost, would like to have lunch with him. The Senate had established its own committee, although it recognized that authority for the decision rested with the Board of Governors. Powell gave Robertson the good advice that it would be worth meeting with the Senate committee, despite its lack of any authority regarding the appointment. The lunch with the committee took place on 11 October at the Faculty Club, and Robertson was subjected to a barrage of questions of a very broad character. Apart from questions dealing with teaching, he had, in many cases, no real opinions and said so in as straightforward and earnest manner as he could, but he had the feeling that he might have appeared to be somewhat evasive, so he was not certain what kind of impression he had made. Later intimations from others suggested that the overall impression had not been particularly favourable. October stretched into November with no news from McGill. He knew there was an important meeting of the selection committee on 12 November, but no rumours had emerged regarding the discussions.

The next Saturday he had lunch at the Mount Royal Club with Powell, who said that the governors' selection committee was going to recommend to the Board of Governors that he be appointed and that the committee had been unanimous in its choice. Powell hoped that the matter could be completed at the Board of Governors meeting on 19 November, although he had some fears that there might be some form of delaying action. Obviously responding to a suggestion from Powell, Robertson delivered a letter to Powell for his use, if necessary at the board meeting, enclosing a standard curriculum vitae and a series of notes that might be helpful in advancing his case. Robertson expressed himself as somewhat unsure regarding what should be included: "difficult to know how bright to make the light and how opaque the bushel." He certainly understood from what Powell had said that there were rivals, but he had a highly developed competitive desire to win, even if he might not be absolutely sure about the challenge that he would have to take on were he to succeed.

The Board of Governors met at 4:00 in the afternoon and started to consider the report of the selection committee. Robertson was attending a dinner meeting of the Alma Mater Fund advisory committee at the University Club. The three governors who were members of this committee arrived to attend the dinner. They knew the outcome but, by common consent, revealed nothing to him nor to any other member of the committee. Even though he studied their expressions and measured their handshakes, he could get no hint as to what had happened. He concluded that either no decision had been reached or that they had selected someone else. It was only when he got home and saw the expression on Roslyn's face that he knew that she knew. Cyril James had called to tell her, and Robertson was to call him back. James, he said, could not have been kinder, wishing him well and seemingly genuinely pleased with his appointment. Lloyd Stevenson also called and was most flattering. Robertson called his brother Bruce to give him the news.

In the end, concluding the usual political manoeuvrings that inevitably surround a search of this nature, the Board of Governors had appointed him with effect as of 1 December 1962. Unlike the current practice at McGill, there was no fixed term for his appointment. He was appointed essentially at the pleasure of the Board of Governors and could, presumably, if the board remained satisfied with his performance and he were so inclined, remain in the position until he reached the mandatory retirement age of sixty-five in 1977. The day of the official announcement was to be 21 November. He made a very brief statement that day to the Board of Governors, whose members were then only men:

Gentlemen –

I am most conscious of the honour of this appointment and of the immense responsibilities that it imposes.

I look forward with the greatest optimism – justified, I believe, by the fact that the University is now in a very sound position

– under the brilliant administration of Dr. James, and of The
Chancellor, – it has reached a point where it is now stronger than it
has ever been in its history.

Surely this is a good base from which to tackle the problems that
now exist and those that will certainly crop up in the future – and
from which to expand in one direction or another as the occasion
demands.

I am most grateful to the Board of Governors, the Senate and
the Graduates for giving me the opportunity to play a part in these
developments. I shall do my level best to justify their confidence.[3]

Robertson was still a member of Senate and attended the regular
4:00 meeting, where he stayed until the item concerning the appointment of the principal came up, whereupon he left the meeting to wait in
James's office until the press conference scheduled for 5:45 to announce
his appointment, at which Chancellor Powell and then he spoke, to be
followed by many questions, some of which were difficult to handle.
There was considerable media interest, with more than forty reporters
and photographers in the room. He and Roslyn celebrated the day with
champagne at home, sharing their excitement with the children. There
were so many phone calls that they eventually left the phone off the hook.
The Ted Eberts – he to see something of a dream come true for his prod-
igy – and the Fraser Gurds dropped in for a visit.

The next day the *Montreal Gazette* included the following observation:

There will be, inevitably, and rightly, some regrets that a surgeon so
gifted should leave the active practice of his profession. But in the
larger sense, there is not a break but a deep continuity. The Medical
faculty is so much a part of McGill ... that his new appointment is
not so much a change of service as a broadening of its scope.

There is in surgery itself a training of the mind that has its value
in other fields. It is study mingled with practice, resolution mingled with caution, compassion with action, judgment with wisdom.
The posts that Dr. Robertson has already attained are such that
not only confer but demand distinction ... In the appointment of a
principal the life of a university comes to depend very largely upon
the qualities of a person ... Dr. Robertson is known as a man whose

liveliness of mind has been combined with an equanimity of spirit. His interests are broad and keen. His integrity and courage are blended with sympathy and attentiveness. He has commanded the loyalty and enthusiasm of his associates.

In the December 1962 issue of *Canadian Doctor*, the editorial comment on his appointment focused on the unusual feature of a medical man heading a great university and included an observation eerily similar to that expressed in the media in Victoria when his grandfather, Alexander Rocke Robertson, had accepted an early appointment to the bench, taking himself out of the active practice of law:

It seems like a big change to go from the stress and strain of surgery to what we are accustomed to think of as the cool, sequestered vale of university life. Probably university life is no longer the quiet backwater it used to be, but nevertheless, it must involve considerable sacrifice for one still young, to give up the absorbing pursuits and interests of a lifetime, and turn to something completely new. Not that Dr. Robertson will lose contact with Medicine. On the contrary, he may now be in an even better position to advance its interests than when he was engaged in active surgery.

Doctors have proved themselves to be versatile in many fields – as businessmen, authors, musicians and what not. The great doctors have necessarily been men of imagination and courage, with ability to organize and improvise, and because of their intimate contact with suffering humanity, are men well seasoned with prudence and charity. The new Principal will need all these qualities, and his selection from a long list of candidates is only one indication that he possesses them in good measure.

A new leader was about to guide McGill University after more than two decades of an extremely competent but very magisterial rule under James. These were new and different times, known only dimly as such, with no developed sense of what was to come, other than that it would likely be quite different from what had gone before, not only for McGill as a university as the academic world evolved but also for McGill in its Montreal, Quebec, Canadian, and international contexts. Robertson was seen immediately as a breath of fresh air, an affable and outgoing person who was, at the same time, a distinguished surgeon and scholar, someone who wanted to do well for the university and the community at large. He had the additional distinction of being the first McGill graduate to hold the position of principal and vice chancellor of the university. One of the university's own had finally made it to the top.

Even before the official starting date of his appointment, he began the entry process into his new job, spending a couple of hours with James on 27 November, attending a meeting of the Council of the Faculty of Arts and Science, and meeting with the legendary J.W. McConnell (who had been approached on Robertson's behalf twenty-three years earlier in the effort to find a surgical position), the university's most generous current benefactor, whom he described as "old and watery in the eye, but he seems to have a keen interest in all that is going on." It was a pleasure to hear him talk about the old days and of his acquisitions on behalf of the university.

HOSPITAL SIGN-OFF AND SUCCESSION

If he had a genuine regret about the change in his status, it was that he would have to give up teaching. In the late stages of the selection process, he had reached the point of wondering whether each round of teaching would be his last. The day after the official announcement of his appointment was somewhat anticlimactic, and the only good part of it was a teaching round with students in their final year. He hated the idea of giving up teaching – in his own mind, if he had any ability, it was in bedside teaching. He revelled in it, and the students gave every appearance of enjoying the rounds. He thought he might have only one more week and would then have to give it up. On 28 November he had rounds again and speculated about whether he might be able to find some way to continue them for a time. On his last official day as professor of surgery, 30 November, he recorded in his diary that he had "a joyful morning of teaching – 3 hours – a packed conference room with a number of the seniors (residents and lab men) coming in to what they thought would be my last appearance. Pictures were taken and I was most touched."

The minutes of the meeting of the Board of Management of the Montreal General Hospital held on 19 December 1962 contained two related and typically laconic items:

12. [Re: Appointment of Dr. H. Rocke Robertson as Principal &
Vice-Chancellor of McGill University]
A letter was received from Dr. H. Rocke Robertson tendering his
resignation as Surgeon-in-Chief consequent upon his appointment as of December 1st, 1962, as Principal and Vice-Chancellor
of McGill University. In accepting this resignation it was, upon
MOTION, duly SECONDED,

RESOLVED:
That in recording with a deep sense of pride the appointment of
Dr. H. Rocke Robertson as Principal & Vice-Chancellor of McGill
University, the Board of Management also expresses its apprecia-
tion of the inestimable service Dr. Robertson has given to this
Hospital.

 During his tenure of office as Surgeon-in-Chief, the Department
of Surgery has become renowned for its teaching and research,
and has enhanced the reputation of the Hospital and contributed
greatly to the welfare of the patients which it serves.

 The Board trusts that Dr. Robertson's interest in The Montreal
General will continue unabated and that under his inspiring
leadership the close historical ties between the University and the
Hospital will be strengthened and enriched.

13. [Re: Appointment of Dr. Fraser N. Gurd as Acting Surgeon-in-
Chief]
Following upon the resignation of Dr. H. Rocke Robertson as
Surgeon-in-Chief, and upon the recommendation of the Medical
Board, Dr. Fraser N. Gurd was appointed Acting Surgeon-in-Chief
effective December 1st, 1962.[4]

Gurd's interim appointment would be made definitive in April of the following year, and he stepped into both sets of Robertson's organizational
shoes, surgeon-in-chief at the hospital and chairman of the Department
of Surgery at McGill. In the ordinary course, this latter position would
have reverted to his counterpart at the Royal Victoria Hospital, in accordance with the established system of rotation of the chairman of the
department between the Montreal General and Royal Victoria Hospitals,
but because the new surgeon-in-chief at the Royal Victoria was Lloyd

MacLean, newly appointed and with a number of significant reorgani-
zational problems to deal with at the hospital, it was considered better to
have Gurd chair the university department, to be replaced after five years
by MacLean.[5]

THE NEW THEATRE OF OPERATIONS

It is one thing to run a department within a faculty or even to serve as
an acting dean, as Robertson did on occasion at the University of British Columbia, and quite another to suddenly become responsible for an
entire multifaculty university. By the same token, it is one thing to speculate about what one might like to do in relation to a university and quite
another to have to balance the many interests that make up the greater
university community. Robertson got a crash course in this complex
subject immediately upon assuming office. About the only cushioning
factor that he had was the Christmas and New Year break, which enabled
him to get his feet under him and be ready to face the onslaught of challenges and decisions that would come at him without respite throughout his entire term as principal. Some of them were entirely predictable
and required nothing more than a decision and management of the outcome. Some were unexpected, requiring careful assessment of the consequences and the design and implementation of corrective or prophylactic
measures. Still others would affect the very nature and existence of the
organization and test the resolve both of the university community as a
whole and of the greater social community within which it existed.

His first official day on the job was Saturday, 1 December. He walked
to his campus office from the hospital, becoming increasingly excited,
and spent a couple of hours again with James, who was most cordial in
the process and who gave him a number of useful hints. After James had
left, Robertson walked on the campus and became excited again. He
hoped he would be able to keep his head in the crises that were bound
to emerge but was comforted by the apparently genuine goodwill of so
many people, for which he considered himself most fortunate. He and
his son Stuart wandered around the campus on Sunday with their dog,
Rab, looking things over and poking around the backs of some of the
buildings. Business began in earnest on Monday with a series of meetings (Robertson always referred to meetings as "interviews") with key
staff, including his secretary, "Mrs. Betty" (Muriel Bett), who gave him
some ideas of how things worked and began the process of establishing a

routine. One conclusion that he drew very quickly was that he was going to be very busy, all the time, and that if he did not deal with the day-to-day issues expeditiously, they would soon pile up and overwhelm him. He would soon develop a regular pattern of meetings with the senior administrative staff, at which the business could be dealt with in an efficient and effective manner. There would be an executive meeting of the Board of Governors that afternoon, the agenda to be reviewed with the secretary of the board, J.H. Holton. He met with Colin McDougall, the registrar, for initial discussions of that portfolio. This was followed by a brief tour of the campus with the gardenmaster, Professor R.D. Gibbs, to discuss the state of the trees and general appearance of the campus, which Robertson thought needed improvement. Typical of the minutiae was that one of the partially dead trees that Robertson thought should come down could not be cut because it housed some brown owls and squirrels. He had lunch at the Faculty Club with Maxwell Cohen, who was entertaining the president of the Hebrew University of Jerusalem.

After lunch he met with P.N. Gross, director of the physical plant, to review the extensive building program then envisaged and found this to be in a considerable state of confusion, something that was going to require a great deal of reorganization and Robertson's personal attention. He met briefly with the chancellor before the Executive Committee meeting and then followed up on two of the issues raised. One was the administration of the Student Union – McGill was the only university whose students ran the union. The new building was in the planning stages, and the students had taken an active part in its design and worked out a budget for its operations. Robertson was impressed with their administrative abilities and particularly so with the academic records of the current and prior student presidents. He delegated the appointment of Health Service doctors who would examine students to J.H. Holton, secretary to the Board of Governors. The next day he faced a concerted complaint from the students in one of the new residences about the lack of sound insulation between the rooms. He investigated and found the complaints to be entirely justified, agreed immediately to measure the sound going between rooms, block the holes for pipes and light fixture holes, treat the wall with different materials, and then retest to see what improvement resulted. The testing was to be done within two days, the holes in the test corridor plugged within a week, and a definitive treatment proposed within two weeks. The cost was likely to be in the range of $100,000.

He met with Dean Stanley Frost, who updated him on the Faculty of Divinity, whence he came, and on the Faculty of Graduate Studies and Research, for which he was now responsible. They discussed the state of the libraries, including personality problems that existed, a proposed visiting committee to assess their status, and the need for fresh resources. McGill University Press was felt to be a great success. Frost said he would stay in graduate studies if necessary but could not do both this and divinity. It was, Robertson concluded, a good and informative meeting. There was a meeting with representatives of the Inter-Fraternity Council (at the time an influential student organization) that required no action on Robertson's part. He then met with Dean Hare of Arts and Science to review plans for the faculty and the lack of support for many of the activities within the faculty. Dinner was with the Senate consultative committee that had looked him over a few weeks earlier during the selection process. Apparently, they now thought it would be appropriate to advise him how things should be run. The irony aside, Robertson thought most of their ideas were perfectly sound.

Wednesday was spent in meetings and inspections: first with the comptroller regarding the budget of the university, then the warden of Royal Victoria College, then the museums committee, to discuss the allocation of museum materials, and last a follow-up meeting regarding the residence sound problems. On it went. The Graduates' Society gave a reception for Cyril James, at which some eight hundred graduates appeared. James was visibly touched by the evident affection of those attending. He spoke, excellently and articulately as usual, and there were some gifts presented. Robertson stayed until 8:30 before going home. At 7:15 the next morning he drove with the McGill comptroller to Quebec City to meet with the provincial authorities on the budget estimates provided by McGill for the 1963–64 fiscal year. He was "instructed" during the three-hour trip but did not feel he knew very much by the time they arrived to meet with the "cold blooded, canny but not excessively intelligent government officials whose duty it was, or so it seemed, to beat us down." He could stay only until lunchtime, but this was long enough to see that the comptroller was quite capable of taking care of himself, and as it turned out he did very well, the estimates being cut by only some $400,000 to $500,000, a not unexpected outcome. He got back to Montreal in time for a dinner at the St James's Club given by the Board of Management for the Medical Board of the Hospital. They presented him, in addition to some fine words, with a print of the original Montreal General Hospital, a framed Stephen Leacock letter, and an early (1656) map of Nouvelle France.

The next morning he was back to business, with another meeting to consider the complications of all the plans for buildings that were under way. The building program involved some nine buildings, all in the advanced stages of planning (if not already started), and in each case there were major problems to be sorted out, not the least of which resulted from the fact that they were dealing with seven different architectural firms. The estimated amount of funds to be invested was, for the university at this time, enormous, in the range of $60 million. While he loved the challenges this entailed, Robertson knew it was going to occupy much of his immediate time. At lunch he met with Lorne Gales, responsible for development, and discussed the general plans for raising funds from benefactors. He instructed Gales to prepare a chart of all schemes and committees having to do with development; it was already clear that some form of consolidation in this sphere of activity would be required. The afternoon was spent with the committee on research to review the nature and extent of these activities throughout the university. While he managed to take his weekend off, thinking optimistically that this might be one benefit of the job compared with his being on constant call as a surgeon, the pace continued and would only increase as time went on. Writing to his mother on December 30, he noted:

The last Sunday of the year – what an eventful year it has been and I find myself at its end deeply immersed in a completely new field – I think it will be exciting but I foresee some very difficult times ahead and I'll have to be very careful to keep far enough away from the trivia and focus on the important things. The trivia are innumerable it seems – and it's hard to know which to ignore – I have already found that my time could be literally taken up with them – many are difficult to hand over to others and some are extremely time-consuming and even interesting and somehow I must learn to dispose of them efficiently and leave myself free to deal with the more important affairs – so much for that.[6]

As an admirer of Sir William Osler, he might well have taken heed of an observation made by the great physician: "There is a tendency for the person in the most powerful position in an organization to spend all of his time serving on committees and signing letters."

OMNIPRESENCE, OMNISCIENCE, OMNIPOTENCE: BASIC TRIMMINGS OF A PRINCIPAL

Principals soon discover that they are expected to be everywhere, to respond to everyone's agenda, to speak at events, to know everything, to make hard decisions without offending anyone, to meet everyone's increasing demands for space and money, to raise all the funds required, and to do so without showing the slightest impatience or fatigue. Many appearances are strictly for form and do not require more than passing attention, while others require the most careful attention and the use of "code" that will be understood by those who need to receive the message without being transparent to those who have no such need. For the latter, a principal needs to have competent and knowledgeable advisors within the administration to help gauge the issues and measure the responses. It is simply not possible for a single individual to manage the complete range of problems confronting the head of a modern university.

Barely two months into the job, Robertson was called upon for a comprehensive report on the state of McGill to the annual meeting of the Graduates' Society of McGill University – now the McGill Alumni Association. McGill's alumni have always played an important role in the affairs of the university. They are formally represented on the Board of Governors, comprise a network that today has representatives in more than 190 countries, were and still are deeply imbedded in the Montreal, Quebec, and Canadian communities, and have led the way in Canada in exceptional eleemosynary support of the university. As such, they have never been shy about expressing their views on how the university should be run, where it should be headed, and what its position should be on a whole range of issues, whether academic or other. Robertson assured the meeting that the reaction of the alumni to any course of action was always a consideration when evaluating any proposal. While generally aware that universities were complex organizations, he had already learned something about the specific complexities of McGill – academic, financial, athletic, moral, and legal – and that no part of it was simple. He had started in January to visit the various departments, faculties, schools, museums, libraries, and offices to meet as many of the staff as possible and to inspect the buildings. He expected this would require about one hundred visits, of which he could do approximately four per week, and had concluded that this would be the best way to get a concept of what was going on. He was already impressed by the talent he had encountered, even when he was not entirely sure about the subject matter, and had a respect for the quality of the work being done, often under very adverse conditions.

He used these observations to comment on the building program for the university, about which there had been some mention that it was unnecessary or overly ambitious. He invited the graduates to come and see some of the facilities he had visited where the staff were working under deplorable conditions, split up in small sections in different old houses or buildings, crammed together in dilapidated rooms, but still somehow managing to do good work in spite of the handicaps. The need for new buildings was very real. He had a great interest in the building program, appalled as he was about its immensity, since he now realized how necessary it was. The new residences and dining hall were already completed. The Allan Memorial Institute Research and Training Building, Mont. Ste Hilaire,[7] and the Eaton Electronics Laboratory and Radiation Laboratories were under way and nearly completed. Nine buildings were planned or ready to start. They included the McIntyre Sciences Centre, Humanities and Social Sciences, Stewart Biology, Chemistry, University Centre, Pathology, the Roscoe Wing, Physics, and the Faculty of Law. There were financial and building-permit problems, but he hoped that within five years the buidlings would be completed. His biggest worry was that by the time they were finished, the university's needs would have outgrown them.

The downtown campus has been a hallmark of the university for generations. Probably no part of the university has the same capacity to generate rumours and speculation about what might happen to it or to galvanize concern about its future. This was as true in early 1963 as it is today. The then current version was that all the trees on the campus were to be removed and replaced by a concrete terrace hiding some formal gardens. His mail had been filled with letters and petitions begging him to do what he could to preserve the natural beauty. The plan in place held none of the apprehended terrors, as the lower campus was to be untouched and there would be more grass and usable space than presently existed. Some trees, mostly unhealthy, would be removed and new ones planted. He pointed out, for the benefit of those who seemed to think that trees lived forever, that in the next twenty years many of the older trees were going to die and that there would be constant replacement of them. The fabled gingko tree might be saved, and the reputed grave of James McGill would be moved to a better place, farther away from the existing fire hydrant that was a constant threat to it. He assured the meeting that the objective of the plans under consideration was to develop an area in the expanding city's centre – which had by then moved up to Dorchester Boulevard (now René Lévesque) from St James Street – of which they could all be proud. The Place Ville Marie complex, along with the Canadian Imperial Bank of Commerce building two blocks to the west, had officially opened the previous year, and Montreal had been designated the host of the international world exposition that would become known as Expo '67.

Certain problems are perennial for any university, and Robertson had stepped in during a period of unprecedented growth in the number of students reaching university age, when the resources of the university would be taxed – perhaps overtaxed – in responding to the demands on its systems and facilities. The previous year a new system for processing admissions had been tried but had not enjoyed success. The current year had operated somewhat more smoothly, but the difficult part was still ahead. The figures, just prior to his speech, showed that as of that date, in the large Faculties of Arts and Science and Engineering, some 3,673 applications had been received, of which almost 70 per cent were Canadian students and just over 20 per cent were Americans. Although the applications had not yet been processed, the administration hoped and expected that every candidate who met the stipulated entrance requirements would be admitted that fall. The great fear was that they would be overwhelmed by students, an outcome that could be met only by expanding the teaching staff or by somehow increasing the range of each teacher.

Finding good teachers involved adhering to the budget available for the purpose and was complicated by the fact that there were insufficient good teachers available, even if there had been no budgetary constraint, and it would be some time before they would become available. This meant that they would have to do whatever they could to retain the existing teaching staff, no easy matter given the raiding that went on between universities. Robertson marvelled at the lack of ethics involved and compared it with medicine (which he had by now discovered was a relatively well-mannered discipline), where they at least tried to inform the other university as they were about to approach one of its faculty. This did not seem to happen in other fields, where often the first one heard was that the faculty member had already received an offer that McGill was unable to match. They would have to exert all their efforts to keep the staff salaries at the same level as those offered by the "pirates" to the west of McGill. They were also considering new teaching methods, such as television and programmed lectures, and were looking at these, as were many others, but he thought this would likely take several years to mature.[8]

At the same time as an overload of students was feared, the university was in the process of expanding the breadth of the programs it offered to improve teaching and research. Some of the projects under current consideration were a centre for marine sciences, a centre for the study of developing areas, a French Canadian studies program, and a centre for research in sociology and anthropology. Many of these involved a new grouping of existing activities and scholarship, with some additional staff to hold the centres together, but all of them involved an immense effort by the staff and a genuine interest not only in local problems but also in the problems of the world. Robertson wanted the graduates to know that the university was a going concern and that it had a splendid and forward-looking and industrious staff. He was careful to point out that many of the plans he was discussing had been developed by his predecessor, Cyril James, that they were going forward with no more hitches than seemed inevitable, and that the new administrators were slowly developing their plans to meet new situations as they arose or, sometimes, as they anticipated them.

It was a good address to this influential community, one that paid it the respect it deserved given its close connection with the university while at the same time demonstrating that the new principal was on the job and in command of the university. He knew where it was going and, having picked up the reins from the James era, had already added his own personality to that of the university. The Board of Governors had sensed that new and difficult times were ahead. It is unlikely that they had any real idea of the pace of change and the developments that would come hurtling at them, but they certainly knew that the educational environment in Quebec had changed dramatically with the all-but-official acknowledgment of the Quiet Revolution through the election of the Lesage government in 1960. This election had followed upon the lengthy Duplessis stranglehold on Quebec life and societal evolution, in collaboration with the then powerful Roman Catholic Church, and upon the succession of a series of short-term Union Nationale premiers after Duplessis's death in September 1959.[9]

At the spring Convocation in 1962 on the lower campus, Cyril James's last as principal, McGill University conferred an honorary doctorate on Paul Gérin-Lajoie, the minister of youth in the Lesage government.[10] If there was ever any doubt that there had been a major sea-change with the arrival of the Liberals under Lesage, it was dispelled during the course of Gérin-Lajoie's Convocation address, when he stated in no uncertain terms (something he might not have been willing or able to do had the honorary degree been conferred by the Université de Montréal on the other side of the mountain) that the church had no place in the educational system of the province. This was a revolution! In February 1962 an informal committee on French-English relations had met at McGill, reflecting the desire of many Quebecers to address issues raised by the Quiet Revolution. Among those in attendance were André Laurendeau, Maxwell Cohen, Pierre Elliott Trudeau, Claude Ryan, and F.R. Scott. Two and a half years after his initial election, two days before McGill's Board of Governors selected Robertson, Lesage was re-elected on 17 November 1962, this time on a platform to nationalize Quebec hydroelectric companies and a political slogan of "*Maitres chez nous.*"

In his chosen profession, Robertson had shown himself to be a superb observer and diagnostician. The same skills were not difficult to apply to the anatomy of the university. It did not require a lifetime to identify the problems that existed, even though there would undoubtedly be more and new indications as time went on. Nor was a prognosis all that difficult: the university faced some overwhelming problems that threatened its ability to carry out its mission of teaching and research and perhaps its very existence. One could see the pandemic – or at least part of it – that was approaching. Many of those most active in the demands for change had had no war experience, had grown up in a culture of entitlement, and lacked self-imposed discipline. French Canada was beginning to shake off the Duplessis yoke and the three centuries of domination by the Roman Catholic Church. In the process, those seeking political power and influence often found it more convenient and palatable to blame the English-speaking minority for creating the situation rather than for merely having filled a vacuum created by the lack of interest within the French Canadian community. The key, for any principal, was to find the right therapy and to apply such treatment as the circumstances and resources would permit. It would prove to be a challenge for which no one could have been fully prepared and one that would push Robertson to the very limits of his ability and stamina.

The year 1963 was significant – not only for McGill but also for Montreal, Quebec, Canada, and the rest of the world. During the same month that Robertson addressed the Graduates' Society, the revolutionary Front de Libération du Québec (FLQ) was founded to support and agitate for Quebec sovereignty and the establishment of an independent socialist state through a combination of propaganda, murder, and terrorism.

FORMAL INSTALLATION AS PRINCIPAL
AND VICE CHANCELLOR

Robertson's formal installation as principal and vice chancellor took place on 2 April 1963 in the presence of Governor General Georges Vanier, as the official Visitor of the University under its charter, and other members of the university community and guests. Chancellor Powell invested him with the office and title, charging that he "may hold the title in peace and in honour and to administer the office in accordance with the Statutes, privileges, liberties and customs of the University." The governor general entrusted the charter and seal of the university to his keeping. There then followed greetings from the academic body of the university, presented by H. Noel Fieldhouse, who assured him of the faculty's loyalty and support in the promotion of those high purposes to which the university was dedicated, and from the student body, presented by Gordon Echenberg, president of the Students' Society, who pledged the fullest cooperation of the students for the future welfare of McGill. Similarly, the president of the Graduates' Society, Dr Newell Philpott, pledged the loyal support of the graduates of the university and their full cooperation in the various activities in which they engaged with the common purpose of enhancing the reputation of McGill University.[11]

In his address in response, Robertson noted that he was as conscious of the honour involved in the appointment to the position as he was of his own limitations and acknowledged, as was inevitable, that the thrill of the one mingling with doubts occasioned by the other created in him that day a state of true excitement. He reviewed some of the challenges faced by his predecessors, particularly John William Dawson to promote the sciences, William Peterson to advance the arts, Sir Arthur Currie to steady the university at the end of the Great War, and James to rally it at the beginning of the Second World War. Robertson contemplated the part that the university might play in the affairs of its own country:

Canada was then, [at the time of the Second World War] and for some time afterwards happy enough as a nation. Externally we were proud to be members of a great Commonwealth, devoted to and still in many ways, dependent upon the mother country, grateful to the United States for its interest and keen that all should participate in the development of our seemingly unlimited resources.

Internally the sectional differences that cropped up from time to time seemed relatively unimportant and their tendency rapidly to subside was reassuring.

In recent years this has largely changed. As we stand now [more] on our own than ever before and relatively unprotected in competition with others we have become aware of the need to control our own affairs and we are resentful of interference, sensitive to criticism and uncertain of ourselves. And just as we as a nation are uneasy about our position in the world so within us is a large and important group uneasy about its relationship to the rest of the country.

I do not propose either to attempt to analyze the reasons for the change or to list what we and others regard as our shortcomings. Nor would I, at this special moment in our nation's history, venture an opinion as to what general corrective measures might be taken.

I feel impelled, however, to express my belief that in the long range solution to our problems, both internal and external, will only be found in the fuller education of our people. I am firmly convinced that concessions, economic adjustments, treaties and constitutional amendments can only act as palliatives until such time as we have raised the levels of our abilities in the various cultural, scientific and economic fields to a point where we can be said to have *earned* a proud position amongst the leading nations.

That there is a connection between the development of a national pride and the improvement of the relationship between the French and English speaking people of this country is a point that is seldom emphasized though it deserves close consideration. Just as it can be held, I believe, that the discontent of our French Canadian brethren is their expression of the whole nation's discontent, so may it be expected that a revival of the nation's spirit will do much to bring our peoples together.[12]

Over the next several months he was in much demand – within the McGill community in Montreal, New York, Toronto, Boston, and elsewhere and within the local educational and business communities. By this time there were bombs going off in Montreal. He had to sound confident and upbeat in public and to be realistic when on campus, a fine line to tread, especially when the shortfalls in expected government support severely limited the university's ability to function and were already driving it into deficit financing. Modest fee increases – but only to just below the 1959 levels (net of the portion to be put aside for increased student aid) – were possible but would produce less than a million dollars, and there would still be a significant deficit.

THE SHATTUCK LECTURE

In the midst of his many duties as principal, Robertson was invited to deliver the 75th Shattuck Lecture in 1965.[13] This lecture, one of the most prestigious in all of medical science, is named after George Cheyne Shattuck, a former dean of the Harvard Medical School. A list of former and current Shattuck lecturers amounts to a veritable "who's who" of medical leaders in North America. The lecture topic is frequently a review of the presenter's scientific achievements in a particular area or, occasionally, an overview on topics such as surgical education, philosophy, or history. Prior to agreeing to give the lecture, Robertson corresponded with the secretary of the Massachusetts Medical Society to explain that he had retired from surgery in 1962 and was currently involved as principal of McGill and would therefore be unable to give a lecture that dealt with a current surgical topic. On 19 May 1965 in Boston, Robertson began by drawing on the relationship between Sir William Osler's Shattuck Lecture of 1893 on tuberculous pleurisy and Osler's presence at McGill.

As for himself, Robertson acknowledged that he was very conscious of the fact that his own surgical experience was comparatively short and that he had done nothing unusual. Even though he concluded that he had nothing to add to the "already toppling pile of literature," he had always found his work to be interesting and had decided, for this occasion, that he would try to analyze what it was that had made each case interesting. He identified four criteria: when the case presents some fantastic or grotesque feature, when it exhibits an extraordinary blunder on the part of someone else, when it runs an unexpected course, and when it illustrates some advance, whether of thinking, technique, or therapy. He used some of his own experiences, primarily from his time at the University of British Columbia, to illustrate each of the criteria, with slides to provide specific details for the audience of professionals. It would have been an interesting and entertaining experience for these professionals, even if they did not leave the lecture with any particular nugget of new scientific or surgical discovery.

He went on to trace the advances in surgical thinking over the years, marvelled at the independence of John Hunter, and then observed how slow the progress was until the time of Lister. He attempted to examine reasons for this. He concluded that the Hunterian approach based on anatomy and mechanical surgical procedures had given way to a detailed examination of the basic elements of surgical science, such as response to injury, the basics of wound healing and infection, blood transfusion, surgical nutrition, and the response of the immune system to operation. He noted the boldness with which surgeons had used the basic-science approach to make an impact on diseases such as ulcerative colitis, peptic ulcers, hypertension, and more recently, the transplantation of organs. He discussed surgical advances in terms of thinking, technique, and therapy. He concluded with the recent advances in the chemotherapy of malignant melanoma and finished somewhat emotionally: "It is for this reason that I am sad to have left the field – and at the same time proud to have been a part of it."

Judging by the written responses and the request for reprints, this was clearly one of Robertson's key publications. Many of the written requests for reprints discussed the eloquence of his oration in making his thoughts on an interest in surgery one of the outstanding Shattuck lectures.

Not all the problems facing a university principal were life and death, even if they were time-consuming. In November 1963, addressing the Women's Canadian Club in Montreal,[14] he gave some examples, including student behaviour, student dress, compulsory physical education (and fines for noncompliance), and the big question of whether they should "let down the bars" and allow the female cheerleaders to do cartwheels. Gradations in the level of problems included building and campus maintenance, population explosion of students, selection of students to be admitted, raising money, and improvement of teaching. The admissions dilemma had always been that of admitting someone who subsequently fails and, in so doing, denying the entry of someone who would have passed. Another growing concern was the loss of postgraduate students, who could get better financial support elsewhere and who, once they left, seldom came back, causing a brain drain and the loss at McGill of additional or replacement teachers for those who would retire.

Only in April 1964 did the chancellor share with Robertson the contents of a note he had received "from the head of a very successful Canadian university" during the search process, dealing with the role of the principal in an institution like McGill. It was probably just as well that Robertson had no idea of the expectations! It read in part:

I doubt if there is a single university, certainly any English-speaking university, which does not feel that a strong McGill is in the best interest of the whole of Canada. Sitting as it does, in the heart of Canada's largest city, it should be a strong, virile university. Situated, too, in the province of Quebec, with its several millions of what may be called newly emancipated people, McGill should be in the forefront in the social sciences and humanities, and giving real leadership in the new emergence of bi-lingualism and in the realization of Canada's bicultural requirements. Great efforts should be made in these facets of university disciplines. The leadership in these fields, almost lost by default by McGill and taken over by the University of Montreal and Laval University, should be regained ...

In selecting a new Principal, I would suggest that vision and personality are far more important assets than scholarly or scientific attainments; that the ability to make decisions – and many unpopular ones will have to be made – and to live under criticism by one's colleagues is more significant than an already attained reputation as a diplomat or a successful businessman. He should be one, in my opinion, who has been "in the academic ranks" and who therefore has had experience at various academic levels. The "American" fashion of appointing non-academic persons to the headship of universities has not been either favourably received by the staffs or even remotely successful otherwise.

Having gone this far, I might add that a critical review of each department within the university would be the new Principal's first major task. Someone who is familiar with the strengths and weaknesses of other universities can certainly do a better job in this connection than a non-academic person could do. Specific concern for the alumni, as well as for the staff and students, is of great importance. The "image" of McGill will in large part be a reflection of its new Principal.[15]

On the other hand, it was a profile that fitted Robertson like a glove, and it is not surprising that the chancellor might want to share it with him, now that he had had some experience under his belt.

In June 1964 Robertson was granted an honorary degree by the University of Toronto, from which both his father and older brother, Bruce, had graduated. His convocation address focused on the relationship between the University of Toronto and McGill.[16] He found it anomalous and somewhat amusing, given the enormous impact on the educational system of the country, that in the official history of the Toronto institution only two references to "McGill" could be found: one to the widow of James McGill's brother, who married John Strachan, and the other, in a mere footnote, to Strachan's having suggested to James McGill that he leave a bequest for the purpose of founding a university. On the other hand, in the somewhat earlier official history of McGill, there was no mention whatsoever of the University of Toronto!

To give some idea of the various challenges that face a university principal, one must avoid the temptation to record them as they occur, day after day. The risk, from the outside, is that it would be very much like trying to drink from a fire hose. From the inside, the principal himself would feel rather like the war surgeon he had been, with an endless stream of patients in varying degrees of distress coming at him one after another, giving no time to rest between operations and no discernable conclusion to the exercise. There were the issues he had already described, and there were others bubbling toward the surface over which McGill would have little if any control. The scene was set and it was known to be potentially unstable. The only choice was to face whatever came and to mitigate whatever serious damage might result. It is often said that anyone can be a good captain in calm waters. The barometer in Quebec and for McGill was falling. The captain of the McGill ship was in for storms that he never anticipated.

UPHEAVAL IN QUEBEC

The times were troubled within Quebec and within Canada. The Lesage Liberals had been elected in 1960 using the *"Maitres chez nous"* slogan, and the status quo relationships that had existed under the Duplessis Union Nationale governments were soon unravelling, as the authoritarian secular and religious regimes, with their unstated agreements of collaboration, faded. They were replaced by an active government concerned with the economic and political development of the French-speaking majority in Quebec. Their objectives led to yet another round of self-examination of the role of French in Quebec and the role, if any, of a French-speaking majority province in Canada, which became increasingly acute as the centennial year of Confederation approached.

On the fringes of the nationalist movement, there were extremists, willing and determined to resort to violence to bring about change. Most of the rhetoric was nationalistic, overlayed with Marxism. The violence needed targets, the main ones being business institutions and those perceived as connected with the English-speaking minority, and these were cast as the sole reason for the relatively undeveloped state of the French-speaking economic community. There was no doubt that the majority of businesses of any significant size were controlled by the minority, due in part to its inclination in the direction of business and in part to a previous reluctance within the French-speaking community's elite to go into business, as compared with the professions. When the majority did take to business in the decades that followed, the francophone entrepreneurs proved to be at least as talented as their anglophone counterparts. In the early years, however, the progress was painfully slow, or at least appeared so to the French-speaking executives and businessmen, as well as to other opinion leaders, who, even where they might not endorse the politics of the extremists, did not assertively disassociate themselves from the violence. Even tacit acceptance by the majority was sufficient to provide cover and encouragement, and the violence proliferated.

The most extreme of the activist groups was the Front de Libération du Québec (FLQ), established in February 1963 by Georges Schoeters, Gabriel Hudon, and Raymond Villeneuve. The FLQ would go on to absorb assorted precursor and parallel groups, such as the RR (Réseau révolutionaire), ALQ (Armée de liberation du Québec), and ARQ (Armée révolutionnaire du Québec). Led by Pierre Vallières and Charles Gagnon and trained by the Belgian-born Schoeters, the FLQ set off a series of bombs, starting in March 1963, when three Canadian army barracks were targeted, followed by bombings in Montreal during April and May. These were the start of more than two hundred violent crimes that it would commit, culminating in the October 1970 kidnappings of the British trade commissioner, James Cross, and the Quebec labour minister, Pierre Laporte, the latter of whom would be murdered. The first death caused by the bombings occurred on 21 April 1963, five days after the first FLQ manifesto was written, when Wilfred O'Neil, a sixty-five-year-old night watchman, was killed.

By July 1963, given the spread of discussions on Quebec nationalism, the Pearson minority federal government had established the Royal Commission on Bilingualism and Biculturalism, co-chaired by André Laurendeau and Arnold Davidson Dunton, to assess the state of bilingualism and biculturalism in Canada and to determine whether the promotion of French outside Quebec might be acceptable.[1] The hearings started the following January in Winnipeg, and a preliminary report would be tabled in the House of Commons on 25 February 1965.[2] Even as the commission pursued its study, the violence continued to increase. By October 1963 some sixteen members of the FLQ had pleaded guilty to terrorist activities. Schoeters was given two five-year sentences, and Hudon and Villeneuve were imprisoned for the death of O'Neil. In December, Mario Bachand was sentenced to four years imprisonment for the bomb explosion on 17 May that had injured Sergeant Major Walter Leja of the bomb squad. Elsewhere, a month earlier on 22 November, the US president, John F. Kennedy, had been assassinated, the day after Robertson had spoken at the Boston branch of the Graduates' Society. The world was rapidly becoming a different, more dangerous place.

These events swirled around McGill University, located as it was in the centre of Montreal, the largest French-speaking city in the country, where it was perceived by the majority of francophones as a beacon of the English establishment, and around Robertson as its principal. Montreal was, at the time, the economic engine of both Quebec and Canada. It was impossible not to be aware of what was going on, what the dangers were, both physical and political, what the impact might be on higher education, and what the consequences might be for McGill, but it was also impossible at the time to foresee the many and diverse outcomes. The future of McGill as a primarily English-speaking institution was inseparable from the Quebec "situation." The political decisions affecting McGill were all taken against the backdrop of how McGill was then perceived within Quebec and, often, against the backdrop of convenient misperceptions as to McGill's position, role, and resources. Throughout his time as principal, Robertson constantly struggled to ensure that McGill was fairly treated and to convince Quebec that McGill was an important part of its past, present, and future and that the success of Quebec was inextricably linked with the education of its youth, both French and English.

Education was also the key, Robertson believed, to a better understanding within Canada. This would take time, and McGill would have to be patient during the difficult times that were already upon it. There was no doubt that the Quiet Revolution (Robertson referred to it privately as the "unquiet" revolution) and the resultant flirting with the notion of independence were challenging the very framework of Canadian federalism and could seriously menace the minorities in Quebec. As to the reality of such a threat, at least in April 1964, Robertson had no answer, other than to say that to dismiss the thought of Quebec independence out of hand would be as unjustifiable as to regard it as inevitable. It was better to admit the possibility and to do everything within one's power to avert it. One thing was already clear, namely that McGill was a target of hate literature, which complained, among other things, about its perceived huge wealth. In fact, the unrestricted endowments amounted to only about $16 million – enough to run the university for eight months if all other sources of funding were removed. Other complaints were that McGill was getting more government contributions than its "share" ought to be, but the figures available made this a hard claim to prove – one way or the other – and Robertson did not think McGill got more than its share. In his public utterances, he was always careful to say that he thought McGill was treated fairly.[3] There were complaints that McGill got more than its share of research funds in comparison with the French universities, a complaint that conveniently overlooked at least two pertinent facts: to get research grants there had to be both facilities and a demonstrated research ability, and the French universities had only recently entered the field. The complaints even went so far as to address McGill's academic program. It was, to some, offensive that McGill would have a French Canadian studies program, the very portion of its academic mission that McGill hoped would help to create understanding and rapprochement.[4]

This criticism notwithstanding, relations were generally good at the administration level among all the universities and reasonable at the academic level, with close cooperation on many projects, all of which should be encouraged. McGill, Robertson thought, should aim to make itself useful and bring credit to Quebec as a whole, not just to the English-speaking minority. On the other hand, McGill must ensure that it retained its identity since it could be useful only if it could be itself. It was important, for Robertson, to stress that McGill had become an integral part of Quebec, was deeply imbedded in it, and was vitally concerned with the welfare of all its people. This was a point worth emphasizing, lest anyone think that McGill was aloof from the current activity or unsympathetic to or unappreciative of the tremendous strides being taken by its sister universities. McGill was, in short, of Quebec and proud to be so. It should remain nonpolitical and nondenominational, preserve its rights, try to cooperate, and not contribute to the confusion. McGill's position should be that it had long been established in Quebec, had grown up with the community, and had contributed considerably to it and that it believed it could best continue to contribute to it by being itself and by improving in every way possible. At the level of students, however, the interuniversity relations were not particularly good. Robertson was determined that, even though the Quebec government chose to do nothing about the unjustified attacks on McGill, the university should not waver under the influence of the heated and thoughtless pronouncements that were occurring so frequently.

Signs of the increasing political tensions could be seen during a visit of Queen Elizabeth II to Quebec City on 10–11 October 1964 to commemorate the centenary of the 1864 Quebec Conference. By the day before the visit, when Robertson arrived, there were police roadblocks in place, although the city looked normal, with no signs of violence and a conspicuous absence of flags – a marked difference from the welcome the queen had received five years earlier in 1959, the year the St Lawrence Seaway was officially opened. During the current official visit, the streets were largely deserted except for a few hundred jeering student protesters, who were attacked by nightstick-wielding police. Robertson observed that the queen had been dismayed at her reception. It would not be until 10 October 1987 that she would return to Quebec City.[5]

This and other manifestations of tensions in Quebec were much remarked upon throughout Canada. One of the problems that Robertson faced when travelling outside Quebec was the barrage of comments and suggestions, seldom helpful, made by people from other provinces on the escalating situation in Quebec. Speaking at the Vancouver Medical Association in late October 1964, as a "displaced British Columbian," he said that anguish was caused by the occasional outbursts of certain British Columbian spokesmen when they expressed their views on the problems of Canada and had suggestions to make as to what might be done to (seldom "with") Quebec and Expo '67. "On the days following these outbursts, I move quietly and carefully with intent to avoid people."

On 20 November 1964 the report of the Quebec Royal Commission on Education, created in 1961 (referred to as the Parent Commission, after its chairman, Monsignor Alphonse-Marie Parent, vice rector of Laval), recommended, to no one's great surprise, a major transformation of the school system, including government control over the Catholic Church-run classical college system.[6] This was clearly one of the most important documents to appear in the realm of Quebec education in many years, with sweeping changes and the abolition of some of the previously existing barriers that had completely separated the Catholic and Protestant systems, coupled with the requirement for a common approach to education. The recommendations included the number of years of scholarity, instruction in second languages, and exchanges between the two systems as well as the establishment of a Superior Council on Education. Barely two years into its second mandate, the Lesage government would almost certainly be expected to act on the recommendations.

At the level of federal consideration of the nationalism issues, there were two members of the McGill community involved in the Royal Commission on Bilingualism and Biculturalism: Frank Scott, who was a member of the commission, and Michael Oliver, who was its research director. Scott often referred to the commission, during his superb classes on constitutional law in the Faculty of Law, as the "Bye-Bye" Commission. Oliver would later be appointed vice principal (academic), in which role he proved to be most capable. Robertson's only concern, prior to Oliver's appointment, had been his New Democratic Party sympathies, which were profound, but these sympathies never got in the way of his duties as vice principal.[7] McGill made submissions to the commission, in which it stressed the basic lack of knowledge of what determines the development of a culture and how an understanding between the different cultures in the country might be strengthened. Neither side, clearly, knew enough about the other. McGill's recommendations, presented in March 1965, included the suggestion that a permanent commission be established to encourage and promote programs of teaching and research affecting biculturalism since the university was convinced that there was a need for a continuing effort of this type.[8] Dealing with the position of McGill and its responsibilities, Robertson underlined the point that McGill wanted to participate in the development of Quebec and stated that the best way to do this was by being a first-rate university working alongside the other universities, which must also be first-rate if Quebec was to progress. McGill's belief was that extension of the interests of all the universities beyond the boundaries of the province and of Canada was fundamental to the development of the country. McGill realized that its relations and cooperative efforts with its French colleagues, while far from negligible, were nevertheless in need of strengthening, which it was eager to effect while continuing to serve the broad community, as it had in the past.

Speaking to the point at a McGill Alma Mater Fund Conference in Toronto in April 1965, Robertson explained:

> I spoke earlier of the challenge of national unity – the one great question concerning Canada as we approach 1967. I would like now to deal with McGill's role in this vital problem, for the accident of our location places us in a strategic position and makes us something more than just one of several large Canadian English-speaking universities.
>
> In our brief to the Royal Commission on Bilingualism and Biculturalism several weeks ago, the point was made that McGill stands ready to act as a willing broker of ideas and sensibilities between English and French-speaking Canada. Indeed, in every respect, our university is ready to play a most active and vigorous role in Quebec.

In a very real sense, McGill is the intellectual and cultural centre of the large English-speaking enclave in Quebec. It would be only natural to think that French Canada may be better understood and appreciated by English-speaking Montrealers than by any other English-speaking segment of Canada.

McGill lives day by day in and with French Canada. The preponderance of its students is reared in this inevitably bicultural city. While its staff is drawn from the world at large, there is an increasing involvement in the Montreal community and the life of the province. The division of "two solitudes" has never been absolute, and at present there is the strongest desire at McGill to break it down. The conviction is widely held in academic circles that the new vitality of this province removes barriers to much more intimate collaboration and intellectual exchange than was possible before.

McGill has seriously attempted to understand French Canada. Years of work by individual scholars was followed naturally by the establishment in 1963 of the French Canada Studies Programme. This is in its infancy and its title does not quite accurately reflect its purpose. It is in reality a French-English Studies Programme looking at our Canadian selves wholly. It makes two contributions. It provides an interdisciplinary mechanism for the study area, and it helps to develop experts in the relationship of French and English-speaking Canada. It can become a major factor in the developing insights into the great Canadian dilemma. Its influence will no doubt be felt over the years in curriculum planning at McGill, and perhaps in other English and even French-speaking universities.[9]

On 11 May 1965, however, in speaking with the McGill staff, Robertson painted a much bleaker picture for McGill at the hands of the Quebec government. The increase in financial support from the government for the following year compared most unfavourably with the increases granted to some other universities. Faced with these facts, McGill should make every effort to become an increasingly important part of the educational system of Quebec. This extended to contributing to the planning – there were members of the McGill staff on practically all of the provincial planning committees that had any relationship to the work of the university – by taking an intelligent interest in the recommendations of the Parent Report, by cooperating in every way to implement those that did not run directly counter to McGill's main purpose, and by cooperating with the other universities in every possible way. Here the efforts still fell short of the ideal and would have to be increased. As to direct actions, Robertson thought that increasing the activities of the French Canadian studies program would help since many of them showed considerable promise of being valuable. And finally, he stressed that McGill should steadily improve its standards so that increasing numbers of French Canadian students would aspire to come to McGill, particularly in the fields of graduate study.

In addition, however, McGill should make the government aware of its position in the matter of unequal distribution. The university administration, led by Robertson, had already done this with Paul Gérin-Lajoie, the minister of education, in a private meeting, during which the minister was presented with documents drawn up from the published government estimates that fully illustrated the point. The toughest question was how far to go in publicizing the complaint. The situation was delicate, and Robertson's own conviction was that, at this time, it would be unwise for the university to make an official public protest. If private communications should fail and if, following the formation of a University Grants Commission, which might soon come into being, and if following the reception of the Bladen Report[10] and actions upon its recommendations, the position was not distinctly improved, McGill might have to resort to a direct confrontation. McGill had, it was clear, all the difficulties that Canadian universities in general shared in persuading their provincial governments to provide enough money for their proper progress. It might be facing an additional difficulty – peculiar to Quebec. If this should prove to be so and if it should be sustained, McGill must then react using every means at its disposal. Robertson said he was putting this bluntly lest anyone on the staff think that McGill was prepared to sit back uncomplaining while steadily losing ground. It would not do this.

On 24 May 1965 a nationalist demonstration was held in Montreal to coincide with the Victoria Day holiday, and twenty-five demonstrators were arrested. With the secret joining of the FLQ by Charles Gagnon and Pierre Vallières, there was a considerable increase in the number of bombs, the lethality of the bombs, and labour unrest. Troubles continued at the Port of Montreal when grain handlers went on strike on 16 June and did not return to work until 10 August. During the 1 July holiday fifty-five people were arrested at separatist demonstrations in Montreal and Sherbrooke. Outside the universities, the politics of extremism continued to escalate. A parcel bomb sent by the FLQ killed an employee at a shoe factory during a strike by the Confedération des Syndicats Nationaux (CSN) on 5 May 1966. Less than two weeks later, on 18 May 1966, Paul-Joseph Chartier was killed, in a washroom at the Parliament Buildings in Ottawa, by the bomb that it was believed he intended to throw into the House of Commons. On 14 July 1966 (Bastille Day) sixteen-year-old Jean Corbo, a member of the FLQ, was killed by a bomb he had carried to the scene of a strike.

Robertson, during a brief escape from the daily battles in Quebec, addressed the Canada Club in London, England, on 1 July 1966, delivering a witty examination of Canada as though done by a surgeon dealing with anatomy – a description of the morphology and function of the country according to the standard anatomical method, using, with considerable licence, he said, the phraseology of an anatomical text:

> Canada is a very large body that stretches for thousands of miles in all directions and is to be found sprawled over the top of the U.S.A., to which it is closely applied, yet separated by a diaphanous membrane known ordinarily as the "Longest Undefended Border," though more recently referred to by those who see some significance in the different drinking habits of the Americans and Canadians as the "Bourbon Curtain." The countries are separated, too, by different loyalties, by certain economic inequalities and by a desperate desire – upon the part of most Canadians – to remain separate.
>
> Canada itself, as may be seen on simple inspection, is a lopsided creature with its circulatory and nervous system each collected in a long bundle stretching in a long line across the continent, supplying the southern part of the country well enough but leaving vast territories to the north relatively unsupplied and hence undeveloped.
>
> The country has ten extremities – or Provinces – held to the main body by bonds of varying strength.
>
> The brain, or control center, of this creature is not always readily to be found by the dissector. There have been regimes when it was easily detectable in Ottawa – but at other times so atrophied has

the structure become that it can only be identified with difficulty, and at such times sizeable nodules of brain tissue may be found in the capitals of the Provinces, and these nodules bear an extraordinary resemblance to the properly developed federal brain.

The central organs – the heart, lungs and liver, are concentrated in areas known as Quebec and Ontario – a fact that is deeply resented by the extremities who feel, justifiably enough, that they should be in a position to do more than simply flex their muscles.

In general, the creature is healthy. The tissues that make up the body are sound – there are immense reserves of strength – growth proceeds rapidly, if in a somewhat haphazard way, its intellect is steadily improving – and its wounds, most of which are self-inflicted, heal kindly.

Thus so far, for the most part, the anatomy and physiology is normal for a developing and still evolving affluent animal that has to share its nest with a restless and somewhat overbearing giant. But one extraordinary feature remains to be described – (not unique in the world, but uncommon enough). It is a congenital anomaly, well developed at birth – (if our Confederation can be regarded as the Birth of the Country) – and probably unalterable. The anomaly consists of the presence of two backbones, firmly fused together yet distinct in nearly every detail. One, derived from a gene of French origin, has maintained its original form almost completely. The other, developing somewhat later in the embryo, was of mixed Anglo-Saxon nature at the outset but, with the passage of time, it has acquired other elements, some of which have acted as buttresses strengthening the structure.[11]

From this unusual perspective, he went on to analyze the current difficulties experienced in Canada and to identify some steps that might be taken to reduce the lack of knowledge of the two cultures of each other and the importance of education as part of the process. It was an upbeat address, filled more with hope than with expectation, but one that might be expected from a man in his public position.

Invited to speak on 20 February 1967 at the 40th Annual Fellowship Dinner, Catholics, Jews and Protestants, organized by the Rabbi Stern Brotherhood, on the subject of the "The Challenge of Canada's Centenary," Robertson again used his anatomical description of Canada, combined with a challenge to combat whatever would impede Canada from reaching the goals that it now, after a hundred years of experience, set for itself. The initial goals had not been all that clear, apart from the fact that the union created by Confederation provided more protection than had been available to the independent colonies. However, having had no defining moment or revolution that articulated aims then reflected in a constitution, such as had occurred in the United States, the Constitution, such as it was, contained in the British North America Act, 1867, contained none of the usual defining language or spirit. It was a functional statute, concerned mainly with the division of powers between the Dominion and provincial authorities. Robertson said it read more like a life insurance policy, expressing no inspiration, hope, or guidance for the beneficiary. So it was hard to tell what the goals may have been and whether they had been achieved.

His diagnosis was that Canada was too absorbed in its problems, choosing as examples the spectre of US domination and the threat to its unity – the very things that haunted and motivated the founding fathers. The obsession with these problems absorbed too much of the national attentions, efforts, and skills, distracting the country from other pursuits that might turn out to be more profitable in the long run. Protective legislation could never be more than palliative and temporary. Perhaps the answer to improving interprovincial relations and relations between the federal and provincial governments could be dealt with by repatriating the British North America Act (which was an imperial statute), amending it, or drawing up a new constitution. This could be successful only if Canada could compete on the world scale in industry and the arts; without this, Canada would inevitably have to submit to the leadership of some other country or countries. The same failure to compete and prosper could lead just as surely to a break-up of the country – discontent feeds on failure. He pointed to Expo '67 as an example of success on the world stage. Robertson was a regular booster for Expo '67, which, as a centennial celebration, showed that Canadians could overcome doubts as to the huge scope of the project, that French and English could work brilliantly together, that all three levels of government could cooperate, that daring and innovative solutions to location, construction, and programming could be found, and that a genuine Canadian élan was generated, seen, and appreciated by the entire world, with the additional benefit that Canadians as well could see the world. Developing the human resources of Canada meant educating the people to do the host of jobs that needed to be done, and a superior form of education was the only means of doing this.

Expo '67 was a huge success and focused world attention on Montreal. It showed, as Robertson had long maintained, that Canada, Quebec, and Montreal could aspire to a place on the global stage and that inspired cooperation between the French- and English-speaking communities was not only possible but had been brilliantly demonstrated. Ironically enough for such a fan of Expo '67, Robertson missed the opening due to the timing of an honorary degree conferred upon him by the University of Michigan, which had caused him to be in Ann Arbor the day of the official opening on 27 April.[12] He made up for this initial absence with many visits over the course of the summer and early fall. The angst or self-doubt within Quebec was much relieved, and the celebration of the centennial was generally incident free. The sourest note of the summer came on 24 July, from the ill-considered blunder of French president Charles de Gaulle and his invocation *"vivre le Québec libre!"* Robertson had been invited to City Hall to greet de Gaulle at 4:00 in the afternoon, but left when the guest of honour had not shown up by 7:30 in the evening. Both Prime Minister Pearson and Montreal's mayor, Jean Drapeau, put the French president in his place, Drapeau especially, who reminded de Gaulle publicly that French Canada had retained its identity and made its advances without help from France and would continue to do so. That said, however, the outburst by de Gaulle had provided support and encouragement to the nationalist and separatist factions.

Universities often wrestle with the problem of whether they should speak out on political matters, especially with the increasing involvement of the universities in society. Robertson had no problem with such actions, especially in matters that might involve the educational structure in the community, the educational process itself, the rights of the university, and such matters as the welfare of its members, things that were of direct concern to it and upon which it had a clear and usually unanimous view. This, he maintained, was quite different from the ordinary issues of the day, on which, owing to the various types of people who make up a university, each with their different approaches and beliefs, there was unlikely to be unanimity. It was in the protection of these very differences that the university's main duty lay. It was vitally important that scholars and students live in an atmosphere in which discussion was uninhibited so that every point of view might be examined, and it was vital that there be no deterrent to the free expression of opinions derived from free debate. If the university (as distinct from its individual members) were to try to develop an opinion on each of the main social or political issues, it would encounter enormous difficulty in finding a consensus, and its members would invest a prodigious amount of time in the search for it – time borrowed from teaching and research. But of greater importance was the inhibiting effect that a "university position" might have on free enquiry and expression. The university as a corporate body, Robertson maintained, has no political role to play. Its members could, and did, enter into the political field. They were completely free to do so, and should be encouraged, but the university as such had, properly, no political view.

During the fall term of 1967 Robertson recorded in his diary his increasing pessimism regarding René Lévesque, then a Cabinet minister in the Lesage government. A month later, in October, a Quebec Liberal convention supported special status within Canada for Quebec, but rejected René Lévesque's "Option Québec," which was, when all was said and done, essentially separatism. Lévesque resigned the following month to pursue a campaign for an independent Quebec through formation of the Mouvement Souveraineté-Association, which merged in October 1968 with the Raillement National to become the Parti Québécois. De Gaulle's France did not cease its advances to Quebec, and in May 1968 Canada delivered a note of protest to the French government for treating Quebec as an independent state during an international education conference held the previous month, to which France had invited Quebec, not Canada. On 24 May the US Consulate in Quebec City was damaged by an FLQ bomb. On 11 July forty Canadian university presidents met in Ottawa to discuss the state of nationwide campus unrest. Not surprisingly, there was no perceived panacea.

On 26 September 1968 Daniel Johnson died of a heart attack en route to inaugurate what is now the Hydro-Quebec Daniel Johnson Dam and was succeeded as premier by Jean-Jacques Bertrand on 2 October. On 7 October students occupied Lionel Groulx College in Ste Thérèse, demanding a second French-language university in Montreal, better job preparation, and a government program to create more jobs. Robertson noted in his diary entry for 8 November that he was very concerned about the "parlous" state of Quebec, with its weak government and hordes of militant youths, burning for action. They had no respect for Canada, thought only of a French Quebec, hated the English, and had no care for the economic penalties that would result from separation. They would riot at the slightest opportunity. The student movement was part of it, and even McGill's activists showed every evidence of playing along with their wild French colleagues. They seemed to want only upheaval and for Quebec to be the centre of it, without thinking at all about the effects on Canada. On 9 December, Bill 85, guaranteeing the right to English-language education, was introduced by the Union Nationale government, but even this minor sop to reassure the English-speaking minority was withdrawn the following March by Premier Bertrand because of continued opposition. On 13 December legislation was passed to abolish the appointed Upper Chamber effective 31 December 1968, and the name of the Legislative Assembly was changed to the Assemblée Nationale.

Violence continued to escalate. On 29 January 1969 the computer centre at Sir George Williams University was occupied by West Indian and Canadian students (to protest the manner in which the university was handling charges of racism directed at one of its professors). On 11 February demonstrators destroyed the $1.4 million computer centre and set fire to the university's data centre. Ninety adults and seven juveniles were charged with conspiracy to commit mischief and arson when the occupation ended on 12 February. On 14 March eight Trinidadian students were convicted of conspiracy to obstruct the use of the computer centre and fined a total of $32,500, with the option to serve up to four years in prison if they were unable or unwilling to pay. They were also ordered deported. On 13 February a bomb explosion injured twenty-seven people and caused an estimated $1 million in damage to the Montreal and Canadian Stock Exchanges, for which the FLQ was suspected. On 7 March FLQ member Pierre-Paul Geoffroy of Berthier, Quebec, pleaded guilty to 129 charges of making and placing bombs, conspiracy, theft, and possession of dynamite in connection with thirty-one bombings in the Montreal area. He was sentenced to life imprisonment on 1 April.

On 28 March some 6,000 demonstrators marched on McGill to demand that the university be made a French-language institution, an extreme example of the current dangerous "zero sum" attitude that progress in French-language education could be achieved only at the expense of English-language institutions. About twenty-five persons were later

arrested and charged with disturbing the peace, carrying offensive weapons, and assaulting policemen. Robertson alerted the McGill community
to the dangers the same day:

> Up to the present, attacks upon the University from whatever quar-
> ter have been relatively subtle but, in recent weeks, there have been
> developing plans for a much more crude demonstration of ill-will.
> Early in February we received the first intimation that McGill
> would be attacked on the night of March 28. Shortly thereafter the
> press started to carry stories of the planning. We have received
> rumours and threats concerning the nature of the attack that have
> ranged from full scale occupation of the buildings with appropri-
> ate destruction here and there, to a simple peaceful demonstration
> outside the campus at which a plea for francization of the Univer-
> sity would be made. We have of course no indication as to what is
> really planned or what may develop – be it planned or unplanned.
> We have therefore made preparations to protect the University's
> property and, in the firm belief that to encourage the student body
> or the staff to resist this invasion if there is to be one, could lead
> to the most serious effects, we are asking all members of the staff
> and of the student body, except for those who have been asked to
> undertake special duties, to keep away from the campus tonight.
> (I shall not reveal the plans that we have for defence but I would
> assure you that they are well developed.) By now the senior officers
> and the building directors have all been fully informed of what is
> to be asked from them. During the course of the afternoon today,
> notices will be sent out and I urge you to comply with the instruc-
> tions that they carry.
>
> There is good reason to believe that some of our students and
> staff members have been involved in the planning of this demon-
> stration. It is conceivable that some of them genuinely believe that
> McGill has not been serving the province or the country well and
> that it would be better if it became a French language university.
> With these I can only disagree completely. For, if they do really
> believe what they say, their right to demonstrate peacefully cannot
> be denied. But there are others whose actions cannot, by any
> stretch of the imagination be justified in this way. As was pointed
> out in a recent editorial in *La Presse*, this sudden interest towards

the Francophones in Quebec and the new-born love affair with
Raymond Lemieux are indeed suspect, and I find it impossible
to believe that the motive here is to help Quebec by these means
any more than it has been to help McGill, its students and teachers during the past year or two. The motive as I see it in both cases
is the same: to create confusion and chaos. Thus one can have no
sympathy with it.

The suggestion that we should become a French speaking university is a stimulating one – in the physiological sense at least. It
stimulates me at once to say 'No,' absolutely 'No' ... That is not to
say that we should remain stubbornly English to the point of com-
municating only in our own language and of failing to seize the
considerable academic and cultural advantages that are open to us
in the French language. To do so would be to deny what we always
have recommended should be the general pattern for Canada and a
particularly prominent pattern for ourselves ...

I wish that it were easier to stand up for oneself without appearing to be against everyone else. I expect that, as I say that I believe
that we must remain an English speaking university, I shall be
accused of being anti-Quebec and of not caring for the welfare of
the majority of its people. This is not the case. I believe that I am
as intent as anyone in this country to see Canada flourish; to see a
real understanding develop between its peoples and I submit that
McGill can best contribute to this by doing what it knows how to
do in the way that it can best do it.[13]

There were some sixty-four recorded terrorist bombings of armou-
ries, public buildings, and businesses in March 1969. On 29 September
the home of Mayor Jean Drapeau was bombed. On 7 October there was
a wildcat strike of police and firefighters in protest against an arbitration board ruling on salary negotiations. This resulted in violence and
looting, two deaths, and extensive property damage. There were broken
windows at McGill, fire and damage to the James Administration building, damage to the Engineering Building and to Dawson Hall, and a
fire-bomb threat. Robertson, disgusted with the wave of terror as a commentary on the state of society and the irresponsibility of the strikers,
was involved in the search for the possible bomb. The following day, the
Assemblée Nationale passed emergency legislation ordering the police

and firemen back to work. A state of emergency was declared, and the government requested assistance from the army, the Royal Canadian Mounted Police, and the Sureté de Québec.[14] On 23 October the Union Nationale government tried once again to broach the language issue and tabled Bill 63, the effect of which would be to allow Quebecers the choice of education in French or in English. This caused riots resulting in the arrest of thirty-four people, but this time the government persisted, and the bill was adopted in the Assemblée Nationale on 20 November.[15] On 12 November, Montreal City Council passed a by-law prohibiting marches, meetings, or public demonstrations on public ground that could result in acts of violence. Violation of the by-law was punishable by fines and/or imprisonment. Two days later the annual Santa Claus parade in Montreal was cancelled because of growing tensions and increased violence in the city.

January 1970 brought with it the selection of a new leader for the Quebec Liberal Party, Robert Bourassa, who beat Claude Wagner and Pierre Laporte on the first ballot. An election, called on 12 March, was held on 29 April, in which the Liberals won seventy-two seats and the Union Nationale took seventeen. Seven seats were won by René Lévesque's Parti Québecois, although neither Lévesque nor his financial guru, Jacques Parizeau, won their seats. The caucus leader of the Parti Québecois in Quebec was Camille Laurin, which often led to confusing signals, emanating normally from Lévesque, who stayed in Montreal.[16] But the Parti Québecois was now a factor, and while most were relieved that there would be more breathing room than they had expected, there was no doubt that the mainline political landscape was now officially altered. The pre-election media, especially in the French press, was strongly supportive of the Parti Québecois, which had led Robertson and the senior administration to agonize about what to do if the anticipated separation were to become likely. They wondered whether they should be planning some form of exit strategy but decided that any such plan would become known and might accelerate separation, perhaps even tip the scales in this direction. So, as on every other occasion when they wrestled with the vexing question, they decided to do nothing. Bourassa was sworn in on 12 May. On 31 May there were five bombings in Montreal, three of which had been close enough to wake up Robertson, prompting the Quebec government to take the unusual step of offering a $50,000 reward for information leading to the arrest of those responsible. McGill was the target of a bomb on 15 June that damaged parts of the Engineering Building. On 24 June, in a Department of National Defence building in Ottawa, a female employee was killed when a bomb went off. In July, Quebec passed the Quebec Health Insurance Act to parallel the national Medical Care Act. Robertson foresaw difficulties, including the level of remuneration of physicians and the interference of government in the practice of medicine and operation of hospitals.[17] The Bourassa government was forced to legislate 40,000 striking construction workers back to work on 10 August.

By this time Robertson's role as principal was nearly finished. He hoped that his successor might have a better time with the Quebec government than he had enjoyed and that there would be more opportunity for positive approaches, of which there had been precious few during his years in office. He speculated that one advantage to the university coming out of his resignation might be that the government would feel that without appearing to be giving in to the pressure that Robertson had applied year after year, they could start to give more to McGill. It was, however, far more a hope than an expectation.

Robertson was already out of office and was in the process of moving to Ottawa when the October Crisis, the most recent nadir in Quebec political history, began with the kidnapping of the British trade commissioner, James Cross, from his home on Redpath Crescent by FLQ terrorists on 5 October.[18] The government refused to accede to the kidnappers' demands. On 10 October the Quebec minister of labour, Pierre Laporte, playing ball with family members outside their suburban St Lambert home, was kidnapped by another FLQ cell. Two days later troops arrived in Ottawa to protect government buildings, officials, and the diplomatic community from possible FLQ terrorist attack. On 15 October, the same day that Robertson and Roslyn were honoured at a dinner hosted by the McGill Graduates Society, troops from the 22nd Regiment arrived in Montreal, at the request of the Quebec and Montreal governments, to bolster civil authorities.[19] The regiment was joined by other armed forces units, which took up positions throughout Quebec. Growing FLQ support culminated in a mass rally of some 3,000 students and unionists at the Paul Sauvé arena. At three o'clock in the morning of 16 October, Prime Minister Trudeau, at the request of the Quebec government, proclaimed the War Measures Act, the first time such powers had been used in peacetime, on the basis that an apprehended insurrection existed in

Quebec.[20] This gave the police extraordinary powers of arrest and deten-
tion in respect of anyone suspected of belonging to or sympathizing
with the FLQ. Even membership in the FLQ became a criminal offence,
and political rallies were banned. Habeas corpus was suspended. Overnight, 465 people were arrested, of whom only 18 were convicted of any
crime.[21]

The next day Laporte's body was found in the trunk of a car at the
St Hubert airport. He had been strangled. Parliament, by a vote of 190
to 16, approved the proclamation of the War Measures Act on 19 October. By the end of the month FLQ member Robert Hudon was sentenced
to twenty-five years in prison for armed robberies and conspiracy to
commit hold-ups to finance FLQ subversive activities, and on 6 November, Bernard Lortie was arrested in connection with the kidnapping of
Laporte. His accomplices escaped after hiding in a specially built com-
partment behind a wardrobe. James Cross was freed by police from a
room in the north end of Montreal on 3 December, in return for safe
conduct and transport to Cuba for the kidnappers and their families.[22]
On 28 December, Paul and Jacques Rose and Francis Simard, suspected
in the Laporte kidnapping, were captured in a tunnel under a farmhouse
near Montreal. They were later charged, tried, and convicted, along with
Bernard Lortie, with the kidnapping and noncapital murder of Laporte.
Paul Rose was sentenced to two life terms of imprisonment, Simard to life
imprisonment, Lortie to twenty years, and Jacques Rose to eight years.[23]
By early January 1971 the troops stationed in Montreal and other parts of
Quebec as a result of the October Crisis were withdrawn. In March the
Quebec government promised compensation for those arrested during
the crisis but never charged, and it ordered the destruction of their police
files and fingerprints. On 13 August the Crown suspended charges laid
under the War Measures Act against thirty-two people, including labour
leader Michel Chartrand, lawyer Robert Lemieux, and teacher Charles
Gagnon.

Robertson thought that the October Crisis would lead directly to the
separation of Quebec from Canada. He believed that the nation had been
brought together by the tragedy and that the governments had worked
together without differences of opinion but under tremendous strain. He
doubted that the country could be made stronger as a result or that a firm
and sympathetic reaction on the part of English Canada would encourage the French Canadians to stay within Canada. He seemed to feel that

the seeds of discontent were beginning to sprout and that the French Canadians would soon feel they could do better alone. Possibly only the economic problems that would be faced might be the deciding factor. He acknowledged that these were feelings he had when he was depressed and that the exhausting events of the crisis may have warped his judgment, but he could nevertheless not avoid this unhappy view.

Even at the end of the year, looking back on what had happened, he could not avoid the feeling of foreboding that had gripped him earlier and in the immediate aftermath of the crisis. It was all but impossible to dismiss from his mind the events of the years when he had had to deal with the treatment of McGill at the hands of successive Quebec governments, the blatant inequalities to which it had been subjected, and the personal feeling of having been regularly beaten down in the fight for equitable treatment on its behalf. His view was, undoubtedly, one shared by many within the Quebec English-speaking community, and the overall pessimism about the future of the country was shared by many outside Quebec. Reflecting on all this, his diary entry for 31 December 1970 notes:

A year end note. It's been an eventful year – starting in Florida where we were holidaying and escaping – not entirely successfully – the cold. I can recall then wondering what was going to happen and I was uneasy in my mind. Amongst my worries were first the normal university ones – what was going to happen – were things going to blow up? As it turned out they didn't – so I might have spared myself this worry. Second I fussed about Quebec – its effects on McGill (starvation and encroachment by the government) and on the English speaking people generally and, in particular on their educational system which I had been trying to defend for the previous 3 months. These worries were, of course, very sure fire and they've not been lightened in any way. McGill was badly treated by the government in the matter of grants – even by the new Bourassa Liberal government from which we might have expected better – and the sight of government encroachment upon the affairs of the University (all universities actually) became increasingly ominous as the year wore on. This assumption – or attempts at assumption – of control here or there by the Ministry of Education is not all bad – it could lead to greater care in the spending of money and in more cooperation – but if it continues to the extreme that people in the Ministry would wish the results could be serious.

The position of the English speaking people was no better – perhaps a little worse at the end of the year. The defeat of [Jean-Guy] Cardinal at the Union National leadership convention and the later defeat of his party and the return of the Liberals seemed, on the surface to augur well for us. But the underlying Nationalism which became more evident during the year and the labour groups more outspoken amongst the "intellectuals" gained strength and, while it's much too early to tell, it seems likely that the Cross-Laporte crisis will eventually be found to have weakened Canada rather than – as many would have it – the reverse. I have become much less optimistic than I used to be about the possibilities of the country staying together – indeed, quite often I think that we would do better to face the fact that the French and the English will never see eye to eye closely enough to make things work smoothly and that we should set about to arrange an agreement between Quebec and the rest which would leave Quebec autonomous and the rest able to communicate with each other.

This is defeatist talk – or thinking – and I only entertain these ideas when I'm feeling depressed – or when the French are being over aggressive – but it is not unrealistic – certainly not to anyone who has been in a position to see the French speaking Canadians gaining by leaps and bounds (from a lowly position in which they had placed themselves) and yelping for more at every leap and, apparently quite unsatisfied with their own progress and totally unappreciative of the very considerable efforts that have been made by the rest of the country to accommodate them. I often feel that the English have given up too much, that they have been too accommodating and have left unanswered too many of the charges of injustice that the French have hurled about with such abandon for so many years. I have even felt that the Separatists (and a very high proportion of Quebecers are facultative separatists I believe) have as a plan to build Quebec up industrially to as high a pitch as possible before making their move – that they will exhaust Federal aid schemes. I doubt very much that this is the case – I doubt that there could be such a scheme for the timing would be impossible

– but I have no doubt that even the most ardent separatist will
bleed the rest of the country so long as he can – and sometimes I
think I see signs of blood in some of the ventures (airport, CBC
building, etc.)

But this, again, is defeatist thinking and I keep it pretty well to
myself realizing that to talk of such things is only to hasten an end
which one still hopes can be averted. And I think it still possible
that the country can hold together – if we could hang on – if we
could develop a generation of intelligent bilinguals – if a basically
English speaking Prime Minister could have the full respect of the
French speaking people and could speak to them in a tongue that
they could recognizes as their own – we could well squeak through
– and we'd be a better country for it – I have always felt that if
the traditional antagonists – the English and the French – could
wholeheartedly work together and if they could share their very
different talents, the result would be extraordinarily potent. This is
still a real possibility in Canada and it is the only objective that we
should set for ourselves.

Robertson was, by then, fully withdrawn from the fray. The situation in
Quebec had a far more immediate impact on McGill than it had, for all
its noise, on the rest of Canada. The politics spilled over into demonstrating the political willingness (or otherwise) of Quebec to provide
adequate funding for a largely anglophone educational institution. It had
proved to be one of the most difficult of the demons with which Robertson had to wrestle in his role as principal, a constant struggle from
which he drew little satisfaction and which drew from him an inordinate
amount of time and energy.

FINANCES AND DOUBLE STANDARDS

McGill's finances, once the Quebec government began to enter the field of supporting the expanding university system, were inseparable from the politics of the day and their linguistic overtones. There was no denying the increasing interest within the French-speaking community regarding postsecondary education nor escaping the fact that the French-speaking institutions had lagged well behind McGill not only in size but also in resources, reputation, and connection with the private sector, especially the business community. McGill's Board of Governors was all but a "who's who" of the national industrial and commercial elite, circles that, if not closed to French Canadians, were not easily accessible to them. The historic and cultural reasons for this were not as important as the then current observation of the existing state of affairs and the related bitterness regarding it.

None of this had anything to do with the obvious needs of McGill, given its size and the breadth of its programs as well as the international standards that it had established and wanted to maintain. The entire educational system in Quebec had to be increased and upgraded as the demands for higher education expanded. Generating the necessary level of awareness among political decision makers and in the public at large was one of the main duties of university leaders, particularly for the principal of Quebec's leading university and the only one with any international reputation. The messages had to be repeated, with shifting emphasis depending on the audience, and as Robertson's understanding of the underlying issues increased, so did his confidence in articulating them. He referred to the various presentations as his "well ground-out [gramophone] records" on such subjects as "The Challenge of Education," "The University as a Force in the Nation's Economy," "The Economic Problems of Education in a Bilingual State," and "The Problems of a Bilingual State."[1]

Ultimately, aside from the routine challenges of running any complex organization, the root of what faced McGill (as well as all other universities) over the next few years was a veritable tsunami of new students as the advantages of a university education became more apparent and as an increasing percentage of an increasing population, especially in Quebec, sought entry. On-the-job training, which had for many years been perceived as the best way to progress in a business career, was shifting to a preference for university-trained individuals who could then be taught the business. The French Canadian community, now released from its ecclesiastical and political bondage, was producing greatly increased numbers of students seeking postsecondary education. There were simply not enough places ready to handle them. Between 1961 and 1964 alone, Robertson's early years as principal, McGill's student body increased by 35 per cent. Every response to such pressures, inevitably, entailed additional costs, which were exacerbated by the increasing costs of living in an expanding economy.

The costs could be defrayed in part by tuition fees, although such fees never amounted to anything close to the total costs of the education provided to the students. Government contributions were increasing, but it was (and remains) inherent in the nature of government-funded programs that monies allotted are never sufficient. The financial concern of the McGill principal was to maximize all sources of funds and then to ensure that the available resources were used as efficiently as possible. Graduates were an obvious additional source of funds, and considerable attention was devoted to making certain that they remained aware of the challenges faced by the university and their financial consequences. Within the university, Robertson centralized and coordinated the approaches to possible supporters. A McGill Fund Council was established to concentrate on fundraising. In previous chapters of McGill's financial history, when there had been a deficit in the operations, the governors, all captains of industry and commerce, had anted up on a personal or corporate basis to balance the budget, but times had changed, as had the magnitude of the sums involved, and such personalized responses were no longer feasible or sufficient.

Prior to the public funding of universities, when no particular community or social expectations affected them, the universities had no need to – and, therefore, had made no effort to – explain themselves and the benefits arising from their presence and activities to the public at large. Now that public funds were directed at universities, there was a new stakeholder that needed to be reassured as to effective allocation of the resources it provided. Moreover, governments needed to be persuaded that in light of the increased expectations of and demands on the university system, the amounts they committed to universities also required drastic increases. The business community had to be educated to acknowledge and understand the benefits it derived from universities and the employees they trained and to support the universities in the development of this essential resource for the community. This was in addition to the benefits of research conducted at universities, which could also produce research on behalf of the business community. All of this made demands on the time and attention of the principal, and hardly a day, and certainly not a week, went by that Robertson was not called upon or sought opportunities to address influential groups on the importance of higher education and the need to provide the necessary resources to support it. And he took a very broad view of the subject. For Robertson, the advancement of education at the highest standards was not just a local or provincial concern but a matter of national priority as Canada moved forward in the world.

THE LIFE OF A UNIVERSITY PRINCIPAL OR RECTOR

In early 1966 the Université de Montréal selected Roger Gaudry as its rector. He was feted by the members of the University Club, to which he belonged, at a dinner on 26 January. Robertson, as his counterpart at McGill, was called upon to introduce him and, in the guise of humour, included the following remarks, which gave some indications, almost a *roman à cléf*, of his personal feelings about the job he had and that Gaudry was assuming:

> As one reads the story of Roger's life to date, a question at once springs to mind – Why would a person who has everything going his way in a career of his own choosing suddenly, as he approaches the peak of his career, drop it all to take up a task that is well known to be difficult, dangerous to reputation and health, ruinous to peace of mind and, to some extent, thankless? For this, in the opinion of most people who have become Rectors, is a very good description of this job ... The man was riding high and would have

gone higher by virtue of his own momentum – and there was no
stopping it – when he was to set it all aside.

My question, again, is why did he do it? Certainly not for personal gain – in any sense. Certainly not as an easy path to retirement, for he knew full well that he was stepping from a relatively
comfortable and manageable frying pan into one of the hottest
of fires – kindled by financial problems, staff problems, student
unrest, and a thousand other flammables.

There can only be, I think, two reasons – first a sense of duty,
for I know that he believed that in the progress of this country the
success of its universities is vital, and his duty, as he saw it, was to
contribute his own efforts to that success. The second reason that
I would offer is that he was confident that he could do the job well
– a confidence based, no doubt, upon his knowledge of universities (he'd been a professor for 14 years and a scholar in two great
universities and a governor of one) – his knowledge of the business
world, in his own Province and the rest of Canada and the United
States – and confidence based on many other qualities and abilities
and circumstance, not the least of which was the fact that his host
of friends in this country were confident, too, that he could do this
job and were solidly behind him. A good testimony of this fact is
this dinner tonight, at which many of his friends are gathered to do
honour to Roger Gaudry.[2]

Shunting interuniversity collegiality aside, the financial problems affecting McGill moved from annoying to serious, and within three weeks
of this event, Robertson had been left with no alternative but to "go
public" with a statement critical of the Quebec government's treatment
of McGill.[3]

POLITICS TRUMP ANALYSIS

The government, ignoring the recommendations of the Gauthier Committee, which had been established to advise on university grants, proposed to raise its allocation to McGill for the 1966–67 year by a paltry
$100,000 despite the proven need for an additional $5 million to bring
salaries closer to the range of those paid at universities of similar size in
Quebec and Canada, the increased costs of operating the physical plant,
and the increased costs of accommodating the swiftly rising numbers of

students. After effecting economies and using all other sources of revenue, McGill was $3.5 million short of being able to balance its budget. McGill's fees were already higher than those at Laval and the Université de Montréal. Dissipation of its free endowments was not a sensible solution and would soon permanently remove a continuing and important source of income. Robertson pointed out that from 1960–61 to 1966–67 provincial grants to McGill had increased by only 47 per cent, while those to Laval went up by 208 per cent and those to the Université de Montréal by 242 per cent. Put another way, the amounts contributed by the province per eligible student were: McGill – $502; Université de Montréal – $1,220; and Laval – $1,290. It was a particularly discouraging time for Robertson, coinciding as it did with the increasing general tensions within Quebec, the deteriorating position of minorities within Quebec, and the uncertainty as to the continuing viability of Canada as a country.

Robertson took the bull by the horns by saying that even more important than the failure of the government estimates to deal fairly with McGill's requirements was the significance of the government's decision as a possible indication of its attitude toward McGill – an institution he believed was important to all the people of Quebec, not merely to the English-speaking community. The government's policy could lead only to a decline in McGill's ability to maintain its standards. If McGill were to decline in any way, Robertson warned, such a development would be deeply unfortunate for Quebec, all of Quebec, and for Canada. The media also attacked the existence of the university's endowment funds. McGill had had much more experience in raising money from its graduates, and this was, extraordinarily enough, portrayed as an unfair "advantage" over the French universities, which had no such tradition. There was a feeling that McGill should be required to disperse these endowment funds before it could obtain government funding. It never seemed possible, despite concerted efforts, to make the point understood that the existence of endowments provided an ongoing source of income that meant the needs from the government could be reduced by the amount of such income. In addition, it proved almost impossible to make it clear that restricted endowments could not be used for purposes other than those the donors had designated and that these restricted endowments also (and to an even greater extent) reduced the need for government funding. McGill was paying, in effect, from its endowment income, expenses that would otherwise have had to be paid by the government.

Robertson challenged the purported explanations of the education minister, Paul Gérin-Lajoie, regarding the adjustment made in respect of research funds received by McGill (that they contributed to the normal operations of the university and should be deducted from the support for such operations provided by the government) as a regrettable misunderstanding of the nature of research funds, on the one hand, and of the university's operating expenses, on the other. The funds received for research purposes, much of which came from the National Research Council, had nothing to do with supporting general operating expenses and activities. Such grants supported, instead, research and postgraduate studies, which were not financed by present provincial grants. This research and graduate work resulted in great benefits to Quebec itself and raised the standards of graduate research and teaching for the whole province. Robertson could only assume that this misunderstanding had led to an error of judgment and urged the government to rectify its assessment of McGill's financial situation and the consequent inequitable approach to McGill's immediate and developing operating needs. It would be a tragedy, he said, if this outside, nongovernmental financing of research and graduate studies should lead to McGill being penalized. The university should be supported in its efforts to maintain high standards while expanding its operating expenses in order to meet the increasing demands of the new Quebec itself as well as of higher education as a whole.

These were uncharacteristically blunt responses, backed by published facts that made a very forceful statement and coupled with direct criticism of Gérin-Lajoie, who clearly did not understand how research was funded (or had been misinformed by his civil servants, who would certainly have known). Evidently, the minister also carried no residual goodwill toward McGill as a result of the honorary degree that had been conferred on him in 1962, and Robertson had sensed that he was deeply hostile to McGill. Robertson concluded his statement by reiterating that McGill considered itself, historically and academically, very much a part of Quebec and believed it had a vital role to play in the continuing scientific, technological, and cultural development of the province. It could not play this role by curtailing its operations, incurring deficits, or allowing its income to dwindle. It was up to the government of the province to protect the deepest interests in higher education of all of its citizens and institutions.

Not surprisingly, the statements produced both public and private reaction. The issue of discrimination was on the table and in front of the government, which would have to respond. Negotiations with the government continued for the next months as McGill officials attempted to obtain a better response to the situation. Faced with the public nature of McGill's protest and the politically charged message, Premier Jean Lesage invited McGill representatives to meet with him and said he was open-minded and would be prepared to make adjustments if he could be satisfied they were necessary.[4] The French media were filled with justifications for the treatment proposed for McGill and even suggested that the province should not support McGill in any way. Why should Quebecers be paying for the education of a whole bunch of foreigners? Perhaps McGill should be nationalized and become entirely French-speaking? Only Claude Ryan of Le Devoir had anything positive to say about McGill.

The McGill Association of University Teachers issued a statement expressing its "concern for the future of the academic community" in Quebec and characterized the political machinations as discriminating against McGill.[5] This was challenged by the Association des Professeurs de l'Université de Montréal, which said McGill should not have acted independently of the other Quebec universities. La Réforme, the French-language organ of the Quebec Liberal Party, charged McGill with being "demagogic" in its protest. In an editorial, it said that the "lack of tact of the Education Department did not justify the demagogic attitude of McGill which presented the problem on the level of an ethnic confrontation." McGill's past growth, it said, had come as a result of both government grants and generous private donations from which the French universities did not "benefit." (No mention was made of the fact that the French universities had done none of the work necessary to generate such donations.) Now that the government was redressing the balance, McGill had no right to act the "martyr," especially since in their period of "deprivation" the University of Montreal and Laval University had not resorted to this tactic.[6] The St Jean Baptiste Society issued a statement that the government should not be contributing to relief of any McGill deficit since it was a private institution that had not consulted the government in preparing its budget.[7] It was an unsettling period, not just for McGill but for the entire English-speaking community. In one of his lighter moments (outside the province), Robertson noted that as Canada was coming up on its centenary, the English and French within Canada were still feeling their way. At the beginning, he said, Canada had had the opportunity to blend American know-how, the British parliamentary system, and French culture but now seemed to be on the verge of a blend of British know-how, American culture, and French politics.[8]

Rumours swirling from Quebec regarding the government's attitude were not good. They suggested that only a paltry sum would be offered to McGill. A meeting was planned with Eric Kierans over the weekend of 12 March, and it was thought that the Cabinet might discuss the matter the following week. Kierans, with his previous McGill connection as professor of economics and director of the School of Commerce, indicated that he would take a strong stand on the "McGill Affair," which was encouraging, that he would refuse to agree to any decision until members of the Cabinet had read the Gauthier Report, and that he would accept nothing less than a return to the funding proportions recommended in the report.[9] Kierans was quite forceful within the Lesage government; the only risk might be that if the rest of the Cabinet baulked and he were to resign, the difficulty would become enormous.[10] In the meantime, the Ford Foundation, which was considering McGill's application for grants of $2 million in support of Islamic studies, developing-area studies, and foreign comparative law, had called, due to the reported problems with the government, and wanted to know whether they had been settled. Robertson was afraid that the Ford Foundation's decision could be affected by McGill's level of financial security and that the foundation might not want to invest in McGill if the university was not likely to prosper, but fortunately the grants came through the next week. Robertson hoped that this good news would not be made public until after the Quebec mess was sorted out. Even though it was all research funding and of no help to the operating budget, Quebec, given the education minister's most recent position on research funds, could be counted on not to understand. It was a strange world, he mused, in which one did not dare rejoice.

It was a period of increasing antipathy and tension between the francophone community and all others. There was much talk and speculation about head offices leaving Quebec, about individuals transferring their money out of the province, and about some leaving the province with their money. Robertson, having recently been the butt of serious discrimination affecting McGill with respect to university grants, was particularly sensitive to such talk but maintained a public face, saying he fully expected that things would turn out satisfactorily. Privately, he was deeply discouraged by the amount of energy that seemed to be required to keep the country intact and, at the university level, to get equitable treatment. If separatism were to prevail and the discrimination increased, it might even be necessary to move McGill.

RETURN OF THE UNION NATIONALE

A change of government in Quebec that would affect McGill occurred on 5 June 1966, when the Union Nationale under Daniel Johnson narrowly defeated the Lesage Liberals, winning 56 seats while the Liberals took 50. This was encouraging, to some degree, since two weeks before the election Johnson had appeared on television to say that the Quebec government ought to support the English institutions and had specifically mentioned the case of the McGill grants. Of course, this was as a member of the Opposition and prior to the election, but almost any straw was worth grasping. Without knowing the outcome of the election and with no decisions emanating from the government in the pre-election period, McGill had been forced to proceed with its budget and the related deficit. It maintained the level of academic activity contained in its submissions to the government, which meant that if there was no improvement on the initial level of funding, there would be a deficit of $3.5 million. The risk had been taken, knowing the serious effects on the university of any retraction at this stage.

In early August all the university heads met first with the new minister of finance to try to get additional funds. The new minister of education was Jean-Jacques Bertrand, who did not impress Robertson favourably, but he agreed to establish a university grants commission and undertook to introduce the necessary legislation. Bertrand read from the report of the committee established by Lesage in February, which had recommended a further $425,000 for McGill, a sum that would have left the university with a deficit of $2.5 million for the year. Robertson gave his opinion of this report "in no uncertain terms," which did not please the minister, who said the government would continue to consider the matter. It would obviously mean another long period of wrangling and recriminations, to which Robertson did not look forward.

Keeping his own counsel, however, for McGill within Quebec, Robertson thought (and his review of the affairs following the August meetings confirmed what he had felt for some time) that McGill's crisis would come within two years. In that time, McGill would have to decide whether it could continue in its present state in Quebec. If the government would not support it as an English-speaking university, McGill would have to either become French or pull out. Neither possibility was attractive. There was still plenty of reason to hope that the government would come around, but he was discouraged, although not terminally so. Each advance that McGill had made toward Quebec, and a number had been made in the belief that its best chance lay in this direction rather than in retrenching, seemed to have turned out wrong. Robertson's feeling on the matter see-sawed, changing from time to time. On balance, however, he was more pessimistic than optimistic about the eventual outcome.

CEGEPS

The educational structure in Quebec was significantly altered in 1966 by the creation of a new intermediate level of education between second-ary school (finishing at grade eleven) and university. The legislation introducing general and vocational colleges, known as CEGEPs, from the French *college d'enseignement general et professionnel*, was passed the following year.[11] This had the effect of putting McGill out of synch with all other universities in North America, and there was great con-cern that its competitive position for good students from outside Quebec would be compromised. The new system added an additional year before an initial degree could be granted, raising the total from fifteen to six-teen. Speculation was rampant as to the effect on McGill, ranging from the pessimistic view that the university's population would drop sharply and never regain its present level to the view that an initial sharp drop would be followed by a gradual restoration in a few years and that enrol-ment would then increase considerably over presently projected levels. Others thought that it would not be possible to get the CEGEPs formed soon enough to cause a sharp drop in the university population and that gradual decreases would occur, to be gradually recovered.

The CEGEP problem, quite apart from its impact on McGill in rela-tion to non-Quebec students, occasioned a further set of considerations affecting McGill. This arose from the Quebec government's desire to establish a CEGEP in the western portion of the Island of Montreal, specifically on property comprising Macdonald College in Ste Anne de Bellevue, which was the home, among other activities, of the Faculty of

Agriculture. The consequences for McGill were unclear, including the degree of disturbance of this important faculty. The government was, however, quite insistent on the location and had the effective means to impose its will, so McGill was fighting what it knew to be a rearguard action. John Abbott College has since been established on the campus, but long after Robertson had left the scene the tensions continued as the Quebec government intervened directly in the governance of the CEGEPs and their financing, which included the financing of the facilities on the Macdonald campus and their subsequent acquisition under terms grossly unfavourable to McGill.

CONTINUING GRIND

On the funding front, despite the apparent interest of the new Quebec government, the initial indications for the McGill grant were particularly discouraging and pointed to a further deficit of more than $3 million for the next fiscal year. The Gauthier Committee was reassembled and began its work on the next budgetary year. In November 1966, as the first study of the situation was being completed, the education minister called for another meeting, during which it became evident that McGill was unlikely to receive sympathetic consideration from the government. There was little alternative but to go public once more regarding the situation, and Robertson held a press conference on 11 December 1966 at the end of ten months of the frustrating negotiations. He pointed out the disastrous consequences for McGill and that the paltry "increase" proposed by the government was in fact a decrease, once the impact of inflation had been considered. He urged a return to the findings of the Gauthier Committee in order to guarantee equity among Quebec universities. He dealt with the suggestion that full provincial support should not be granted to McGill until it had dissipated all of its other resources as a thoroughly unsound principle from the perspective of financial management, a suggestion that could not be considered as remotely fair unless the government declared a policy of treating in the same manner the endowments of all institutions that it subsidized.

McGill's fees were already the highest in the country. Education Minister Jean-Jacques Bertrand said that the problems of operational grants to universities, including McGill, were still under study and that no report was expected until January. He rejected the idea that McGill should be treated as an "isolated case" while affirming in the Assemblée Nationale that "the government intends to treat all Quebec institutions, universities and others with equal justice."[12] He also huffed and puffed that he was surprised by Robertson's declarations since the university principals and their advisors had met with him and Finance Minister Paul Dozois on 18 November to study the financial situation of the universities for the current and succeeding fiscal years, adding that the problems were common to all universities. The federal government, ducked the issue, not wanting to get into any further confrontations with the Quebec government. Prime Minister Lester B. Pearson commented that the government planned no special action regarding McGill and threw in a Pontius Pilate-like statement that McGill "does undoubtedly receive assistance from the Federal Government in the manner provided by the arrangements we have made with the provinces."[13]

Within three days Premier Daniel Johnson acknowledged that he was embarrassed by the government's announced decision and by the fact that the reasons for it were never revealed to McGill, which had added insult to the injury.[14] The St Jean Baptiste Society of Montreal once again waded into the fray, strident and dusting off earlier rhetoric but unburdened by fact, asking by what principle the state should be forced to balance the budget of a private institution that did not consult in preparing it and that chose to ignore – at its own risk – the decisions taken in the matter by the minister of education. The society called on the directors of this institution (McGill) to have the courage to suffer the consequences of the policy that they themselves had adopted. To proceed otherwise was, it said, using demagogic means to force the government to modify the criteria then in place to ensure a rational financing of higher education in Quebec. It continued, darkly, to state that the administrators of McGill should show greater prudence and see that they were "advancing on particularly dangerous ground."[15]

This was a time when the "discrimination" card could be freely played only by the Quebec francophone majority (on the basis of its own minority position within Canada and in North America) and never by the anglophone minority within francophone Quebec. As it played out in the educational portfolio, there seemed to be a discouraging attitude that progress could be made only by the emerging Quebec universities at the expense of the existing universities. Instead of all aspiring to rise to even higher levels, there was a previously identified "zero sum" approach, which would become particularly overt during the "McGill Français" demonstrations in 1969, that called for the aspiring universities to rise to the diminished level of the former leading institutions – a distressing Lilliputian perspective in an area so important to the community as a whole.

Perhaps some good had come from the confrontations over funding in 1966 because the initial auguries from Quebec for the next year's grant, derived from a meeting with the ministers of finance and education in January 1967, seemed quite positive for McGill, including an agreement to pay three-quarters of the previous year's deficit over three years, plus a considerably larger annual grant, even though it did not keep pace with the grants to the other universities. There was, however, no such thing as pure good news since other indications were that the grant increases might be coupled with a requirement to reduce tuition fees by about a hundred dollars, which would put McGill back almost to its previous position. If the fee reduction was not imposed, the grant increases would improve the relative position slightly.[16]

A particularly sour note was the news that former education minister Paul Gérin-Lajoie was reportedly disgusted with the French universities for not raising a fuss about the discrimination against the French universities in the budget. There was, of course, no such discrimination, and the French universities had got more than their share, even applying what was meant to be a purely objective analysis. Robertson had concluded that Gérin-Lajoie was not just hostile to McGill but violently anti-English, which made things particularly difficult. Quebec still chose to regard private donations to McGill from its supporters as though they were grants made to McGill by the government and reduced the grants it would otherwise have made to McGill on a dollar-for-dollar basis. Even with the indications of better treatment, Robertson discussed the possibility of McGill becoming a federal institution with Carl Goldenberg, who said he did not think it was impossible, although it is hard to imagine on what basis a university could become federal under a constitution that assigned responsibility for education to the provinces.

The budgetary woes continued in 1968, this time apparently designed to remove benefits achieved by McGill the previous year.[17] Robertson was in Quebec in late February to learn that the government was not willing to spend the Gauthier Committee's recommended amount of $90 million for universities, only $85 million. The difference was to be deducted from the preliminary allocations to the English-speaking universities, while the French universities were to have their own allocations increased, a decision that ignored, once again, the recommended distributions proposed by the Gauthier Committee, which had been created by the government precisely to advise it on an objective basis. Remonstrations with the education minister seemed to produce no result. As soon as the meeting with the government had ended, Robertson approached Laval's rector, Monseigneur Louis-Albert Vachon, then president of the Conférence des Recteurs et des Principaux des Universités du Québec (CREPUQ), to convene a meeting of the organization to discuss an urgent problem. He wanted to tackle all the rectors. Vachon canvassed them and said that they were willing to meet but that Roger Gaudry of the Université de Montréal would meet only on condition that they not touch on the question of money!

Robertson said that this was absurd and that the sole purpose of the meeting was, precisely, to discuss the financial situation. It bordered on the surreal to pretend that the financial situation could not be discussed. Gaudry relented and they met at Laval that afternoon. He found the other rectors grinning, as he noted, "like Cheshire cats," having, Robertson suspected, engineered the whole thing themselves. They let him talk. Gauthier, whose committee had recommended allocations based largely on objective criteria, also attended the meeting. Robertson's main argument to his colleagues was that the universities should not sit back and allow the government to make purely political decisions on the allocation of funds. Sooner or later, one or other of the French universities might fall out of political favour, or some other university might emerge that had more political appeal than any of them, and then there would be cries for an objective (as opposed to political) approach to the allocation of grants. The French rectors were not, at the time, impressed. It would be only a few years later, when the Université de Québec system was developed and became, in time, the government's pet, that they would suddenly change their minds and began to insist on objectivity as the only fair way.

Trying to obtain equitable financial treatment for McGill at the hands of an unsympathetic series of Quebec governments remained a constant and debilitating struggle that required a disproportionate amount of Robertson's time and energy throughout his time as principal.[18] The costs of providing the educational services required from the university increased every year, and each year the Quebec government found new ways not to provide McGill with what was required, despite being able to provide for the requirements of the French universities. Regular consultation and communication with the public servants merely confirmed some of the subterfuges that were developed to achieve the desired outcomes. This continued up to and including Robertson's last year in office. A proposal had been made, for example, that college-equivalent students not be included for purposes of calculating the grants and that graduate students (for whom the costs of providing the necessary education were considerably higher) be weighted equally with undergraduates, both of which would have the effect of reducing the McGill grant and which Robertson thought had probably been a proposal designed to achieve this very purpose.

The CEGEP issue was still current. Robertson had spent considerable time preparing comments and positions on McGill's behalf regarding proposed legislative changes affecting education (Bill 62 at the time) and the indifference with which the Quebec government seemed to treat English-language education in the province. During a budget meeting in Quebec on 29 January 1970, a representative of the Ministry of Education made a statement attacking the McGill spokesman on the question, which Robertson took as an attack on himself, and he retorted that the bureaucrat's comments were unacceptable. In addition, Robertson said that while he was quite interested in the question and would be willing to pursue the matter in depth on another occasion, the statements made by the official were not the purpose of the present meeting and urged the chairperson to continue with the set agenda. Although civil on the surface after Robertson's chastisement of the ministry official, several members of the CREPUQ were hostile to McGill. It seemed to the McGill administration that every effort would be made by the other universities to develop justifications that would produce less for McGill than would result from any reasonable formula that could be devised. By early May it appeared that McGill's deficit for the forthcoming year would be at least $3 million and might well rise to $5 million.

Quebec governments never seemed to understand, nor appear, to this day, to want to understand, the difference between levels of funding that merely provide access to some form of higher education and the need to have increasingly higher standards of education to keep pace with the rest of the world. The ability of Quebec to compete on world levels is not just a matter of access to universities within Quebec but is inextricably linked to the quality of the education the students receive and the quality of the teaching and research available to the students and the community at large. Linking low tuition fees and government support is well and good but only provided that the total amount of financial support for the universities is sufficient to generate the necessary quality to allow society to develop in competition with other countries that are investing in high-quality education.

The best model is one that achieves a balance between the public, which needs the societal outcomes of a university system, the students, who benefit personally from the education that they receive (and that no one "owes" them), and the private sector, which draws on the product of the universities, be it educated talent or the increase in knowledge derived from university-based research. Everyone has a stake in the outcomes. It is a matter of reckless self-deception to believe that all this can be achieved without investment in the highest-quality education. The mantra intoned by the proponents of low or non-existent fees that low tuition fees lead to greater accessibility has consistently been shown to be wrong. The data show precisely the opposite. "Free" education has never been a success at the postsecondary level. One has only to look at the chaos and diminished quality of the education based on this model that is provided today, for example, in France.

STUDENTS, FACULTY, AND GOVERNANCE:
SHEPHERDING RADICAL CHANGE

Few, if any, could have had sufficient foresight to predict the extent of the changes that would occur in society and in relation to universities in the 1960s. It was a generation of protest, rejection of authority, demand for participation in decision making, disruption, and occasional violence. It was the Viet Nam era. Robertson was unacquainted with the extent of the currents and with the full platform of university life, having been sequestered in what he described as "a relatively isolated and unworldly department." He was unaware of what should perhaps have been his biggest problem and worried, in effect, about the wrong things. He had come to the job as principal only to be overwhelmed by problems of finance, construction, and university business in general that haunt and possess the would-be educator:

> But, even if this is true, I should subsequently have been more
> impressed than I was by what happened in Berkeley in the fall of
> 1964 and alerted six months later by the reaction of our own stu-
> dents to the announcement of a fee increase. There was something
> about the way they responded to this bad news that should have
> tipped me off and I should not have been lulled by the poor organi-
> zation and short lived enthusiasm of this particular uprising. Nor
> should I have felt that their battle cry which was "Free Education"
> really expressed their discontent – for it ran far deeper and wider
> than such a slogan would suggest – in fact it wasn't "Free" educa-
> tion that they wanted, it was "Better" education or, as the most
> critical of them were to say later on, just "Education" which, they
> felt, they were not getting.[1]

It was only by looking back, which he could do in March 1970, that he had a clearer picture of what had transpired. In 1964 McGill had been on the brink of a revolution, in which, even six years later, they were still deeply involved. Robertson recognized the tactics of the revolutionaries (control of the student press and government; assassination of the character of anyone thought to be standing in the way of their demands; the use of obscenity for shock purposes; the trumping-up of issues; parades, placards, occasional violence) for what they were, although the tactics could not simply be ignored. The objective underlying the tactics was to get power – in order to liberalize the institution, to remove sources of suspicion, to allow the students a wider range of choice than the traditional curriculum permitted, to make courses more relevant, and to make the university more useful to society. To achieve this, it would be necessary for those in a position to do so to reshape the whole governance structure of the university, from the Board of Governors, down through the Senate, to the policy-making bodies of the departments. Places for students would have to be made on all these bodies and all their committees.

There was probably not much doubt that universities needed to change as postwar society evolved and demands on them increased. There were many irresponsible, although not unintelligent, agents of change, particularly among the students. For them, change was low-risk (in some measure because they did not understand the possible consequences), but it was very much high-risk for the institutions. The Marxist techniques of agitation, control of the media, and disruption of process were too new for conservative institutions and those in control to deal with, except by reaction (which was, of course, one of the objectives of the tactics), so they were always on their back foot as they responded. Where control of the university media was in their hands, there was a constant leveraging of the apparent levels of support for the political agenda and a disproportionate impression as to the level of support for the agenda, whether on the campus or elsewhere. Within the institutions, the faculties were often not much more responsible; they simply wanted more control and more money – in the latter case, without accepting any responsibility for raising it. The eventual result was to place in the hands of the teaching staff the effective control of the Senate (the majority of which was composed of elected professors), to give the Senate the right to elect a number of its representatives to the Board of Governors, to place students on the Senate (to the extent of about one-seventh of the body), to place students on practically every committee in which they could reasonably have any interest, and to leave the governance of the departments to be worked out by the departments themselves.

It was a long, bitter, and often ugly process. With the benefit of experiencing several decades of the results, one can almost wonder what the problem really was since it now seems perfectly natural that staff and students should be involved in university governance and that they should behave responsibly in the course of exercising their duties. At the time, however, the process leading to the changes was confrontational, and those advocating for change were often extreme in their demands, strident in their attitude, and objectionable in their conduct. It reminds one of the adage that there are two things that are best not observed while they are being made: sausage and legislation.

GETTING FROM HERE TO THERE

Signs – although by no means the first – of some of the troubles to come with the student newspaper, the *McGill Daily* (already in the control of the activists), appeared on 12 February 1965 with what Robertson referred to as two "outbursts": one "a perfectly foul article describing a speech of the editor of *The Realist* – a filthy New York magazine"; and the other a large advertisement calling for the students to demonstrate in front of the US Consulate in protest against the bombings in Viet Nam. The former had drawn protests from parents and the latter a hail of protests, mainly from American students attending McGill. Robertson called in the *Daily* editors and "bawled them out" and then tried to make peace with the US consul. Although the *Daily* would soon stop publishing for the rest of the academic year, giving him some peace from his worries every time he opened an issue, he constantly wondered (showing how little he understood as to their objectives of confrontation and disruption) what sensible things he could do to cause the publication to be more reasonable. The times were such that the *Daily* fully intended to continue its tactics of trying to provoke the administration in the constant hope that the administration would react, thus providing yet another opportunity to escalate the tensions between it and the students.

A month or so later, on 22 March 1965, there was a student "Day of Protest" that began with a mass rally in the early afternoon to which René Lévesque, then minister of resources in the Quebec Liberal government of Jean Lesage, arrived some forty minutes late. Robertson had little regard for Lévesque, whom he described as a "volatile, unreliable sort of fellow." He was, by reputation, a rabble rouser, but as far as Robertson could tell, he did not succeed in rousing the rabble at all, which seemed to disappoint the students, who then marched down from the campus to Place Ville Marie, where they were addressed by some New Democratic Party faculty members, before returning to stage a sit-in at the Arts Building, filling the corridors. The purpose, they said, was to indicate their earnestness and support of the Board of Governors, and they presented Robertson with a petition containing 5,500 signatures. The Board of Governors, blissfully ignorant of the irony of such enthusiastic "support," met in another building with little concern regarding the sit-in and decided to form a committee to talk with the students. Matters limped along until the end of the academic year, with the near certainty that they would pick up the same confrontational character in the fall.

FROM THE PULPIT

Robertson was invited to deliver an address at St George's Church on Peel Street in Montreal in mid-October 1965, appropriately enough on Medical Sunday.[2] He chose as his topic, no doubt in the context of student and other unrest he was experiencing at McGill, the youth of the country. The address itself was somewhat ponderous but expressed a genuine interest in trying to determine how to respond to some changes that were, on the whole, probably worthwhile. He defined youth as that portion of the population old enough to recognize and to define the issues that confront the world and themselves yet not old enough to have assumed responsibility or to have gained experience. It was an issue, he said, that he could easily perceive from his vantage point as a university principal and one that would have an increasingly direct impact on him in this role and at a personal level as well. The problems he identified were twofold: those that the youths discern in the world and those that they create by their actions to protest against or to correct the faults that they see. He did not think that they exaggerated the importance of the problems they perceived; if there was exaggeration, it lay in their reaction to the problem. The current uprising of youth was probably universal since within the past year everyone had seen one form or another of student revolt in, among others, England, Italy, France, Germany, Japan, Korea, South America, and North America. Nor was the reaction something new, although there was some novelty in the means of protest they had adopted. Important also was the fact that the strongest reactors among the youth were not numerous in proportion to the total youthful population.[3]

As to the cause, he argued that the main cause was loose discipline, starting from poor parenting, loose family ties, and permissiveness. This was, he said, a view he had come to based on his age and particular family background, together with the experience he gained during the war. It was a regrettable fact, he went on, that the very word "discipline," which in their minds was the antithesis of freedom, evoked, like the word "establishment," complete disdain among the militant youths of today. The ability to administer discipline was rapidly declining not only in public institutions such as schools and universities but also in the home. The lack of discipline led to considerable freedom of action on the part of youth, and this freedom, unimpeded by responsibility, gave rise at times to alarming results. Add to this, he said, the impersonality of the whole social structure, heap upon this the patent dishonesty, both intellectual and moral, that is to be seen on all sides in politics and the markets, accentuate the whole by the extraordinary new means of communication that were now available, and cap it all with the normal lust for gossip, excitement, and the public eye, and one could identify most of the factors that were involved.

He then turned to some of the forms that the reactions took. "Eccentric dress and total disregard for the proper attentions of the barber," he said, were interesting phenomena, usually taken to be characteristic of protest. Indeed they were, but they were of relatively little importance in the overall picture, and surprisingly enough, in most instances these eccentricities were not displayed by the prototype of the student leaders. During the past fifteen years or so there had been three main forms of reaction, the first of which could be described as withdrawal, a traditional form of resenting society that became particularly popular in the early 1950s when groups, with the works of Rousseau, Jefferson, and Thoreau tucked in their knapsacks, would escape from it all to lament and to sneer from the sidelines. This was the "beat generation." In the mid-1950s, however, there had emerged a new generation whose alienation took new forms, which were active as distinct from the passive grumblings of their beat predecessors. Youth became, as they put it, "committed." Nonviolent for the most part, they tried to assert themselves in the great issues of the day – human rights, peace, free speech, and others – using mass action as the technique. These activists could be divided into two groups, one as rebellious as the other. The smaller group had decided that the structure of society must be broken. Like the escapists, they were romantics at heart and would not come to terms with the real world. They would rather destroy it. The other group, with a much more sophisticated solution, did not attack the structure itself but believed that the levers that operate it were in the wrong hands and should be replaced so that politics would be managed by the citizen, industry by the worker, and universities by the student.

He went on to ask whether these reactions were irrational. Certainly, the out-and-out radical youth – the type that withdraws into his own beard and blue jeans – was ridiculous. There is a ridiculous fringe on nearly every human activity. But the central core of reacting youth, he believed, was basically sound, at least (speaking in medical terms) in its diagnosis of the world's ills, if not in its proposed therapy. If the only effect of the furore of these days was that adults would be inspired to reappraise their position and to strive for improvement, youth would have served their world well and might, with satisfaction, pass on, eventually, to reach middle age and become criticized in its time. But something more than reappraisal was now demanded and would, he had no doubt, be delivered. Action was called for – and it was needed – and one could be certain that unless in years to come successive waves of youth were to see effective action, they would continue to demonstrate, to sit in, to march – and if these tactics did not work they might adopt more strenuous means to embarrass their lethargic, compromising, selfish elders. There was to be no thought of brushing this matter aside; nor did he think it should be brushed aside. Whatever argument he might have with youth's desire to take over the reins of management, whatever views he might have on the more extraordinary aspects of their behaviour, he believed that they had done well. Their observations on society were valuable, and their insistence on action would produce action that would otherwise not occur. Immediate steps had to do with the humanizing of organizations, large and small. There would have to be a positive effort to bring this about – it is not natural to all people to pay attention to their fellows – but it was important because only when a personal element could be reintroduced into society would reiteration of the basic values of integrity, honour, industry, and loyalty begin to be effective. To the isolated student, such teachings currently had little substance. Even more important was the feeling among many of the youth that there was a lack of personal future for them.

This brought Robertson to his final point, that of long-range plans or prospects, where he acknowledged that he was on far less secure ground, namely the possibility that something useful might emerge from research in the expanding fields of psychology and sociology. Given the changes that had been wrought in the physical welfare of humanity in the last hundred years as a result of research in medicine, agriculture, and engineering, was it too much to hope that the psychologist, the psychiatrist, the sociologist might, by the relatively newly begun research, achieve considerable results in the field of human behaviour? He thought there was some hope that current studies in animals, both human and nonhuman – in which observations on frustration, aggression and its inhibition, the value of sublimation, the causes of tension, and related matters were being recorded – could eventually point the way to some improvement in individual behaviour, to appreciation of values, and above all, to appreciation of the needs of others.

Robertson adapted the same theme to several different audiences over the years, but without significant change, as he wrestled with behavioural issues, particularly with the behaviour of youth. It was a hallmark of Robertson, perhaps derived from his professional training, that he never stopped at the symptom but always looked behind it for the cause in order to get at the root of the problem. Another was that he remained open to change and was genuinely interested in the views expressed by the students, especially once the substance could be extracted from the form and manner in which the views had been expressed. In this respect, despite the heavy personal toll exacted from him in the course of his duties, he was the ideal principal for his time, and McGill fared better under his leadership than the great majority of other universities.

At the end of September 1967, after the Duff-Berdahl Report[4] had been issued and McGill had formed its own committee, which was within a couple of months from issuing its commentary, he addressed students at the McGill Conference on Student Affairs, first doing his best to assure them of his interest in the problems that they identified, especially those pertaining to the system of education and its subject matter, as well as to its improvement, before concluding with a touch of steel:

Well, Ladies and Gentlemen, I have tried to convey to you the very real facts that we – the much maligned "Administration" – are thoroughly interested in your welfare, that we are not content with things as they are; that we have made some constructive changes and that we shall make more. I know it is difficult for some of you to believe that there is no quick cure for our academic ills and I have not asserted that our illness is not so severe as to prevent a very large number of students from acquiring an extremely good education, for to do so would beg the question.

My purpose is simply to indicate a genuine interest in you. If I am less impatient than most of you, if I have not resorted to returning the insults that some of you toss out with reckless abandon, it is because I believe that such tactics can only delay the development of the sort of co-operation between all elements of the University that is necessary if we are to move towards the goal that we all want to achieve.[5]

This sober and balanced analysis generated a mixed reaction. There were students who were spoiling for trouble, some of which erupted in a spectacular manner barely a month later.

THE MCGILL DAILY

In the turbulent times of Robertson's administration, it was not surprising that the student newspaper, the *McGill Daily*, would be critical of the university authorities, often focusing on the principal and the Board of Governors, the more obvious symbols of authority within the university. That the university staff were also pressing for radical changes in academic, as well as university, governance allowed the students to be even farther ahead and more provocative. In common with many other campuses, there was a strong doctrinal component in the student positions, and it proved to be a simple matter for special interest groups to hijack the *Daily* and use it for propagation of their own agenda. This was not popular with the vast majority of the students, but the arrangements for collection of the funds allocated to the paper were tied up with collection of student-related fees by the university and transfer of these fees to the Students' Society. The discontent was sufficient to lead the university to consider the possibility of refusing to collect the fees, but nothing concrete ever came of this. In the result, the *Daily* continued to collect the necessary revenues and to thumb its nose at the administration.

Indeed, its objective seemed to be to find ways to try to provoke the administration into some sort of response that could then be used as the basis for further reaction and protest by the students, who, however little regard they might have had for the editorial content of the *Daily*, were also looking for ways to confront the administration. Robertson had recognized the tactic for some time but was finally goaded into action as a result of the reprint, in the 3 November 1967 issue, of an article from an American publication by the name of *The Realist*. It was an offensive and obscene article purportedly based on the John F. Kennedy assassination and the subsequent conduct of Lyndon B. Johnson,[6] and Robertson, after consultation with senior administrative staff, laid charges against the editors involved, Peter Allnutt, Pierre Fournier, and John Fekete. The charges would be heard by the Senate Committee on Student Discipline. He called the students the following day to advise them of the charges, in the presence of invited members of the Students' Council.

Having informed the students of the charges on 4 November, Robertson addressed the Students' Council on 6 November to advise them formally as to what he had done and why.[7] He reminded them that since the inception of the Students' Society of McGill University, it had been customary for the society to run its own affairs and for the university administration to intervene only when it was judged that the Student's Society, or one of its elements or members, was acting in such a way as to affect adversely the integrity or the proper functioning of the university. With rare exceptions, the students had shown an admirable sense of responsibility, and the university shared in the pride that the Students' Society had felt in its ability to manage its own affairs.

He reminded them that one of the student activities of great importance was the newspaper published by the Students' Society and produced by a group of students appointed by the Students' Council. This newspaper, the *McGill Daily*, had wide circulation within the university itself and a considerable circulation in the surrounding city and elsewhere. While the opinions expressed in this paper were those of the authors of the articles or the editors or contributors and while the university administration played no part in the editing or production of the paper, there was, in the eyes of the members of the university and of the public, an intimate association between the *McGill Daily* and the university. When, therefore, an incident occurred that was of such importance as to appear to have contravened the standards of decency generally accepted in university circles, the university had no other course of action to follow than to intervene. In such situations the administration did not judge the case

but was bound to indicate clearly when it believed that a university judgment was required. This they had done after much consideration in the
case of the recent article that appeared in the *Daily*. Three students had
been charged, and they would appear in due course before the Senate
Committee on Student Discipline. Robertson would make no comment
on the incident nor make any reference to the committee's proceedings.

His reasons for making the statement went beyond the present incident. There had been, as the students knew, for some time a tendency
on the part of the *Daily* to publish occasional articles that he believed
had raised questions in the minds of some student and staff readers of
good taste and sometimes of good judgment. Robertson wished to say at
once that the administration had no wish to censor or to control student
publications and in particular the *Daily* itself. The *Daily* had had a long
and important, if often controversial, role in the life of the university,
and it must always retain its character as an independent student voice
on the campus. This role must and would continue. But the university,
Robertson said, could not stand aside when its own reputation might be
harmed by student behaviour, whether in the *Daily* or in other activities, particularly when there seemed to have been a gross abuse requiring
immediate attention.

Editorial freedom, he continued, did not mean the right to be unaware
of consequences. And if these consequences seemed to bring the university's good name into disrepute, then the authorities must take whatever
action is necessary to see that the university was protected and to bring
any serious breach to the attention of the whole university community.
Robertson said all of this not to threaten the Students' Council or the
Daily or any student or group but only to put the issue clearly and frankly
to them for the better understanding of the present problems and in the
hope that more effective preventative and corrective measures could be
developed by the council itself. He invited their cooperation not merely
to determine better solutions for those issues of student self-government
that arose but also to establish the means whereby the integrity of the
university might always be safe-guarded. He knew he could look to the
Student Council for a determined effort to deal with its own problems
– and the *Daily* was primarily its responsibility. Robertson would make
no recommendation to the council as to how it should act and, at the
moment, would not make any statement as to what steps the administra-

tion might find it necessary to take with respect to the long-range solution of this general problem. He was seeking cooperation and was ready at any time to discuss these matters with the council.

He concluded his statement by emphasizing his own respect for the fullest artistic, literary, and journalistic freedom that was in the classic tradition of the *Daily* and the university as a whole. He did not stand in judgment, as principal, of the literary merits of controversial materials published in the *Daily* or elsewhere. What was objectionable to one generation was often genius to another, and in the present time of changing values, marked by an abundance of means to express these changes, older forms and boundaries were reshaped, and activities crossed over into new areas of boldness and experiment. Indeed, with these evolving standards in mind, he was suggesting to the Senate Committee on Student Discipline that they invite two students as observers to sit with the committee during the enquiry. But in the end, all were bound by certain minimum canons of decency in public discourse, and a regrettable but necessary moment might arrive when they believed those standards had been ignored and when, as a result, a self-respecting university would have to decide and then to act.

It was a case of damned if you do and damned if you don't. On the one hand, the article was clearly obscene and had received wide circulation within and outside the university. McGill was identified with it despite the fact that the university exercised no editorial or other control over the content. On the other hand, the matter provided the much sought after opportunity for the students to protest, and they took every advantage of it, including occupation of the principal's office, teach-ins, and ultimately, break-ins, necessitating that the police be called to the campus. Robertson, addressing the staff, was entirely unapologetic about having called the police. The situation had been out of control. The prime reason for not calling the police on campus, in general, is because they might be seen to interfere with academic freedom. There was nothing academic about breaking down doors and breaking into offices. He had called the staff meeting to explain the events of the past week but was not seeking any approval. The meeting was for informational purposes only.

One semi-amusing moment occurred during the sit-in, in which Robertson's office and the corridor leading to it were occupied by students, when the university solicitor, Peter Laing, arrived for a meeting with

Robertson. Laing had been a forward-observation officer during the war, directing artillery fire. Those on the receiving end of artillery fire know that such observers are nearby and devote considerable energies to locating and removing them. Laing had been badly wounded and lost both legs, but after recovery, he had learned to walk very well with the prostheses provided by the Department of Veterans' Affairs. He surveyed the mass of students sitting in the corridor, announced in his trademark deep barrister's voice that he was going to visit the principal in his office, and stated that although he could not speak to personal experience in the matter, he had been reliably informed that it was extremely painful to be walked on by a man with two wooden legs, whereupon he started forward. This produced a veritable re-enactment of the parting of the Red Sea and unimpeded access to the principal.

FRATERNAL CONSULTATION

For all his personal determination in the matter, Robertson was interested in what his brother Bruce might think and on 13 November wrote to describe the events, enclosing a copy of the *Daily* article. He was enjoying the matter in a way, relishing a fight, and although he was confident that he was right, he was not confident that he could lick the opposition, which consisted of an organization called Students for a Democratic Society (SDS), a branch of the Students' Society but not a popular one and, generally speaking, supported by the Students' Society in this affair. The SDS was, he suspected, a communist-inspired organization with branches in many universities. He had seen the article the afternoon of 3 November, was duly shocked, called together some senior colleagues and the university solicitor, and decided, after discussion, to lay charges against the editor, the editor of the supplement, and the "writer." They all knew at the time that it was a plot designed to drive them to action, but he had felt very strongly that he could not back away from what he regarded as a clear responsibility. He had no reason to hope that the opposition would desist since it was a heaven-sent opportunity, and they proposed to exploit it to the full. The main concern was that they would continue to raise hell and keep the university in a turmoil until people wanted to start giving in – to make some kind of compromise – and this he would not do. His only way out might be to resign in order to relieve the situation. He thought he would let Bruce know about it because he would hate for him to hear of some drastic news in the papers. He said that he was very calm and calculating about the whole thing – no emotion other than "downright outrage" and certainly no regrets about his actions – and that he should not be ashamed to have to resign on an issue of this sort. His only disappointment was that he hadn't been able to bull it through to victory, Although he still thought he might be able to.

Bruce's reply, dated 17 November 1967, was a model of an older brother's advice and legal experience:

In warfare of this kind, two things are particularly important, one that you take a consistent position through the piece and that your position be on sound ground, legally and factually.

1. If the University makes [facilities] available to the students in which all or some of the activities of the Daily are carried on, people are likely to think that the university has some responsibility – as indeed it does morally and perhaps legally also – for the activities of the paper.

2. Apart from the fact that the article is disgusting it is a libel on President Johnson and probably on Mrs. Kennedy.

3. McGill's relations with the U.S. and people in it are of great importance to it both financially and culturally. As to finance there is the help that you got in HARP[8] and the grants you are getting or hope to get from the Ford Foundation. If the university allows its facilities to be used for the publication of stuff like this, its relations with the US and people in it may be jeopardized.

4. To have left the discipline of the students to the Students' Society would have been to shirk the responsibility which you had. I agree that you had to act and that you were right in referring the matter to the Senate Committee. If the article was nothing but a reprint from The Realist, no question of freedom for students to develop creative writing can be raised.

He hoped that Rocke was not letting his personal involvement affect his judgment too strongly. It was as principal of the university and in what he considered (rightly, Bruce was sure) to be its interests that he had done what he did, and he should continue with the same interests in mind. It was most unlikely that any precipitate action on his part in resigning would advance McGill's interests:

> You must try to make time your ally and not let it bring about your downfall. You expect that the students will delay matters by taking the affair to the courts. Well, let them! If your legal position is sound, you will win out there. If it is not, the sooner you find it out the better. Your purpose is not to get the guilty students suspended or expelled as fast as possible, but rather to establish the principle that there must be decency and responsibility in the publication of The Daily with the help, and bearing the name, of McGill. It may take a long time to do this. In the meantime your position will be maintained and eventually, I hope, will be established, and other people may grow even sicker than you of the whole affair.
>
> I can imagine how you are loathing the whole affair and how anxious you are to bring it to a conclusion and be rid of it. Undue haste to this end may warp your judgment and result in the cutting of corners which you will eventually find you should not have cut. Much as it is against your inclination, I would rather see your administration's policy and its image that of an authority implacably determined to see that, no matter how long it may take, those responsible for harming the university are properly dealt with by due process of law (meaning university law as well as provincial law) than that of a body bent on wreaking vengeance with all possible speed.
>
> Some or all of the things that I have said may appear to you, in the midst of things and knowing so much more, to be utterly idiotic. Still, I hope that you may find a few good grains among the chaff.
>
> I am so sorry that you have become involved in this as you have, but I do not see how you could either have ignored the article or have passed the buck to the students, who, as you point out, could not have acted as effectively as the circumstances may warrant. If there is any more information than what will appear in your dia-

ries that you care to pass on to me, I'll be most grateful to receive it. Any help I can give in the meantime is, of course, yours for the asking.[9]

SENATE COMMITTEE ON STUDENT DISCIPLINE

The original charge of publishing an obscene libel[10] had been dropped and replaced on 7 November with one that read: "Participating in the publication on campus of an article which contravenes standards of decency acceptable by and in this University: namely, an article in the column entitled 'Boll Weevils' appearing on page 4 of the supplement entitled 'Flux' of the McGill daily of November 3rd, 1967, the whole incompatible with your status as a student of this University." There was some initial difficulty in getting the Senate Committee together, which met for the first time on 13 November and agreed to a request by the parties that separate hearings be conducted for Fekete, on the one hand, and for Allnutt and Fournier, on the other. Fekete was already represented by a lawyer, Claude Armand Sheppard, who was armed with a plethora of motions attacking the jurisdiction of the committee, asking the committee to recuse itself, and requesting a public hearing, all of which were heard and rejected. The Allnutt and Fournier cases were disposed of by the committee on 24 January 1968 with formal reprimands. Assisted by his lawyer, the Fekete matter naturally dragged on longer. Having rejected the motions presented on 13 November, the committee offered the arrangements for closed-circuit television that had been offered to Allnutt and Fournier, an offer refused by Sheppard, who was advised that unless his client changed his mind, the next meeting of the committee would be held in private on 21 November.

This led Fekete to institute proceedings in the Quebec Superior Court (asking the court to review the record of the proceedings of the committee), which meant that the committee was unable to proceed with the case until the court proceedings were completed. The action was, not unsurprisingly, dismissed by the Superior Court. Unsatisfied with this judgment, Fekete appealed to the Quebec Court of Appeal, which dismissed the appeal on 2 February 1968.[11] On 7 February, apparently unembarrassed by the outcome of the court proceedings, Sheppard requested closed-circuit television for the first time, something that he had refused when initially offered and that he had strongly opposed before the Superior Court and Court of Appeal. The committee rejected the request. Sheppard then indicated that his client would not participate in the hearing, and after being warned that withdrawal would result in immediate administrative suspension, Fekete withdrew. The suspension was imposed immediately.

Three days later, after representations had been made by the Students' Council, the committee reaffirmed its position that Fekete had waived any right that he may have had to a televised hearing but, because of the request and in view of the widespread student interest, agreed to a televised hearing. Fekete was advised that the suspension would be lifted as soon as he provided an undertaking that he would appear before the committee and testify, which was provided on 16 February. Eventually, on 29 February, the hearing took place, not without another barrage of motions and objections. A letter from Robertson to the chairman of the committee dated 19 February, drawing attention to yet another "Boll Weevils" column, did not, ruled the committee, constitute the laying of a new charge. Sheppard made more motions requesting that the committee decline jurisdiction, that its members recuse themselves, that a public hearing be granted in place of a televised hearing, and that the charge be dismissed as unfounded on its face. All the requests, at least three of which had already been dealt with prior to the court proceedings, were denied, and the hearing got under way. The only evidence was given by Fekete, and Sheppard did not call any other witnesses. The basic facts, of course, were not much in dispute.

Fekete admitted that he had taken the initiative in publishing the article, that he had anticipated that it would produce a shock effect on the campus, and that he had indeed intended that it should have such an effect.[12] He also acknowledged that he had made the deletions from the original article, which had appeared in *The Realist* in May 1967. Although he attempted to justify the publication on several grounds, he also admitted that he had been warned by the editor of *The Realist* that publication might lead him into conflict with others on the campus. Fekete recognized that both the editor of the supplement and the editor of the *Daily* had the authority to veto the publication, but he accepted responsibility for it. The committee concluded that Fekete's responsibility was, by his own admission, just as great as that of Allnutt and Fournier and, for the reasons given in disposing of their cases, decided that the publication contravened the standards of decency by and in the university. He was

given, as had been given to the other two, the penalty of formal repri-
mand. In the circumstances, it was not much of a sanction, but at least
the point of principle had been established, precisely the essential point
that had been identified by Robertson's brother Bruce. The students who
had occupied the principal's office were charged for the disruption and
were equally gently sentenced to conduct probation by the same Senate
Committee.

Ten years after his eventual retirement, Robertson would address the
James McGill Society, looking back on the stressful days of student unrest.[13] He recalled the two-day occupation of his office by students who
were protesting the measures proposed for dealing with the Fekete situation. The students were eventually removed, one at a time, by the police.
They remained, apparently pursuant to some strategy they had devised,
completely limp while being carried from the office by the police, but
the moment they were outside the building, they began writhing and
screaming, undoubtedly to try to attract television and media attention
and to claim police "brutality." There had been none, but the Marquis of
Queensbury rules did not apply to student politics of the day.

THE TEACHING STAFF

The first formal step toward academic staff involvement in the governance of matters within the university had come in 1923 when the Senate
was formed.[14] In more recent, postwar years and especially in the Viet
Nam era, there had been a marked change of attitude, with staff and students wanting substantially increased participation, occasionally bordering on a desire for complete control. A committee of the McGill Association of University Teachers (MAUT), chaired by Maxwell Cohen of the
Faculty of Law, urged that teaching staff should have more say. This led
to an invitation to the staff to select some members of the Senate, but by
1962 it was clear that further changes would have to be made. McGill had
joined with other universities and the Canadian Association of University Teachers (CAUT) to set up the Duff-Berdahl Commission, which had
reported in March 1966, following which McGill had set up its own committee of representatives of the Board of Governors and Senate to study
the report and to suggest how McGill's governance should be changed.
This internal report was completed by November 1967, and after discussions with staff associations and students, amendments were ratified

in the summer of 1968, to come into effect at the start of the new academic year.

The initial changes included several provisions: an absolute majority of the Senate was to consist of elected members of the teaching staff; there was to be student representation on the Senate (eight out of sixty-two); five members elected by the Senate would sit on the Board of Governors; students would be added to practically all committees of the Senate; and a membership committee of the Board of Governors would be created with equal numbers of representatives from the Senate and Board of Governors.[15] These changes, revolutionary in their time, were designed to place academic control of the university with the teaching staff rather than with the Board of Governors, to provide student representation in the upper echelons of the university governance, to create better liaison between the Senate and Board of Governors, and to ensure a more "representative" Board of Governors.

As principal, Robertson had essentially three major issues with the teaching staff. The first was to ensure that they were adequately paid, the second that the ratio of teachers to students be improved, and the third that the level of teaching be commensurate with what the standards required and the students demanded. The 1960s were years of massive expansion of universities, and there was widespread competition for talented staff, who were, not unrealistically, anxious to earn as much as they could. For McGill, this meant there was a much bigger potential to lose or to fail to attract staff, who had the entire continent and beyond as potential employment opportunities. It also had to compete within Quebec to ensure that its salaries matched as closely as possible the salaries at Laval and the Université de Montréal, not always a matter that could be determined with accuracy because of differing conditions of employment and a general lack of transparency that would allow such comparisons to be easily made, including differences in methods of reporting, variations between what was reported and what was actually done, problems in determining the significance of averages, medians, and minima, differences in promotion policies, and differences in fringe benefits. All the professorial staffs at the other universities were unionized and militant. McGill was and remains the only university in Quebec that has only a staff association, the MAUT, and that does not have "collective bargaining," as this term is understood in unionized proceedings. This is not to say that there were no tensions between the administration and the professoriate, but salary and other matters pertaining to conditions of employment have traditionally been less confrontational and divisive at McGill than within its sister institutions.

In his regular meetings with the teaching staff, Robertson was at constant pains to assure them of the efforts being made on their behalf and of the priority that he attached to their equitable treatment. A significant portion of every budgetary increase was allocated to salary increases for the academic staff. This was a particularly difficult issue due to the refusal of the Quebec government to provide McGill with sufficient funding, driving it into continual deficits that would eventually force the university to expend its unrestricted endowments, a penalty it suffered for having had the initiative not to have relied solely upon government financing.[16] Despite the fact that McGill had always been blessed with loyal staff, both academic and nonacademic, who understood the pressures on the budget, the negotiations, from time to time, were frustrating to Robertson, who wanted to do his best for them but whose hands were tied by the financial strictures. One example was recorded in his diary entry for 20 April 1967, where he regretted that McGill's teaching staff should act exactly like a trade union, demanding to reopen concluded negotiations since they felt they were not catching up with the Université de Montréal fast enough. Robertson said that he would reopen the negotiations the following month, without commitment and, equally, without prejudice.[17]

Teaching and teaching methods were perhaps even more complex problems to be resolved. The magisterial method of the lecture by a professor, who was in a position of complete superiority to a class, whose duty was to write down whatever the professor said and be able to regurgitate it come examination time, was about to go the way of the dodo bird. Frank Scott was known to have described the lecture process as an exercise by which the notes of the lecturer were transferred from the notebook of the lecturer to the notebooks of the students without passing through the minds of either. The students made it clear that this pedagogical approach was no longer acceptable and that teaching had to improve. The early activist descriptions of university teaching were undoubtedly exaggerated and their blanket indictments of goals, teaching methods, professors, and curricula wild overstatements, but knowingly so, in order to get attention and to cause people to think. They served their purpose, with the result that those responsible began thinking, acting, and experimenting. Recalling a discussion of curriculum at a Tripartite Committee meeting on 28 June 1968, Robertson noted in his diary that the students were thoroughly unhappy about the teaching and apparently genuinely so. He thought that the chief fault lay with the professors, who were not intent enough, as a group, on teaching. He speculated that perhaps a good number of them were not competent to meet the students' great expectations and that some of the better ones were, he suspected, too busy with "other things." He could only suspect the latter because he could not find out without "raising an awful fuss" since to approach professors to obtain information as to how they spent their time would be positioned as an encroachment on, or at least a threat to, academic freedom. He resolved to think about the issue over the summer. The issues were "hot," and something would have to be done about them. The status quo was not acceptable, and the potential for direct action by students was a genuine risk.

The 1968 fall term started uneasily. On 19 November, James Ferrabee wrote an article in the *Montreal Gazette* pointing out that none of the threats of violence on the part of students had been fulfilled, suggesting student activists were getting tired of it. Nothing could have been more a proverbial red flag to the bull, with the result that the same afternoon some thirty students entered the Arts Council room during a faculty meeting and refused to leave. Matters of importance were being discussed, they stated, and they felt they should be permitted to hear what was being said. The faculty discussed the problem for a few minutes, then moved that the meeting adjourn, the decision carrying by 64 votes to 49, and it ended peacefully. There seemed to have been no particular rancour involved. Robertson thought that the faculty should have decided, one way or the other, whether the meeting was open or not. If it was an open meeting, that would have been fine, but if not, then there should have been a more united position on the episode. The same day, Robertson was advised that students in the School of Architecture were on strike regarding one of the professors and would not go back until he was gone. They had spoken to the director of the school some time ago, but nothing had been done about it. They had also spoken to the dean of engineering, who was now retired, but he had done nothing about it. They were now complaining to the new dean, George L. D'Ombrain, who reported to Robertson a day or so later that the matter had been settled.

Some of the steps taken to respond to the students included adjusting the curricula, setting up a centre for instructional communications (which provided an extensive range of teaching devices that were widely used, including television, taped lectures, films, slides, and other teaching aids), and experimenting with various types of approaches to courses, such as offering students a choice of ways to take a course – by seminar, by student group, or solo. They put on full-length courses in which students could choose (within certain wide fields) what they wanted to study and how they wanted to go about it – completely unstructured courses. The university added courses in which early undergraduate students could devote their full time to research projects. They encouraged law and medical students to work as undergraduates in clinics established in the city in order to add to their educational experience. Privately, Robertson was not convinced that some of the "new" methods were necessarily improvements over the traditional methods but was realistic enough to recognize that they needed to be tried and that, in time, there might be a return to earlier approaches.

THE STANLEY GRAY AFFAIR

In a university there is a remarkable degree of autonomy and independence among members of the teaching staff. The role of the university is to encourage new ideas, to challenge the established order and thinking, and to provide an environment in which students and faculty are free to express whatever they believe to be a defensible perspective on what has gone before or what may come to pass. It is an extraordinary environment, one that attracts exceptional scholars and exceptional students. Many of the quantum leaps in knowledge and the paradigm shifts in social evolution can be traced to universities. The concept of tenure, that no one can be discharged from an academic university position just because of the eccentricity or unpopularity of his or her ideas, is a fundamental tenet of the university community. If there is a professor who insists that the world is flat, this cannot be the basis for terminating the employment relationship. If a professor embraces Marxist principles, to the exclusion of all others, this is a matter of academic freedom, and the long-term test will be whether students (or colleagues) have any interest in the teachings of the professor. Students can be, to some extent, "consumers" of education and can vote, like other consumers, with their feet. Colleagues, who have their own ideas, are seldom restrained in expressing their critical judgments on other academics. The unkindest cut of all is to be judged as unscholarly or, worse, irrelevant.

McGill in the 1960s was not immune to the flavour of the month, particularly in the field of political science. It sought out and hired its share of the fashionable Marxist scholars. It is not the purpose of this work to express an opinion as to the quality of their academic work. Indeed, it is fairly arguable that students should have been exposed to such views, especially in the time of the Cold War, when political and other choices had to be made in the context of East and West. Students played an important role in the hiring of many such academic staff, including, at the time, Pauline Vaillancourt, a professor of political science out of the University of California (Berkeley), and Marlene Dixon, a doctorate in sociology from the University of California (Los Angeles) who was hired, after having been dismissed by the University of Chicago, because the Department of Sociology was worried that students might strike. Dixon taught the first women's studies course at McGill. There was some effort to deny their reappointments, perhaps because of their involvement in radical activities and even because of their Marxist views.[18]

Stanley Gray

The most notorious faculty member, however, was a lecturer in the Department of Economics and Political Science. Stanley Gray was a self-described "shit disturber." Few would disagree that he got the description at least half right. Armed with a degree from McGill and a bachelor of philosophy from Oxford, the omniscience of youth, and a serious "attitude" with regard to authority, he was embraced by the department and given a teaching position in 1967. There does not seem to have been much concern regarding the quality of his teaching, and he was, apparently, well regarded within the department. He taught the fashionable Marxism of the day.

It was not his classroom activity that led to a confrontation with the administration but his interference with the business of the university. There were three occasions in particular: attempting to disrupt a meeting of the Senate Nominating Committee on 24 January 1969, disrupting a meeting of the Board of Governors on 27 January, and disrupting a meeting of the Senate on 5 February. During the first meeting, Gray had led students into the meeting room and later into the principal's office and refused to leave despite a specific request from Robertson that he do so. They came back a second time, Gray remaining at the back of the group. They came back a third time and occupied the principal's office, interrupting the meeting of the committee in the adjoining room. The committee, obviously feeling the pressure, voted to recommend opening up its meetings, but the Senate later rejected the request. The next action was forcible entry into the meeting room (including overpowering security guards) and disruption of a meeting of the Board of Governors by about a hundred and fifty students, led by Gray in a disorderly and noisy demonstration that prevented the transaction of the meeting's business. There was no doubt as to their refusal to leave the meeting room when required to do so by both the chancellor and the principal, acting in the exercise of their duties. Robertson had got up from his chair, walked over to the crowd of students, stood in front of Gray, and advised him and the group that this was a serious matter and that they should withdraw. The crowd refused and shouted back that the governors' behaviour was incorrect and disgusting. Robertson ordered the group to leave and to terminate its demonstration. Gray replied, "We will terminate you." The chanting continued, and various students and Gray exchanged insults with various governors. The chancellor declared the meeting terminated, and the governors left amid further chants from the crowd. There was a similar disruption of the Senate meeting a few days later, in which Gray was also involved, although the degree of his involvement was less clear than on the other occasions.

This culminated in a decision by the university administration to fire him, a confrontation that must have been a dream come true for Gray and his activist followers.[19] It provided an opportunity, not seen since the Fekete and *McGill Daily* matter a year or so earlier, for disruption, protest, and vilification of the university administration. The firing of a university teacher, even one as junior as Gray, is unusual and potentially complicated. The academic concept of tenure, given the intellectual freedom that it protects, is one of the basic tenets of academe, jealously and vigorously protected by all academics, even though Gray, as a very junior lecturer, did not yet have the protection of academic tenure. For the most part, universities themselves are active supporters of the concept as well, even while recognizing that it can, on occasions, be abused and be transmogrified into a form of job security that is unrelated to academic freedom, becoming merely a sinecure, regardless of the degree of effort produced by the academic staff member. The Canadian Association of University Teachers had developed a policy statement providing for a process of independent arbitration, should a dismissed faculty member wish to have access to it. In its letter to Gray dated 18 February 1969 recommending that he be dismissed for having willfully impeded the business of the university on three occasions, the university invited Gray to submit the question to arbitration under the CAUT policy, an offer left open until 25 February. Gray immediately wrote to the university Senate, care of Robertson, to protest against Robertson's recommendation of dismissal and the institution of the CAUT-type proceedings.

Gray had his supporters in the Senate and among the faculty, but Robertson was ready to defend his decision. He refused to discuss the details but spoke generally of disruption and the use of forceful tactics in the university. There had been a special meeting of the Senate on 1 February, at which Robertson had presented clear evidence of organized efforts to disturb the orderly process of business – indeed, to disrupt the normal workings of the university.[20] He had outlined the disruptions and reminded the Senate of its own statement the previous September that "regardless of sincerity no individual or group of individuals has the right to disrupt or to interfere unreasonably with the workings of any part of the university." At the same time he had assured the Senate that if the use of force and disruptive tactics were not settled, there might be no opportunity to debate other issues and that even if there were debates, the shadow of force would influence every opinion. Nothing in the debate then nor in what had happened since had given him any reason to change his view of the urgency of the issue – quite the reverse, for there had been another disruption since then, in the same room during a Senate meeting, and there were other signs to suggest more to come.

> Thus, when it is suggested to me by such bodies as the Students'
> Council of this university, by the Political Science section of our
> Department of Economics and Political Science, by a portion of the
> Tripartite Commission and by a Syndicate of Professors of another
> university that I should take no action, indeed that I should retract
> what I have already done, I have to wonder how aware these groups
> are of the facts of the situation and how great their concern is for

the welfare of this university. And I have to reject their advice. In doing this I am encouraged by the expressions of support from a great many members of the staff and by the action of several thousand students who have signed a petition addressed to their Students' Council urging it to resolve to move to outlaw students' attempts to bypass existing constitutional channels.

There is a large part of the university that is alert to the significance of these disruptions and a time must come when everybody realizes what will happen if power tactics of this sort continue. Of all the signs that point to the firm intentions of these disrupters to keep on disrupting until they get their way I would choose one and I select it because it appeared in Senate at that special meeting on the first of February. One of the student Senators speaking on the subject of the prevention of disruptions said, in effect, "It's simple, all you have to do is agree to our demands!" He didn't say this jokingly – he meant it. It was a highly significant statement and I predict that if this sort of thing continues we'll eventually reach a point where we shall have no alternative but to agree to the demands of any group that is determined to get something done. Can there be any doubt in any reasonable person's mind that we should call a halt to it now?

A disciplinary action, as has been taken, is one thing – in my view an absolutely necessary step – but much more important is the opinion of the mass of members of the university. The only thing that will put a full stop to tactics of force will be the massive disapproval of the vast majority and this I believe is developing. Anyone who makes a move to check these 'mini-fascists' as they were dubbed in today's Daily, can expect a reaction that will follow a clearly defined pattern including: character assassination, rumours, falsehoods, protestations of outraged virtue, threats and, above all, diversionary tactics – tactics that divert the mind from the simple question, "should we allow people to force their will on others?" I was expecting all these – and I've already had a large dose of each of them – but I won't be distracted from pursuing a course which I believe must be followed.

I intend to pursue it – I'm quite conscious of the risks involved in proceeding – but I'm equally aware of the risks of letting things go in the hope that they will somehow or other right themselves,

and I think the latter risk is by far the greater. If Senate, the Board
of Governors, the bulk of the staff and the bulk of the students
show themselves willing to take a firm stand on this general issue
we have nothing to fear – and I propose to do everything I can to
persuade them to take this stand.

It took lengthy negotiations between Robertson and Gray before Gray
would agree to proceed using the CAUT process. For one thing, he insisted that a majority of the three-person panel must be French-speaking,
which reflected bad judgment on his part that such members, simply
because they were French, would support him in his position and was
insulting to their intellectual independence. Robertson got permission
from the Senate and Board of Governors to support these negotiations,
and on 20 February an agreement to arbitrate was signed and was later
confirmed on 26 March by a submission to arbitrate. The chair of the
panel was Walter Tarnopolsky, dean of law at the University of Windsor,
and the other two members were from the Université de Montréal, Noel
Mailloux, professor of psychology, and André Morel, professor of law.

The matter dragged on until July. In his diary entry for 11 July Robertson noted that it was a black, humid, and threatening day, which he
hoped was not prophetic for the last day of the Gray case. Gray continued
his argument all morning, speaking for three hours, not an extraordinary performance for him, as Robertson noted, but it would have been
for everyone else.

On and on he went saying the same things in a dozen different ways. He has considerable cleverness of a sort – he's quick to
spot weak points in his opponents' arguments and to exploit his
discovery to the full and he disguises his real nature very well and,
to hear him for a short time, one would be hard put to believe that
he was anything other than an earnest social reformer. He's that all
right, but he's also ... ready to use any means, destroy any person
or anything in order to achieve his goal which, although he claims
it to be "a better world" goes little beyond self-glorification – he is
very vain – that trait keeps cropping up and is amusing to observe,
and God knows during the past few months I've had plenty of
opportunity to watch him in action. One of his gambits that I enjoy
– in an acidic sort of way – is his insistence on the democratic prin-

ciple in the university. It is pretty clear that his only reason for supporting this view is that he believes that he, or his like, can sway
or manipulate enough voters to support him on his views. If he
couldn't do this, or thought that he couldn't, he'd be dead against
the principle.

The court will now retire to consider. The chairman (Tarnopolsky) said that he hopes to have the report out by the end of the
first week in August. I find it hard to believe that this group of
three can find any other decision than that Gray should be fired
– if they do, I shall have to confess that my sense of values is very
different from theirs. Whichever way they go will have an important effect. If they excuse Gray the stage will be set for mayhem –
it will be very hard to put anyone out of a university in Canada
– even harder than it is now.

Should they recommend his dismissal, the general situation will
be less affected I think – there will certainly not follow a wave of
suppression. But the hands of the administration will not be weakened as they otherwise would be – and this is important.

It would be a masterpiece of understatement to say that Robertson had
the slightest respect for Gray.

Judgment Day

To make a long, noisy, and expensive story as short as possible, the panel
ultimately concluded that McGill was within its rights to dismiss Gray,
whose actions were unjustified disruptions of the business of the university. It took the panel some thirty-nine legal-size pages to reach its conclusions.[21] In many respects, like cases decided in the ordinary courts
during times of war, the reasoning of the panel, in the social and academic
context of 1969, was somewhat suspect. These were, after all, university
professors deciding on the conduct of a fellow academic (no matter how
junior he was and how objectionable his conduct may have been) during
a time of unrest and significant change in the entire university community, not just in Canada. They were clearly looking over their own shoulders to make certain that they could not, as academics, be perceived as
favouring any university administration. The arbitral award was filled
with sidebar journeys of speculation on points that had not been argued,

the nature of universities, possible retroactive legitimization of currently illegal acts, and the requirement of institutions to respond to demands for change. It fell decidedly short of a model of rigorous legal analysis.

On the other hand, despite its many detours and stretches of fuzzy logic, the panel had managed to get to the proper final outcome on the main issue of whether Gray should be dismissed. The conduct that Gray had organized and in which he had participated as a leader could easily have resulted in the laying of criminal charges, but the university had not fallen into this political trap. There was no doubt, however, that the conduct of Gray and his supporters had been intended to threaten and to coerce, first, the Senate Nominating Committee, then the Board of Governors, and finally, the Senate, all constitutionally established bodies for the carrying on of the university's activities. Gray had eschewed the regular means of expressing critical views of the university and its governance as being too conservative for his taste. Resort to so-called direct action was not justified on any of the grounds raised by Gray, who also argued that direct action could be resorted to as a first step unless the university discussed the issues faced by it and was either democratically constituted or met the needs of its constituents. His demands were for greater representivity in the university's governing bodies, open meetings, student housing, abolition of the Faculty of Management, removal of certain individuals from the Board of Governors, and a new initiative, not yet fully defined, known as "McGill Français."

The panel observed that progress on such issues within McGill had been no slower nor less fundamental than at other universities and that some measures had, indeed, preceded those made in other universities, so there was no justification for direct action going beyond speech. Demands for open meetings had not come from the community at large but mainly from within the academic community, and McGill's Board of Governors was the first in Canada to hold such a meeting (ironically, the very one that Gray and his followers had disrupted) and its Senate was one of the first to do so. The meeting of the Senate Nominating Committee had been the first of a new committee, and there was no evidence of any intransigence that would justify, as a first step, an action clearly intended to be physically coercive. Student housing was on the agenda of the disrupted Board of Governors meeting, and there was evidence of conscientious and expeditious efforts to solve the problem. It was unlikely that the university would accede to the demand to abolish the

Faculty of Management, to be used as a site for co-op student housing or a "socialist" faculty of management (whatever that might be). There was no evidence that any democratic majority wanted this, whether from within the faculty or Quebec society. As to removal of governors and McGill Français, even Gray acknowledged that a majority within McGill was opposed to the concept, despite its having just been formulated, and there was no evidence that any majority wanted to remove any governor. Among the hundred and fifty students associated with Gray, there was no strong feeling on either of the last two issues, which had not been included in the jointly prepared list of demands.

The panel concluded that the demands presented, the evidence of the amount of support for them among students, faculty, and the "people of Quebec," and the nature of the response to them by the decision-making bodies at McGill did not justify the type of direct action resorted to at the time. The events of 24 and 27 January, particularly as they involved a faculty member, were not justifiable. There were fundamental distinctions between the responsibilities of a faculty member and those of a student. More than in the case of a student, a faculty member must show that the times and circumstances were such that rational persuasion was ineffective and, therefore, that violent and direct action had to be resorted to. Almost from the time he started teaching at McGill, Gray had worked his way into leadership roles within student groups to prosecute policies of confrontation through them. There was no evidence of any restriction on him to express his views and to advocate for his programs. He had rejected his own association, the McGill Association of University Teachers (MAUT), as too conservative for him. The panel concluded that this was arrogant and unacceptable.

Disposing of the case, the panel decided that Gray had impeded the business of the university, adversely affecting its wellbeing because the manner and the circumstances in which he had acted constituted gross misconduct. There had been no waiver on the part of McGill. The repeated warnings to Gray had no dissuading effect whatsoever, and Gray's statements at the hearing had made it clear that no future admonitions would dissuade him from the course of action he adopted. There could be no doubt that he had deliberately ignored statements made by persons in the exercise of their authority, and he had asserted at the hearing that he would decide for himself whether their statements, requests, and orders were worthy of consideration.

Although the panel acknowledged that McGill had been scrupulous in following the CAUT Code, it felt that the Code should require the principal and/or dean to discuss cases such as these with the head of the department concerned prior to the first formal meeting with the faculty member, a meeting required under the Code. This may have been a perfectly sensible recommendation for CAUT to consider for future occasions, but the panel then continued with the unwarranted conclusion (having already acknowledged that no such step was contemplated in the Code) that it was incumbent upon the principal

> not to be satisfied merely with public warnings given in the heat of action. We feel a Principal owes enough respect to a faculty member to discuss their differences in private and thus to emphasize the seriousness of the course of conduct adopted by the faculty member. The Principal should have called Mr. Gray into his office at some time prior to February 11th. Although we cannot conclude that this would have deterred Mr. Gray from the course of action he chose, and which he does not repudiate, in other instances this might prevent a situation as serious as the present one from developing.

The panel was obviously playing to some off-stage audience with such an extraordinary statement, which only further underlined its often dubious reasoning, but it did at least pull the legal trigger on the principal matter before it and conclude that there was sufficient ground for disciplinary action. It would have been naive, in view of Gray's declared intention to go on, for the panel to conclude that he could be persuaded that his course of conduct was unacceptable and that he should instead resort to his powers of intellect and expression to achieve his aims. The panel concluded, "reluctantly," that there was sufficient ground for Gray's dismissal.

The important point was won. Gray was gone and Robertson felt that he had sufficient basis to continue as principal. He had been concerned that, had the University been unsuccessful in its litigation with Gray, he would have been forced to resign since he would be perceived to have had no moral authority to continue in office. His biggest concern had been that the entire senior administration might follow suit, and he had spent some considerable effort to persuade them that the only possible resignation should be his own. This was a far more serious issue than his worry that he should resign over the Fekete matter (which was, when all was said and done, little more than the antics of a wilful child smearing symbolic feces on the wall), and even though by this time he had already determined that he would retire before the normal retirement age, it could have had a material adverse impact on his ability to run the university.

In a letter to his brother Bruce on 16 September, Robertson wrote that Bruce's views on the judgment coincided with his own. Robertson had read it only once, under strained circumstances, when the judgment had been delivered by hand by one of the arbitrators. He had been with Peter Laing and James Hugessen at the time, and they had set the judgment up on a lectern to read together. Like good lawyers, Laing and Hugessen had first turned to the last page to see that dismissal had been ordered and only once they knew the result started at page one. Robertson said that, had he not known the outcome, he would have been dismayed by the reasoning and opinions expressed by the panel and assumed that the matter was going to be decided in Gray's favour. Knowing the bottom line, he shrugged his shoulders and had never again looked at the decision.

> Several things disturbed me – the most important was the point
> which you raised, viz. their suggestion that if a university does
> not respond rapidly to popular demand it would expose itself to
> disruption by those whose demands had not been met and that
> these disruptions would be justifiable. As you said if that were to
> be taken as "precedent" by future courts, universities would simply
> have to move with the breeze no matter how unsavoury it might be
> and chaos would result. The other annoying part was that which
> had to do with my warning Gray – the court felt that I should
> have had the courtesy to warn him privately that if he continued
> to behave as he had been behaving, I would have to move for his
> dismissal. I had pointed out in the proceedings that (a) the Senate
> had published a statement and the Board had approved it to the
> effect that anyone interfering with the functioning of the university
> would be subject to disciplinary action and (b) that on both of the
> first two occasions (Nominating Committee and Board of Gov-

ernors meeting) I had pointed out to the mob – of which on both
occasions Gray was clearly the leader – that it *was* interfering with
a university function and that if it did not disperse serious action
might be taken.

The timing was interesting. The Nom. Committee meeting was
a Friday afternoon. Following that, during the weekend, I debated
with myself as to whether or not I should act – whether, indeed,
I should call Gray in and warn (or threaten – as he undoubtedly would have put it) him. I was still thinking it over when on
Monday he led his noble band in to the Governors meeting and I
decided then that I would lay charges. It took a good many days
of work with the lawyers to frame the charges, to get authority
from the Board to sign a contract with Gray to submit the case
to arbitration along the lines of the CAUT procedures (which, I
was convinced, was the only way of arriving at an unchallenge-
able decision. The Board of Governors have the power under
our statutes to fire a member of the staff, but I think that had we
brought Gray before it and had it dismissed him we would have
been submerged and, eventually, drowned by charges of "Kangaroo
Court" – "Star Chamber" etc.) While we were still working on this
Gray invaded the Senate a week later – this was a sort of encore and
we simply added it to the charges we had already prepared. Thus
I had little opportunity to "warn" him before he had committed
the crime a second time, after which time the decision to charge
him was immediately made. Perhaps not an important point to
anyone but me – though other presidents may feel constrained
by the Board's reasoning to warn when otherwise they would act
more positively. I do not feel that I should criticize this judgment
publicly, much as I would like to, but I may have some things to say
about the procedures in general which are much too cumbersome,
time consuming and expensive (about $60,000 in this case!).[22] I
think that a university should make its own decisions by establishing its own court made up of members of the faculty, but it's a long
story and it's going to take months of argument to put across such
an idea. If we get into another jam in this year, we'll have to resort
to this same procedure because we certainly can't set up our own
court once a crime here has been committed.[23]

THE SMOKE BEGINS TO CLEAR

Writing for the 1970 volume of *Old McGill*, Robertson summarized the progress that had been made across the broad range of university issues, at the level of students, staff, teaching, and university governance, the latter being regularly monitored by a joint committee of the Senate and the Board of Governors, which would undoubtedly recommend further changes as technicalities were addressed and as those involved learned how to operate a Senate that was twice as big as its predecessors and made up of a much wider range of people. On the whole, however, he thought that the sudden change from one form of government to another had gone surprisingly well. He concluded, however, with this observation:

> [B]ut the disturbing thing about it all is that while obviously the contributions that the students and teaching staff have made have been considerable, the amount of time that they have had to spend in Committee work at Department, Faculty or Senate level is very great.
>
> Committees tend to breed Committees and it takes longer and longer to make decisions. Our great task is to determine the extent to which democratization and widespread participation are compatible with the true academic life. Neither the students nor the Professors, if they are to progress academically, can afford to invest as much time in the business of University government as they have been doing in the past year or so. We can only continue to experiment, but the considerable experience that we have had so far suggests to me that our experimentation should be directed along the lines of making our government more efficient rather than making it more representative.

As William Blake observed in *The Proverbs of Hell*, "You never know what is enough unless you know what is more than enough." Perhaps there had been a surfeit of reaction and demands, with people on both sides growing tired. For whatever the reasons, the level of violent and confrontational activity seemed gradually, although not without the occasional flare-up (such as the October Crisis in 1970), to diminish over the next few years as the noisy 1960s became absorbed in the next and following decades. Gray, the noisiest of the diversions, continued his own political struggles but moved away from academic life, much to the relief of the McGill administration.[24]

Robertson had been able to temper and rein in the most extreme suggestions for change, while nevertheless remaining responsive to them, and had always been willing to explore new solutions. Whether they would be lasting solutions was a matter of opinion, but there was experience to be gained: it might be proven that there was no shortcut to learning, that a fair degree of supervision was necessary, that the teacher might not be replaceable by a machine, or that there might be some merit in many of the traditional methods. On the other hand, the efforts to challenge, to stimulate, and to engage the interests of students made the whole process more productive and satisfying. The biggest worry for Robertson was the possibility of disillusionment. One of the worst things that could happen would be for the enthusiasm of the students to die out. In spite of all the discomfiture that such enthusiasm had caused, it had enormous potential for good in the university and in the world at large. Stanley Frost, who was part of the administration throughout Robertson's tenure, remained in awe of his patience and flexibility. Writing to Robertson years later, Frost said that Robertson was the ideal man for the circumstances, better than any principal in the history of the university, and that he would rank Sir Arthur Currie only a distant second to Robertson. As a result of Robertson's work, Robert Bell, his successor, would be able to enjoy eight years of relative calm. Robertson's steady presence at the helm of a ship that was constantly tossed on stormy seas and that, from time to time, may have appeared to be in danger of foundering was a tribute to his character and to his remarkable ability to bring about consensus, even in the most difficult of circumstances.

RESIGNATION FROM McGILL

Events had taken their toll, even on someone with the stamina and devotion of Robertson. He had begun to think that he would retire well before the normal retirement age of sixty-five. The bloom was off the rose. Where major change occurs within institutions, there may not be much discernible pressure around the edges, but it can be enormous where the incremental changes are being forced, forged, or negotiated and where the catalysts are reacting with the existing elements. This pressure fell on the senior administration and, ultimately, at McGill, on the shoulders of Robertson as its principal. There was a limit to what he was able to endure, which he recognized, and this led him to begin to think of getting out. Once thoughts of this nature start to be entertained, even privately, the outcome is merely a matter of time.

His first diary entry on the subject was 4 September 1967, in which he recorded that he had been giving a lot of thought as to how long he should keep on in the job.[1] An earlier inkling of the nascent thought may be gleaned from his diary entry on his birthday, 4 August of the same year, where he wrote, "55 years old and feel every minute of it." In many ways, he noted, he loved it, but the pressure was great enough that he did not think he should keep at it for very much longer. He did not expect to stay on for a further ten years, until he reached the retirement age of sixty-five, and if he were to retire before then, he should do so well before so that he would still be young enough to take up something else, although he had no idea what that might be. He began to think that 1971 would be a good plan. He would be fifty-nine, and it would be the 150th anniversary of McGill. This would leave him only four full academic years to go, and there was much to be done.

His first written effort to communicate the decision was a letter written on 1 September 1968, addressed to Chancellor Howard Ross.[2] It was in his own handwriting so that it would be secret. The letter obviously followed upon discussions he had already had with the chancellor and reflected a considerable effort on his part to bring some form of closure to the events that had developed during his time as principal. The enormous expansion in terms of students, staff, and physical aspects of the university that had occurred during the past six years, while striking in itself, was less significant, he believed, than the evolution of a new form of university governance (he called it "government"), an evolution that had already progressed considerably and would, he had no doubt, accelerate with great rapidity in the near future. They had seen in recent years a marked ascendancy in the power of the academic staff, for powers vested in the departments, the divisions, the faculties, and the Senate had all increased as the process of "democratization" initiated by the staff itself had gradually been effected. Robertson had concurred in this development. As the academic staff had approached their goal, the students had, within the past two years, started their drive for a voice in the "decision-making process," with an objective that he thought was natural and proper if it remained within reasonable limits. The combined efforts of staff and students, although they were not yet united, would, he was confident, soon lead to further changes that would be more radical than those that the university had already experienced and that would in fact completely alter the position of the principal and the senior administrative officers of the university. He did not deplore these changes; indeed, he intended to continue to work to assist in bringing about such changes as seemed sensible in an orderly fashion.

The other aspect that had led him to review his position concerned the relationship between McGill and the provincial government. Since 1960 McGill had become more and more dependent on the Quebec government for financial support, and as a result McGill was now beginning to experience the government's as yet poorly defined, but powerful, influence on the university's affairs. This he did deplore and he had done – and proposed to continue to do – all that he could to prevent or delay this tendency. Thus far he had had little success in this respect, and he was not confident that he would be any more effective in the future, for he thought that the forces there, too, would not be denied. It was natural, therefore, that he should now consider his own position in this rapidly changing scene. If he were to continue as principal until the normal retirement age of sixty-five, it would mean that he would remain until

1977. He doubted very much that his strength would hold out so long, but he was, in any event, convinced that it would be undesirable from every point of view, for if anything had become clear in the past few years, it was the need for an increasingly youthful approach in the direction of the university. Indeed, he thought that he was already beyond the ideal age.

If, then, he were to retire before he reached the statutory age, the moment should be chosen carefully rather than left to the turn of events. To this choice he had given the most serious thought during the past many months and had come to the conclusion that he should retire from the post of principal at a time to coincide with the introduction of the greatest changes in the university government, which he judged would take place some time within the next eighteen months. This would make it possible for a new principal, probably appointed by a new technique, to take up the post under a new form (probably bicameral) of government. He therefore felt he should advise the chancellor that it was his intention, in the near future, to tender his resignation. The precise timing would depend on the rapidity of developments, and he proposed to continue their conversations with a view to finding the appropriate moment. He concluded by saying that all of this involved absolutely no rancour on his part. No one could have had more cordial, sympathetic, and coop-erative treatment than he had had from all parts of the university from the moment that he arrived at McGill. If goodwill were the only factor involved, he would undoubtedly stay on indefinitely. But the matter was much more complex than this consideration, and his decision was entirely dictated by the issues that he had already summarized.

It was a typically articulate and graceful piece of work, one that left very little scope for negotiation over and above the timing of his depar-ture. That it produced huge consternation within the small circle privy to the discussions and correspondence can well be imagined. Robert-son was in continual touch with Ross, who waited until 24 September to respond in writing. Ross acknowledged that there had certainly been great changes since they had become involved in the university's affairs (Ross became chancellor in 1964) and that he was sure the principalship had proved very different from what Robertson had expected it to be. However, if events had made the work less satisfying than it might have been to him, they had also made his contribution all the more important. No one could have steered McGill through these difficult days, he said, with better balance or more wisdom. Ross was not sure the principalship would decline in importance. He hoped that it would not and that all those involved would be wise enough to see that it did not. On the other hand, he had some appreciation of the unfair pressures and strain that these bellicose times placed on those in authority and could therefore understand Robertson's decision to limit his term as principal. He concluded that when Robertson did decide he should go, it would be a sad, sad day for McGill and that for Ross personally, it would be the end of one of the most perfect working relationships any man could have had.

Robertson wrote to Ross on 10 October to record the gist of their recent conversation regarding his proposed retirement and to say that having considered the progress of events and the rate of change, he had come to the conclusion that he should retire in 1970, by which time most of his own objectives, which he had discussed with Ross, should have been achieved. He felt he should advise Ross formally that it was his intention to retire during that year. The precise time of his effective retirement was not easy to fix at the moment, as a variety of circumstances in the university might affect the decision, but he would like to plan on completing his term as principal at the end of May 1970. He felt bound to tell this to certain of his close associates, such as the vice principals and deans whose appointments were terminating and might be renewed, but he thought that it would be unwise to make this decision public until the time came to commence the search for a successor, which might be in the spring of 1969. One of the many regrets, indeed one of the greatest of these, that he would have at the time of retirement from the post of principal would arise from the breaking-up of their association as chancellor and principal, which, Robertson said, had been for him a glorious experience in every respect. It was therefore with reluctance that he was writing this letter to him now, a reluctance that was only relieved by the belief that Ross appreciated his reasons for taking this action.

Somehow or another, some word of this proposal appears to have leaked, at least within the university circle. On 30 November 1968 George Dion at Macdonald College spoke to Robertson to say that he had heard from several people that he was resigning soon – indeed, at the end of the year. Robertson assured him that he had no such intention and then went on to tell Dion what he planned to do. Dion said he would put pressure on him not to follow through with his plan, which, Robertson noted in his diary, gave him the only satisfaction of the day. The general esteem in which Robertson and his work were held continued to grow, and he received two additional honorary degrees: one from Memorial University of Newfoundland in 1968 and another from Jefferson Medical College in 1969.

Whether prescient or not, the *Montreal Gazette* published an editorial on 4 March 1969 entitled "Dr. Robertson's example at McGill."

Amidst all the insolence and abuse directed against him by some of those at McGill University, Dr. H. Rocke Robertson has added still further to his stature by the way he has retained his dignity, courtesy and restraint. None of his predecessors in office at McGill through all the university's long history, ever had to face those with so little regard for the standards of conduct that have been – and ought always to be – essential to university life. No principal's patience has been so sorely tried; none has been so deliberately and insistently provoked.

Yet at no time has Dr. Robertson departed from the standards of conduct that a principal owes to his university as a community of scholars. He is well aware that part of the tactics in a minority on this, as on other campuses, is to wear the principal down and drive him out. He has remained calm, and unshaken.

In all this there has been something more than a man who is acting naturally in accordance with the standards that he owes to himself as a gentleman. There is also the conviction that, as McGill's principal, he cannot allow abusive arrogance to be respected by a similar reply.

As the protector of McGill's life, he is rightly convinced that freedom is possible only if there is no intimidation or disruption. While welcoming reforms, he has had, at the same time, to be certain that the university is not being delivered into the hands of those whose aims may not be the university's reform but its disintegration. While encouraging and enlarging freedom, he must be certain that it will not allow the university to become terrorized by a minority whose aim may not be freedom but domination.

McGill University embodies the devotion and work and generosity and loyalty of thousands of teachers and students and graduates down through many generations. It is a precious heritage.

Dr. Robertson, as principal, cannot allow anything of such value to be tugged and pulled about by the most aggressive minority of the moment.

At a time of short tempers, arrogant tauntings and impulsive recommendations, Dr. Robertson, at the very centre of the turmoil, has set the example of the better values of university life. He has retained his confidence that, whatever the stresses now may be, the standards of a university as a place of study, teaching and research, a place free of violence, must endure. He knows, by standing for these values, that he is fighting the winning, not the losing, battle. Universities must change, but they must not be allowed to sink.

It is impressive to observe how many of the teachers at the university are supporting him – and what he stands for. In their statement, above their signatures, they realize that "in these times no university administration is likely to follow an error-free course." But they "recognize the integrity of Dr. Robertson and his earnest desire to serve the university." And they add: "Under the most trying circumstances, he has retained a sense of balance, and has accorded his critics a degree of courtesy that has not been reciprocated."

By his unswerving loyalty to the high standards of dignified and courteous conduct, Dr. H. Rocke Robertson has honored himself, honored his university, and will be honored in the future in the record of these critical days.

Robertson announced his intention to resign the office of principal at the Board of Governors meeting in May 1969, but the announcement was not made public. At the end of August he wrote to Cyril James to advise him of his impending retirement. He had to keep working on the chancellor to set up a committee to search for his successor and, as late as 2 September 1969, still thought the chancellor was not enthusiastic about the idea and was being somewhat evasive on the subject, but Robertson prevailed. He gave some thought to staying on until May 1971, perhaps as a form of trade-off and because it was possible that the graduates would add their own pressure, in which case he might feel that he was letting the side down. However, at the Board of Governors meeting on 15 September 1969, the chancellor asked the board to establish a committee to advise on his successor. There were many nice comments made, and a couple of the governors who had not been aware of what was in the wings suggested that he should stay until 1971, but Robertson was firm about sticking to his plan of leaving in 1970. He would not let the university down but thought that the sooner they found a replacement, the better for all concerned.

Robertson settled on 1 September as the date by which he wanted to leave. This would be the start of the new academic year, and he thought there should be a new leader of the university at that time. Even if the search committee had not finished its work by then, there could be an interim principal. There was, as well, another search committee at work, this to find a replacement for Howard Ross as chancellor, who had been persuaded to accept the appointment as dean of the Faculty of Management. The outcome was something of a surprise, when Donald Hebb, one of the university's – indeed the world's – foremost scientists, was elected by the Board of Governors on 9 March, beating out Stuart Finlayson and Carl Goldenberg.

That he would be stepping down then became public knowledge. Both of the English newspapers commented on the situation, the *Montreal Star* on 19 September and the *Gazette* the following day. The *Star*'s commentary was headed "A vast change in principal's role" and read:

"The use of a university," Woodrow Wilson once declared, "is to make young gentlemen as unlike their fathers as possible." It almost seems quaint to read these words now, but essentially they are as applicable today, as when they were uttered 55 years ago. The difference, of course, is that the usual generation gap has been accompanied by more than the usual expansion of a university's knowledge. Progress was leisurely and easily absorbed in Wilson's time. Now we are flooded, and often overwhelmed, by an outpouring of writing, teaching and concepts. We are caught in revolutions that go beyond education and information; they delve into social and moral values on a scale that is virtually unprecedented.

Dr. Rocke Robertson was understating it yesterday when he suggested that the pressures on a university principal are much greater than they ever were. In his own tenure at McGill University, which began little over six years ago, more of a cataclysmic nature has happened in the academic world – in terms of expansion, of student assertion, of public involvement – than perhaps in

the six centuries that went before. Dr. Robertson set out to make
necessary adjustments at McGill, and succeeded to a considerable
degree. But in explaining his decision to retire, he may have hit the
key point: no man should stay too long as president or principal
of a contemporary university with its immense and diverse and
changing demands.

Dr. Robertson, typical of his decency and sensitivity, has left
time for a successor to be found by next year. But the job of heading a university, despite the challenges it offers, no longer is quite
the agreeable one it was in the era of Wilson. In the United States
today scores of universities are on the lookout for a capable man
or woman to fill the top position which remains vacant. McGill's
selection committee has an unenviable assignment.

The Gazette repeated its earlier title, "Dr. Robertson's example at
McGill."

Dr. H. Rocke Robertson has announced his retirement as Principal
and Vice-Chancellor of McGill University, which may take place
in the spring. Though the period of his principalship has not been
long it has been critical. He has seen the university through some
of its worst strains and dangers. He has guided the transition. His
place in the long history of McGill will be unique – and uniquely
important.

During these last seven years – and especially during the last
two – no man could have been more insistently harassed, more
frequently provoked, or have had to endure more insolence. The
triumph of these years is that he has used only the honorable
weapons; spoken only the considered opinion; adopted always the
moderate attitude; cultivated always the wise and rational course.

He has had the most difficult task of all – that of realizing that
some valid need for change may lie at the heart of even the crudest
and most extravagant demands. The duty of a principal in such a
time is not to fall back on the old academic rule that nothing must
ever be done for the first time. He has to welcome in the university
the process of self-examination and to promote significant change.

Of the demands for change that have confronted him in his
principalship Dr. Robertson has said: "Nor can this be regretted,

for if it can be claimed that the complaints are exaggerated, that they are presented in a barbarous fashion, and that few concrete proposals for correction are offered, there is unquestionable substance in them, and a need to search for improvements."

At such a time a principal has to take up the forbidding, and longsuffering, and tedious task of sorting out the demands for change, evaluating their meaning, separating the wheat from the chaff, the genuine from the absurd. It is not a process in which anyone is likely to be entirely pleased, or should be. It is a principal's thanklessly necessary duty.

The aim has been clear enough. "Our obvious task," says Dr. Robertson, "is to preserve what is good while effecting the necessary changes." But this has required his exemplary patience and self-control. "In the heat of the contemporary academic world," agreement has been hard to reach between the conservatives, on the one hand, who resist any change, and the radicals, on the other, who would promote change for its own sake.

Nor has the task been only one of reconciling the well-intentioned differences. There is a third force with which the principal has had to contend – those who have no concern for the welfare of the University, and ... seize upon the confusion and turn it, wherever possible, to their own purpose: to destroy the University in its present form.

In the midst of all this turbulence, Dr. Robertson has the faith that the future will always be on the side of the moderation that must always prevail, in the end, in university life. Fairly soon, he is convinced, the time will come when it will be clear that real progress in the universities – as in all our institutions – will be delayed, if not nullified, by violent actions. The use of force – so tantalizingly effective in the short run – can never solve complex problems.

Only last week, speaking at the Alma Mater Fund dinner, and looking forward to the future, Principal Robertson remarked: "The aim as I see it is not to have a peaceful campus, but one where sensible and civilized rows are going on."

To be sensible and civilized even in the midst of rows may seem exceedingly difficult. But Dr. Robertson, as McGill's principal, has shown that it can be done. He has set his example because he believes that the future of universities will belong not to crudity or intolerance, not to violence or to hate, but to the courtesy and the forbearance, the reason and the wisdom that are the only true freedom.

Writing to his brother Bruce on 16 September 1969, the day after the Board of Governors agreed to form the search committee, he said he felt greatly relieved that the affair had now progressed to a practically irreversible point because he had become powerfully sick of the endless petty (and not so petty) bickering that seemed to be such an inevitable part of the job. He told Bruce that he had no plans for himself and would not consider any until he knew for certain when he was to be "freed." In his diary he had noted there was a continuous and monotonous parade of any number of things, to the point that he despaired of doing anything else with his time but patching them up, there being no hope of ever getting rid of them. All of this made him rather glad that he would not be doing the job much longer. Robertson received many letters of support, but now that the announcement had been made, his own thoughts about the decision had clarified:

For personal reasons I am, of course, relieved – I simply do not want to carry on much longer and R[oslyn], I don't believe, could. The hardships, criticisms, vitriol and tensions all affect her more, I think, than they do me. But going beyond the personal side and thinking of the University I think that the timing will prove to be good. We need, badly, to have a shakedown period. I suspect that this move to change of leadership will tend to quiet down the radicals while they wait to see who is to follow as Principal.

The day of the announcement was a hectic but very pleasing day for Robertson. There was a reception at the Faculty of Management to honour the new dean (and former chancellor), Howard Ross, and this was followed by a dinner, organized by Carl Goldenberg and law professor Jacob Ziegel, at the Faculty Club to celebrate Frank Scott's seventieth birthday. Robertson declared it to be one of the best functions he had ever attended. Like many, Robertson was very fond of Frank Scott. He noted, not long after he had retired, that he had encountered Scott at the Ottawa airport, finding him full of anecdotes, one of which he noted in his diary: "(Poet, of sorts, to Bernard Shaw – 'There's a dreadful conspiracy of silence about my book of poetry – what do you think I should do about it?' G.B.S. 'Form it')." The guests included Prime Minister Pierre Elliott Trudeau, poets, and former politicians (mostly, observed Robertson, former members of the Cooperative Commonwealth Federation, CCF-ers). The tone was exciting and the speeches excellent, led off by an extemporaneous and clever address by Trudeau that set the bar for the rest of the evening.

It did not take long for Robertson to start thinking about what he might do once his appointment came to an end. He and Roslyn began talking about it within a matter of days, and others within the community approached him with a variety of suggestions. Justice G. Miller Hyde, a governor and president of the Montreal General Hospital, suggested that he might take on the job of coordinating the teaching hospitals.[3] Fraser Gurd wanted him back in the medical field, although Robertson thought that having been out of the practice for eight years, there was no possibility of catching up on what he had missed. Someone suggested that he might write a history of McGill, a prospect that he considered, at least long enough to note that he would have to stop any such history as of 1962, when he had become principal. Other ideas included becoming an overseas executive. His inclination, however, was to look for something in Ottawa. He knew that it would be difficult, having been so prominent for so many years, to remain in Montreal, much as he loved the city, and particularly difficult to be in any way connected with McGill or its teaching hospitals, one reason why he decided against the hospital coordination project.

In the middle of January 1970, still trying to avert the resignation, the chairman of the Board of Governors, Stuart Finlayson (later, in 1975, chancellor of the university for a year), and Howard Ross enlisted no less an icon than Wilder Penfield to intervene with Robertson. Penfield called him on 13 January and was at his most persuasive in expressing what they thought, reading from a letter addressed to Robertson. After seven years as principal and vice chancellor, in this most difficult time of strain and stress, he and Mrs Robertson now proposed to lay down the heavy load that they had carried. The letter asked that they reconsider and look, with Penfield and the others, at the whole situation. Perhaps the harness should be shifted; perhaps they could make his leadership easier, happier, and more effective. Penfield suggested that they both needed and deserved a sabbatical rest and that everyone knew they both needed it. Indeed, probably every university would be well advised to schedule recurring sabbatical periods for leaders. Freedom, with the opportunity to study and travel and gain distant perspective, is what they needed in these days of change and growth.

He went on to say that Robertson had not failed (obviously a message that the chancellor and others thought they had detected from Robertson's decision) but that he had succeeded where so many presidents of other universities had not. He had built a strong team. They could carry the load if he were to take a sabbatical leave. What were his terms to tackle the job afresh? In the years ahead, faculty leadership and student understanding may constitute less of a problem since the lines of academic evolution are more clearly drawn. Robertson had helped to draw them. Patience and repeated demands would bring full justice from Quebec in the end. English Canadians needed him more than he realized – not in the field of politics but in this place of science and culture and academic confusion. Robertson had done so much. He was in the best position to do more. Could Penfield and the others be of assistance to the Robertsons in planning their way of life, give them greater protection from the demands of the office, or provide more supporting services for them? Did he want a formal vote of confidence from the faculty? There was no one who had the experience, the patience, the strength, and the universal respect and affection that Robertson had. No one was as well qualified as Robertson to lead the university into its next decade.

Penfield reported to Finlayson that he had expressed these thoughts to Robertson. Robertson had said he was agreeable to meeting with Finlayson, Howard Ross, Anson McKim, and Penfield to discuss the prospect of his retirement but had also said that his mind was pretty firmly made up. And so it was. He recorded the event in his diary entry for 13 January 1970:

At dinnertime Wilder Penfield called on the telephone. He had been talking with H.I.R. [Ross] and Stuart Finlayson and Arnold Heeney and they want to come and talk about my continuing as principal. Wilder read me a very flattering letter that he had composed. This disturbs me deeply. I made up my mind in 1968 that I would retire in 1970 and I had thought over the situation very carefully before deciding. One of my reasons was the very adverse effect that my difficulties have had on R[oslyn]. Much of the stuffing has been knocked out of her – she feels very deeply the criticism that has been levelled at times against me and the university, the exasperations, the difficulties etc. etc. and when I reported to her my talk with Wilder her immediate response was a firm "no" and as we talked on she didn't relent. I think that she is right. I dread the thought that I am letting the university down but I honestly think that I have given all that I possibly can. For this job, I am quite convinced, a man has to be younger than I am. After 7 1/2 gruelling years I feel, at 57 1/2, exhausted and ancient. I find that my memory is not retentive enough any more to enable me to keep up. This may be a manifestation of fatigue but it worries me nonetheless and I fear that it will lead me in to serious difficulties sooner or later. Nor do I think that a long holiday (Wilder suggests a sabbatical year) would solve the problem. I'd be nearly 60 when I returned and, if I get deeply involved in affairs again as I would have to, I'd soon be exhausted again. At the moment the university is in good shape administratively and I feel no guilt in leaving in that respect. It is hard to analyse one's own feelings. One thing I know (and cannot say to anyone but R.) is that I do not believe that I (nor anyone) can stem the tide of Francization that will involve the whole of Montreal and, of course, McGill. I loathe the prospect, and my life, were I to stay on, would be one of fighting a rearguard action. I see very little chance of working out a good saw off with the French who are enormously militant and, with their total control over the government, powerful.

On days like this I wonder if separation of Quebec isn't the best course for the country.

This did not mean the governors just walked away from their idea. They had a great principal and wanted him to continue. A month later, on 13 February, Finlayson, Penfield, Hyde, and Ross took him to lunch at the Mount Royal Club to continue their efforts. Robertson was steadfast and they were pleasant about it. They offered him any sort of terms and made tempting suggestions, all very difficult for Robertson. He thought they believed his reasons for being so stubborn were rather thin – he was doing well and could continue to do so. Robertson doubted that he could. He was tired beyond belief and felt that he could not stem the very difficult tides of student, staff, and government problems that he knew were coming. Someone else might, although he was not sanguine about it, but he knew he could not. He thought it was wise to withdraw and hope for the best about what another person could bring to the situation.

The attitude of Roslyn played a much greater role in his resignation than it had in any part of the job itself, where she had no meaningful role to play, other than as "wife of the principal." With her limited higher education, she was not comfortable with the academic and other notables who were constantly on the university scene. While it is unlikely that she would have initiated the idea, once Robertson had put it forward, she embraced it with great determination and would not countenance any backsliding or extension of the time he had decided upon. As he noted many times in his diary, she had suffered more from the tensions and attacks than Robertson himself. Robertson was discouraged by the Quebec situation and had a persistently gloomy outlook as to what he considered would be the end game. If he stayed, even in Quebec, he would be involved in what he regarded as a continual reactive action in defence of the rights of English-speaking Canadians. Roslyn had, in addition to her general lack of enthusiasm for his continuing the job, a far more visceral perspective and was worried about him being an obvious target for the Front de Libération du Québec (FLQ), a worry that was brought into sharper focus only a few months later with the kidnappings of James Cross and Pierre Laporte, followed by Laporte's murder. It even got to the point that Robertson thought it might reach the stage of an ultimatum: if he stayed on as principal, she would leave. This was, given her loyalty and unswerving support of him, unlikely and out of character, but he was obviously far from sure, something that had an important impact on him and his thinking.

On 21 April 1970 Robertson was one of nine inducted into the Order of Canada as a Companion of the Order, the highest rank, one reserved for those whose contributions as Canadians have been extraordinary. The investiture ceremony was at Rideau Hall and was attended by Governor General Roland Michener, Prime Minister Pierre Elliott Trudeau, Chief Justice of Canada Gérard Fauteux, and many other "notables." The Robertsons drove up to Ottawa from Montreal in time to check into their hotel, change into formal wear, and climb aboard the bus that took them to the ceremony. He found the whole exercise to be well organized, dignified, and impressive, and the governor general spoke to each of the inductees. The ceremony was followed by drinks and a dinner, a brief speech by the governor general, and drinks with some friends. It was a long and tiring day, but he was impressed with "the whole show," and while he felt wholly undeserving of the honour, he was nevertheless very pleased. It must have seemed to him and Roslyn to have been at least a partial vindication of all of his efforts over the past few turbulent years.

By mid-May, Robertson was advised that the search committee for a new principal had narrowed the search to eight persons and was ready to start interviewing. Reportedly there were seven outside candidates and one internal, but he did not know the names, and it was not certain that all would agree to be interviewed. Robertson and Roslyn started to focus on Ottawa as their new location. At 2:00 in the morning of 16 June a bomb exploded against the south wall of the Engineering Building, blowing one wall into the internal combustion laboratory in the Department of Mechanical Engineering and breaking many windows. Fortunately, no one was hurt. The same day, Finlayson told Robertson that the Executive Committee had agreed with his departure date of 1 September but wanted the Board of Governors to approve it as well.

On 24 June, Finlayson called Robertson to say that the committee had settled on a unanimous recommendation to propose the eminent physicist Professor Robert Bell as principal. Robertson was immensely relieved on two counts: first, that he thought Bell would be good and, second, that the decision appeared to have been reached peacefully. Robertson had had the usual dealings with Bell, a respected member of the university faculty. He had also had a talk with him, recorded in his diary entry for 16 January 1967, when Bell – McGill's top physicist, recently elected to the Royal Society of London – was being courted by Dalhousie University, which wanted him as a Distinguished Professor and was offering $10,000 more than McGill's best offer. "Extraordinary to find the Maritimes with enough money to do what they have always cursed Upper Canada for doing." Fortunately for McGill, Bell elected to remain where he was. Robertson thought the search committee had had some doubtful moments and that it had not fully pulled together until that evening. A third element was that he could have a clear conscience about sticking with his retirement date. Recommendations of search committees are, in most cases, followed without too much discussion, especially when their recommendations are unanimous, but the process of presenting the recommendation to the Board of Governors was a formal requirement since it is the board, not the committee, that makes the appointment. Robertson spent the whole of the following day (even missing a regular corporate board meeting at Bell Canada) planning the process for conducting the meeting and notifying people who needed to know, but the plans were upset by a leak to the media well ahead of the scheduled time. The official view of the most likely suspect was a student on the committee. A ferocious debate ensued at the meeting – not against the recommendation of Robert Bell but as a result of some junior members of the board wanting to know who else had been considered. The committee refused to disclose any of the names, and there was great difficulty, which was effectively settled when the staff members supported Bell's nomination very strongly and, in the end, reached a unanimous decision to appoint him. He was expected to take over on 21 August, which delighted Robertson, being both earlier and easier than he had planned.

As Cyril James had worked with Robertson on the transition, so Robertson worked with Bell over the summer as his own term ran down and Bell geared up to take over. Robertson continued to think he would do well in the office. On 10 August he organized a meeting between Bell and Roger Gaudry, rector at the Université de Montréal, to help keep intact whatever interuniversity solidarity had been generated. Two days later he arranged for some of the student leaders to have lunch in his office so that he could introduce the new principal to them. On his last day as principal, Robertson spent the day in his office, apart from a brief shopping trip to get some cigars for Bob Shaw, and had several visitors. Bell came for lunch and spent the entire afternoon, until the close of business at 5:00, when he officially took over the mantle. The Canadian Television (CTV) network came for an interview with each of them. Watching the eleven o'clock news, Robertson thought his own efforts were entirely uninspiring. He brought the staff who were closest to him to his home for the evening, where they shared a happy time, some gifts, and a few tears. They gave Robertson some cufflinks engraved with his initials, one with the date 1 December 1962 and the other with the date 21 August 1970, marking the term of his office, as well as a pipe, both of which touched and pleased him. He and Roslyn celebrated the start of their new lives by watching the late movie on television, something they had done only once before. It was the story of the German pocket battleship *Graf Spee*, and having often recalled the excitement of the Sunday in December 1939 when she was expected to break out of the harbour near Montevideo, they could not resist watching the show.[4]

Not surprisingly, he had not fully collected his thoughts at this stage, and his diary entry for his final day in office included some contradictory thoughts and observations:

I had little time to think, during the day about my Principalship and my future. I think I felt a bit dazed and that I shall only get down to reasonable appraisal after I've started to write my annual report and at the same time have commenced my preparation for my new job. In the meantime my immediate feelings are of sadness (because I have enjoyed so much of my work and am so devoted to so many people with whom I have worked). I feel strangely little "relief" – the word that most people have used in connection with my retirement. I have not, I think, been greatly affected by the load. I have been bored with the repetition of troublesome things to an extent that I felt that I would sooner or later come to disregard them which would have been disastrous, and I have sometimes wondered how much longer I could keep up the pace but, I realize fully now, my feeling of relief is not very strong – indeed, as it is turning out sadness rather than relief is by far the stronger emotion. Perhaps the certainty, now, of my retirement – or rather the fact of it and the certainty that I shall not be called upon to deal with financial problems, parking, pensions, fringe benefits, internecine strife of various sorts, etc., gives me room to be sorry to be missing the good things.

Today as I wrote letters to the Chancellor, the Chairman of the Board and to several henchmen to whom I had not already written I realized how strong the group is that is continuing and I am quite satisfied that Bob Bell is an excellent choice – he shows good promise.

All in all I'm pleased – I think that McGill is in good shape – we've made some important progress in the last 8 years – people have been extraordinarily kind – even the newspapers!

Within the university, Stanley Frost had drafted a flattering resolution that was discussed with enthusiasm and passed unanimously by the Senate:

The Senate of McGill University marks with profound regret the resignation of Dr. H. Rocke Robertson from the office of Principal and Vice-Chancellor of the University, and by that act from the Chair of Senate. When the Board of Governors in 1962 announced the appointment of Dr. Robertson as Principal, Senate passed a resolution expressing its great satisfaction that a member of the University's teaching staff, and one who had recently been elected by his colleagues in the faculty of Medicine to represent them in Senate had been chosen as Principal and that the new Chairman of Senate was thus to be for the first time one who was already a member of this body. After the eight years in which the meetings of Senate have been chaired by Dr. Robertson, Senate places on record its recognition that during those years he never ceased to be in every sense of the word a member of Senate and indeed he very quickly became far more than simply its presiding officer.

It was in large measure he who planned and encouraged the new form and the new role of this body, which emerged during the years of his Principalship; by his own regard for Senate he at all times enhanced its stature and prestige; by his unwearied patience, his constant courtesy and unswerving integrity, he more than any other set the tone and established the standards of conduct and debate; and at a time when Senate could have fallen into frustration and ineffectiveness, it was he who fostered and achieved the stability of Senate, so that in a period of rapid change the senior academic body of this University has been able increasingly to give the leadership for which the situation called. Other bodies in this University will doubtless record the contribution made by Dr. Robertson in innumerable other areas of its life and activities; Senate affirms that it recognizes with admiration and gratitude the immense debt which it owes to its presiding officer during the most important years of its development, and wishes him Godspeed in all his future undertakings.[5]

The new organization of the Senate has stood the test of time quite admirably, and McGill has a genuine, functional, bicameral system of governance, with the Senate the acknowledged master of matters academic and the Board of Governors responsible for the business and financial aspects of the university. There is crossover membership, with Senate representatives on the Board of Governors and members of the Board of Governors on the Senate, and each has tended to defer, in the final analysis, as appropriate in the particular spheres of responsibility. Students are now represented on both bodies and have generally been active and responsible participants.

On 10 September 1970 Robertson was invited to the Hermitage Club, where the deans and vice principals had been meeting all day, discussing, as usual, the budget and how it could be cut back. The discussions had apparently gone well, tempers had not been lost, and everyone seemed quite cheerful. There was a splendid dinner, with much to eat and drink, followed by some presentations, a cake from Margaret Thomson, and from the deans and vice principals a book, magnificently bound and printed, called *The University* and containing an extract from the speeches of each of the principals, starting with Bishop Mountain and ending with Robertson. He was most touched and noted that "I spoke for a long time and said a number of laudatory things – all fully meant – about the people. It was a grand affair I thought."

About five weeks later, on 15 October, after the kidnappings of Cross and Laporte, the Graduates' Society held its annual meeting and dinner, at which the Robertsons were guests of honour. They had by now just moved to Ottawa and drove to Montreal during the afternoon for the occasion. Robertson was particularly pleased with the recognition given to Roslyn, which included the society's gold medal and a beautifully bound and illustrated book for her own collection. The event was gratifying to him, but he was more delighted by the recognition of Roslyn, who so thoroughly deserved it and whom everyone was thrilled to see get it. He noted ruefully in his diary that there had been times in recent years when he had thought it likely that he would be drummed out of the principalship in disgrace, notably in relation to the Fekete and Gray affairs. He wished, at those depressing moments, that he could have foreseen this evening, which was laden with good spirit, fine citations, and standing ovations.

A special Convocation was organized for the afternoon of 30 October 1970 in the Sir Arthur Currie Memorial Gymnasium for the sole purpose of conferring an honorary doctorate on Robertson, where he was presented by his friend and former chancellor Howard Ross.[6] Robertson delivered a gentle and largely positive address, recounting some of his early experience at McGill and summarizing the progress that had been made in the governance of the university, a difficult process in which much effort had been needed to sort out the good from the bad, the practicable from the fanciful, and the sincere from the malicious. The process had been demanding and had forced the university not only to ask some fundamental questions about itself, about its role, and about the extent to which it should respond to political issues but also to accede to demands of "relevance" and to direct its teaching and research along certain lines. He thought the university had emerged from this difficult period with more confidence and determination and with structures that were stronger and better balanced than before. He complimented the Senate on its ability to deal with the questions before it, now that the heat of earlier debate that had interfered with its work had diminished, and complimented those who had kept their heads during the tumult. He remained unsatisfied with the political treatment of McGill at the hands of the Quebec government, which regularly turned aside the recommendations of its own special committees that studied the needs and merits of the universities as a whole, always to McGill's disadvantage. He expressed his confidence in the new principal, wished everyone well, and concluded with "May God bless McGill."[7]

Typical of his internalizations, Robertson was less than enthusiastic about his own efforts. He had had great difficulty preparing his Convocation address and finally had written out the notes for it only on the morning of the event, getting up early and finishing by noon. He walked the notes up to McGill from the hotel where he and Roslyn were staying and had someone type the speech, which he received shortly before leaving for the Convocation. Despite what he may have thought about his own remarks, it proved to be a very pleasant day:

> There was a surprisingly large crowd in the gym – the ceremony
> was simple and nice. Howard Ross presented me – my speech
> seemed to go alright though I was not pleased with it – I didn't
> get the real punch that I had hoped to achieve. Next a reception
> in Redpath Hall. A huge turnout of staff of all types – all so kind.
> Hugh McLennan spoke and we were presented with magnificent
> things – R[oslyn] a picture by [Robertson left a blank in the diary,
> evidently not remembering the name of the artist] and me a beau-
> tiful print by Peachey (Quebec 1784) and a cheque with which I am
> to buy books – $2500! Hard to believe. I was tremendously touched
> by the whole thing. There have been times when I felt that I might
> be leaving the university with my tail between my legs but today's
> celebration was beyond my wildest hopes and I seem to be leav-
> ing on the best possible terms if the appreciative words are meant.
> R. and I were made thoroughly happy by it all. Next move was a
> dinner at the University Club given by all the Governors who had

been in office during my term – nearly all of them were there and it was a fine dinner. Donald Hebb spoke for a moment – Bob Bell followed, then Stuart Finlayson whom I followed – I was tired and I don't think my speech was good – can't remember what I said. Home at about 11 exhausted. It has been a wonderful day – I've dreaded it for a long time but now it's over I'm simply delighted.

CONCLUSION

There could be little doubt that Robertson had left an important imprint on McGill and that he had ushered in many important changes in university governance, achieved in a shorter time and without some of the huge upheaval that occurred in other universities. Part of this was the result of his character and of his ability to accommodate change. After all, this attribute had marked a good part of his professional life, and he himself had been an agent for sweeping changes in medical care. Another factor was that he genuinely believed that many of the governance changes requested by faculty and students made good sense, especially once the useful ideas could be separated from the impracticable and the venom removed from the presentation of the demands. By the time he left his position, elected faculty members made up the majority of the Senate, and there were eight student representatives on this important decision-making body as well as on twenty-two of the twenty-seven standing committees, where, as a practical matter, most of the decisions were actually made. Management of the huge increases in student population – enrolment shot up by 70 per cent, matched by an 85 per cent increase in staff and crowned by an explosion of 187 per cent in expenditure – would have tested any institution and exhausted any leader even without the vitriolic nature of student demands and the overt discrimination of the Quebec government's funding. Coordinating the construction and coming on line of ten major buildings and three new research facilities was only part of the daily workload. Add to this the complete renovation of the education system in Quebec, which threatened the alignment of the English-speaking system in the province with the rest of North America, and the profound disinterest by the Quebec government in matters of English-language education, and it becomes difficult to imagine the pressure that weighed on Robertson virtually twenty-four hours a day.

Robertson's was a well-earned and honourable retirement.

RETIREMENT YEARS

Welcome as release from his burden of leading McGill may have been, there were a few adjustments that did not come as automatically as Robertson may have hoped. He noted that his first day of retirement was rather unproductive, hoping it was not to be prophetic. He got his diary in shape and arranged for delivery of it, covering the years 1961 to date, into the hands of the McGill archivist for microfilming. He set a limitation on the use of the microfilm, permitting use by an official university historian at any time but not by anyone else until thirty years after his retirement, 21 August 2000. His intention was to keep it out of the hands of irresponsible people until it would be of no further interest. At the same time, he speculated, perhaps on the basis that there is nothing as past as a past principal, that it might not have any such value even now.[1]

The next day he worked a bit on his final annual report, after which he and Roslyn went for a sentimental pre-dinner walk, through the neighbouring property, to the herb and scent garden established in Roslyn's honour at the entrance to the McIntyre Sciences Building, through the Stewart Building courtyard, around the main campus, and along Sherbrooke Street, admiring the flowers and mourning over the fast-disappearing elms. He found it strange not to have any responsibility for what was now going on at the university and was dejected by this. Still in Montreal, he was generally aware of what was going on, including tensions regarding proposed cuts to the budget and the complaints within the Senate as to the work of the hapless task force charged with finding the areas to cut. Over and above the McGill problems, there was a confrontation looming between the doctors and the Quebec government, which seemed to be getting increasingly ugly. He also had to spend time sitting for his official portrait that would be hung in the Redpath Library, along with those of his predecessors and the former chancellors of the university, a process that he found as boring as it was time-consuming.[2]

Having decided that it would be best to move from Montreal to Ottawa, to have a complete separation from McGill, the first step was to find a new home, for which they began to look during the summer of 1970, settling on a place at 301 Buena Vista Road in the Rockcliffe Park area of Ottawa, a former home of Lester B. Pearson. It needed some work, so once Robertson concluded that his finances were equal to the cost of the house and the work, they made their deal and began to get ready to move at the beginning of October. Moving day proved to be 9 October – their furniture arrived in the midst of the crisis caused by the kidnapping of James Cross and shortly before the additional kidnapping of Pierre Laporte, and they spent the weekend settling in and beginning to unpack the dozens of crates, arrange the furniture, and hang the paintings. Both Robertson and Roslyn had extensive collections of books, which added to the pleasurable complications of sorting and shelving their treasures. Flowers had to be dug up in Montreal and crammed into the car for transport and replanting at the new home. They were not fully clear of Montreal, however, until after the special Convocation scheduled for the end of the month, making several day or overnight trips for the celebrations already noted.

Robertson had one more professional experience at the Montreal General Hospital the week after getting his honorary degree, this time as a recipient, rather than provider, of services. On 6 November he had an operation – a left radial meniscectomy – performed by his friend and orthopaedic surgeon Jim Shannon. His next six days in hospital were something of a blur, during which he had "some great pleasures and some tiresome moments – the latter mostly concerned with trying to sleep at night." His pleasures were found in the letters, flowers, and visits, of which he felt he had more than his share, as well as books sent to him by several people. Among those who visited were hospital personnel and volunteers, as well as a number of the medical staff, including Fraser Gurd, Alan Thompson, Jimmy Martin, Doug Cameron, Shaun Murphy, and Fred Greenwood, five members of the McGill football team, some McGill colleagues, Bob Shaw, Bob Bell, Alex Hutchison, and several others. Shannon took good care of him, and the knee seemed to come on quite well, so by the time he was ready to leave on 12 November, he was

doing well on crutches and was getting back pretty good quadriceps function. There was still a fair amount of effusion, but at no time was there
any severe pain, although the discomfort was quite persistent. He found
it difficult to read over the continual throb and so watched a good deal of
television, deeming it a godsend for the patient. A possibility of diabetes
that had concerned him was ruled out by a normal sugar tolerance test,
much to his relief. It was, however, a condition that would develop over
the years. Doctors are no better patients than any other class – many
are worse – so he found that his recovery after being released from the
hospital was slower than he expected and had to have the knee drained
of fluids that had built up due to overexercise, a medical process that
he observed with some professional reservation, unvoiced, however, to
the performer of the procedure. Thereafter, he took the recovery process
more seriously and had a full recovery.

IF YOU REALLY WANT TO GET BUSY, RETIRE

The title of this chapter is somewhat misleading, implying as it might,
that Robertson's years after McGill were spent smelling the roses (which
he loved and grew with great passion) and in quiet reflection. There were,
it is true, some elements of this, especially with the family, since, in reality, his life had been far from "normal" from the time he agreed to take
over the Montreal General Hospital position and create a huge change in
its approach to surgery. This situation was exacerbated by the demands
put upon him during the turbulent years at McGill, in the crucible of
government, student, faculty, public, media, and graduate stresses that
broke many in similar positions in Canada, North America, and elsewhere. He had done his best to keep these family contacts fresh and had
done well in the circumstances, but after McGill, it became possible for
these to reblossom, and he and Roslyn rejoiced particularly in this aspect
of retirement. But he was still an active and vigorous man, filled with
ideas and energy. It was not as though he were ready to be put out to pasture – even an attractive pasture. He had a demonstrated ability to tackle
complex issues, get a team of people together that could coalesce, and
produce a useful result within a defined time parameter and budget.

Robertson had been approached, even before his retirement from
McGill, by the Science Council of Canada to see whether he might be
willing to take on a study of the delivery of health care services in Can-

ada. It was the kind of project to which his organizational talents were well suited and which appealed to him, provided he could get his mind around a methodology that would make such a study useful. He was given a small staff and a small but adequate office at the Science Council and then began the task of determining how to produce a meaningful outcome. This included discussions in mid-September with the Ontario deputy minister of health, Ken Charron, who outlined the province's plans, from which Robertson observed that Ontario had done little thus far but had a good base for delivery of health services and plenty of money to spend. The more he read and thought about health care, the more he found that his confusion increased. Fortunately, there was a delay in getting the first formal meeting of the committee together (at which Robertson was to put forward a recommended course of action), so he had some additional time to think. As far as Ontario was concerned, he found it to have a massive health organization "machine" that was not moving very much and about which he suspected there was far more talk than action.

By the end of November, as work on the survey progressed, he noted in his diary that he had read a good bit of Thomas More's *Utopia*, wanting to see what he had said about the health delivery system in his ideal world. He found quite extraordinary both how close More's description had come to what now existed in the Soviet Union and what More had to say about the health system, including having large hospitals on the outskirts of the city, attended by "cunning phisitians" who were constantly present. The eventual report, *Health Care in Canada: A Commentary*, was delivered in 1973 and contained a number of useful observations and recommendations relating to the public health system.[3] This was followed by a study for the Ontario government on the effects of lead pollution.[4] There were more two major studies: one performed for the Traffic Injury Research Foundation[5] and the other for the Association of Universities and Colleges of Canada (AUCC).[6] He continued his presence on the Board of Directors of Bell Canada, through to its becoming a subsidiary of Bell Canada Enterprises Inc.,[7] as well as his active participation on the Royal Bank of Canada Award Committee, on which he served for some twenty years. Coincidentally enough, the first recipient of the award had been Wilder Penfield. He maintained his connection with the Gault estate at Mont. Ste Hilaire, which he, with the help of his friend Howard Webster, had been instrumental in establishing, and was honorary president of the research institute located there.[8] He was a member of the board at the Hospital for Sick Children in Toronto and at the Ottawa General Hospital. He wrote the entry for the fifteenth edition of *Encyclopedia Britannica* in 1974 on "wound" and had a lifetime position at the Osler Library, where his interest, contributions, and graceful diplomacy were recognized by all concerned.[9] He was constantly involved attending functions, giving speeches, and raising money on behalf of McGill.

One pleasure of retirement, in addition to making oneself useful in a variety of ways, is the opportunity it provides to look back and to reflect on events that were lived in the hurly-burly of the present tense. Such an occasion occurred in the week before Christmas 1970 when Robertson and Roslyn were discussing a trip to England in 1958. Roslyn was certain they had seen Salisbury Cathedral; Robertson had no recollection at all, so he dug out his diary of the trip, which proved Roslyn correct – they had stopped on their way back to London from Bath (during the trip when Robertson had met Robert Milnes-Walker, who had recommended him to Cyril James as a worthy surgeon-in-chief for the Montreal General Hospital).

Once launched on diary reading I took up my diary written during the war and sent home to R[oslyn] and the family. I was surprised by two things – first my constancy in writing – I had not actually recalled writing a diary – I thought that I'd just written letters – but last night I read a fairly faithful (I think) account of our doings between the day we sailed from Montreal in July 1940 and mid-March 1941 – hardly missed a day. My second surprise was the abandon with which I described some of the warlike things – I gave the name of the ships conveying us across the Atlantic – the site of the R.M.R's camp – the site of our hospital, etc. – many things that would have been censored had they been seen.

On the whole the diary was quite dull I found – I, of course, knew that those to whom I was writing had immediate access to the news and I made all too few comments on the events as I heard about them and all too seldom gave my own opinion on affairs – a lack still quite apparent in my current diary. Only once or twice did I write, in the part that I read tonight, what I thought was going to happen in the war. One outburst, however, was perceptive enough – in Feb. 1940, I said that although everyone else seemed to think that England would be invaded in the spring, I was sure that there would be no invasion this war and that instead the Germans would move to the East – I wonder where I got this firm conviction which was so very right as things turned out.

His other concerns were personal ones: Should he have resigned from McGill? Had eight years been a long enough term? Was he letting the side down? Could he have contributed more by staying on for a bit? He had been tortured by these questions even in Florida earlier in the year and still was – to a degree that lessened steadily but that was still considerable. He thought, when he wrote to the chancellor in August 1968, that by 1970 he would have done all that he could do, and he thought that this was probably correct. Still, he felt guilty, and the glorious way in which Roslyn and he had been treated by all and sundry at the time of his retirement, all the kind things that were said, was not sufficient to fully ease his mind. He was greatly pleased that a good successor was found – and so easily, as it turned out – for which he felt much the less guilty.

But what was I going to do? Immediately and later? This was another worry. I couldn't go back to medicine – I've been out too long. I would hate to be an administrator in a hospital or government, I'd loathe Industrial work – I couldn't loaf. The offer of a "surveyorship" from the Science Council was timely, allowed me to explore a field in which I had some expertise, perhaps, and permitted me to set aside my concern about the long run for a while. As things have turned out I've enjoyed my first 4 months of the study. I've read a great deal, have assembled a good team of research assistants, have outlined the study fairly well – now for the fact finding and later the report. On the whole I'm quite cheerful about this.

Our own immediate affairs are very good. We love our house in Ottawa – it is absolutely right for us in every way and our only hint of discontent comes from the fact that spring is so far away and we shall have to wait so long to get at the garden! Rolly seems well. She is still much too thin and I often worry about her but every evidence is that she is quite alright. Our children are all blooming – Tam and his family seem to be ecstatic in Geneva. Ian etc. happy and doing well in Ottawa and looking forward to going east (Phillipines) in a few month's time. Bea apparently happy in her devotion to Joel. Touie a question mark still – nice as can be but no drive, no goal, no work – he's 23 – perhaps soon he'll catch on.[10]

Taken all in all we've an enormous amount to be thankful for – a little to worry about – extraordinarily little really – it's been a good year and prospects are bright.

Work continued in the new year on the survey project, the principal initial challenge being how to approach the "Problem," as Robertson referred to it. He and the team alternated between confidence and doubt that they could produce something useful. During a trip to Switzerland in February, he called in at Lausanne to meet with the director of the public health service, with whom he spent a couple of valuable hours. Driving back toward Geneva along Lac Léman, they stopped for a visit at the *lycée* in Coppet, at which he had studied briefly in late 1925 and early 1926 and which, he said, looked just the same as it had forty-five years earlier.

THE DICTIONARY PROJECT

Robertson's collection of dictionaries was quite remarkable and may well have been unique as a private collection. In addition to the joy of searching for and acquiring these items, Robertson had long thought of publishing some form of study of the dictionaries and of trying to place them in context as to their importance and contribution to the development of the field. This thought had occurred to him long before he retired from McGill, and from time to time, when he had a few moments of breathing room, he gave some thought to how he might tackle the job. He was well aware that he was no lexicographer and that whatever he might produce would undoubtedly be sneered at by the professional lexicographers (as it eventually was), but he was determined nevertheless to proceed. The time would come only during his retirement. Going back to 1967, he had recorded some thoughts in his diary while on holiday for 19 August and the days following:

Worked on the dictionary book materials. I am amassing my notes (I am surprised at the number I have collected over the years) in a loose-leaf notebook and am slowly getting myself into a position where I can start the actual work on the dictionaries themselves. I now have a rough idea of what I want to do. The general plan is to produce a book describing my own collection (I've not decided yet as to how far I'll go with the description of each book) and showing how it illustrates the development of the English dictionary. At the present I am planning to reproduce the Title page of the earliest edition of each dictionary with a bibliographical description and to interleave these pages with a text dealing with the general aspects. I shan't be able to work out the actual relationships between the bibliographical pages and the text until I am much further advanced in the preparation of the data. I feel that now I have made enough headway to say that I am over the hump – that very real barrier between thought and action which consists mainly of a sense of horror at the prospect of an enormous amount of work and which can be overcome only by doing some of the work and discovering that it is not at all unpleasant – in fact (or one knew away down deep all along) it is exciting.

20 August. Nevertheless I did a good bit of work on my dictionary effort today – morning and afternoon. I spent my time writing out new cards which I shall arrange in order of the date of the first edition, which order I shall use in producing the book. On this same card I shall write various other essential data – Author – Title – editions – and some, as yet undecided bibliographical details. At one moment I think that I should give a full bibliographic description of each book; in the next I consider that this would be presumptuous and highly risky for I am no bibliographer. The decision will depend in part upon whether or not the descriptions have been done by someone else – Kennedy is my current hope and I plan to look him up as soon as I get back to town.

23 August. This is our last day of holiday this summer – it's been a short holiday but one of the best we've had. I feel disgustingly healthy physically and I'm delighted to have made so much progress with my work on the dictionaries. I am now quite determined to produce a book and thus to risk the scorn of "experts." Clearly I'm acting in response to a challenge and the pleasure that I shall have during the years of searching and sorting will probably be the only good result.

His eventual plan was to donate his magnificent collection to the University of British Columbia. Part of the "deal" was that the university would publish the work that he put together with Wesley, one of his grandsons.[11] Robertson was right: he was no lexicographer, despite his love of the books in his collection; the principal value of the grandfather-grandson work was to give an indication of the depth of the collection, while providing little if any academic value-added in the process. There was sufficient osmosis from the books to endear them, and the idea of them, to Robertson but not enough to enable him to fully understand their importance as academic works.[12]

THE ROYAL COLLEGE CONNECTION RENEWED

The demands of the job as principal at McGill had meant that Robertson's active involvement with the Royal College was curtailed. He had, of course, continued his connection while he was at the Montreal General Hospital and was the Royal College Surgical Lecturer at its 1960 annual meeting in Montreal, speaking on venous thrombosis, an interest that had commenced with his research work at the University of British Columbia and that he had brought with him to McGill.

It was not until Robertson sold the Rockcliffe Park home and moved to his farm in Mountain, Ontario, in 1975 that he began to become active again at the Royal College, although by 1974 he had been persuaded to become its third Honorary Archivist-Librarian, a position that he would occupy until 1992. He was delighted with the position, and it formed one of the most enjoyable portions of his entire professional career. The job involved a weekly commute to the college's offices, initially still at 74 Stanley Street in Ottawa, where Tuesdays were spent working with Ruth H. Clark, the official college librarian, from 1962 to 1992. Robertson became the chairman of the Archives and Library Committee and immediately took on the task of upgrading the Roddick Library, established in 1961 as a memorial to Sir Thomas Roddick, the founder and first president of the Medical Council of Canada. It was then located in the college offices and is now in an expanded state in the new college building at 774 Echo Drive. Robertson considered that an academic institution representing medical specialists should collect books written by its fellows and locate them in a special section of the Roddick Library. He began by donating his own memorabilia from the Second World War and encouraged all

other military veterans in the medical profession to make similar donations of their own publications, an initiative that has resulted in a significant collection of the military experiences of Canadian surgeons during
that conflict.

Robertson was also instrumental in establishing the D. Schlater Lewis
Library Fund, endowed for purposes of funding acquisitions for the Roddick Library and the archives of the college. He worked with Ruth Clark
to compile and prepare a catalogue of books in the Roddick Library, an
invaluable tool generally, as well as to arrange exhibitions of books or
artefacts at the college offices and at annual meetings. He played a major
role in producing the 50th Anniversary book in 1979 and was on the
committee that selected Dr David A.E. Shephard to author an account of
the Royal College from 1960 to 1980.[13]

Both Robertson and Ruth Clark retired from their positions in 1992.
Their contributions were recognized at a special luncheon during the
April 1993 meeting of the Royal Society Council. Some insights as to the
respect, bordering almost on reverence, in which he was held emerge from
the tributes paid to him on this occasion. Clark herself described him as
"a wonderful raconteur, a good judge of people, considerate of their feelings and rarely critical." On their mutual love of books, she said, "What I
remember best about Dr. Robertson was his love of books. He had a way
of holding a book in his hands as though it were a precious jewel." Dr
James Graham, secretary of the Royal College,[14] during his own remarks
at the luncheon, raised the legitimate question of why such a remarkable
Canadian, serving eight years on the council, had never been elected to
the presidency of the college. The answer lay in the restrictive nature of
the college by-laws of the time that governed the election of officers. The
presidential term at the time was still two years. The president had to
be elected from active council members and the office rotated between
medicine and surgery, to which were added linguistic and geographic
considerations and, probably, although not explicitly stated, seniority in
academic and professional worlds. Graham said: "I believe I am correct
in stating that the example of Rocke Robertson was the major stimulus for Dr. Mackenzie to initiate by-law changes approved by Council
in 1966 that permit candidates for president to be nominated not only
from among serving Council members, but also from among those who
have served two full terms on Council. This was a highly significant new
policy that has been utilized to great advantage over the past thirty years.

Circumstances were too late for practical implementation in the case of Rocke." Concluding, he recounted how he had developed a great admiration for the rare and exceptionally gifted gentleman – tall, handsome, genial, articulate, forceful, witty, charismatic, all combined with a superior intellect. His distinguished service would place him among the great fellows of the college.[15]

Another speaker was Dr James A. Darragh,[16] who reiterated how pleased the college had been that Robertson had resumed his college activities and had become its Honorary Archivist-Librarian. He also noted the many other activities that Roberston had assumed in his "retirement" days. Several of the commissions on which he had served produced formal reports, and the signed copies of the reports occupied prominent positions in the Roddick Library, as did selected case records from many of the Canadian war surgeons, including Robertson, Frank Mills, Fraser Gurd, and Douglas Cameron. Robertson's and Mills's cases were, of course, from their experiences in No. 2 and No. 1 Canadian Field Surgical Units in Sicily and Italy. Darragh described Robertson's interest in books, especially from the eighteenth century, which had led to his prized collection of dictionaries. He echoed Ruth Clark: "If you have had the opportunity to observe Dr. Robertson examining a rare book, inspecting it from all angles and scanning the contents, you have seen a scholar and bibliophile in action. He shares his interest in books with Mrs. Robertson, who has her own collection. This common interest must have contributed to their happy marriage of more than fifty years."[17] Robertson's Royal College contributions have since been collated in the *H. Rocke Robertson Memorial Book*, located in the Roddick Library.[18]

THE OSLER LIBRARY

For someone with a consuming interest in books, history, and medicine, it would be a natural attraction for Robertson to turn to the collection of Dr William Osler's books in the Osler Library. Osler had left a lasting imprint on the study of medicine at McGill, and Robertson himself had brought about a new focus during his time at the Montreal General Hospital and in the medical faculty at McGill. He did much the same for the Osler Library, organizing the Friends of the Osler Library in 1972, over which he presided for many years. It did not take long, under Robertson's leadership, for the friends to expand, and they soon became a significant source of the library's annual funding. He organized, as president of the class of 1936, that the 50th Anniversary gift of the class would be directed to the library, creating an endowment that pays for most of the purchases of rare books and for the Osler Library fellowships. Dr Faith Wallis noted that Medicine '36 made possible for the twenty-first century what Osler's bequest had made possible for the twentieth: the acquisition of new resources for the history of medicine and the provision of means for their scholarly use.[19]

He donated a set of the famous *Encyclopédie* of Diderot and d'Alembert to the Osler Library, one of the jewels of his collection, along with many others and worked to get other much needed sources of funding. Faith Wallis had a further description of Robertson:

> But he also gave of himself. His commanding common sense enlivened many meetings of the Curators, and his acute awareness of financial realities kept us alert to the necessity of investing as well as spending. But for me, speaking very personally, Dr. Robertson represented an ideal of scholarly integrity and personal nobility that matched perfectly the Library he had done so much for. I recall that at one luncheon following a Curators' meeting, we were talking over coffee and I let fall a remark about an absent third party which, I immediately realized, was quite mean-spirited. Dr. Robertson responded with a quiet expression of sympathy for the object of my spite, and the sword of shame went through me. The gesture was typical: he would not connive in malice, but instead of reproaching me directly, he simply called upon my own better feelings. The moment remains engraved in my memory as one of the greatest moral lessons of my life – doubly memorable for being so subtle and gentle. They say that large animals are seldom fierce, and in my experience, large men are very tender and kind. Physically, but in so many other ways as well, Rocke Robertson was definitely a man of stature.[20]

LOOKING BACK: SURGICAL PUBLICATIONS

Robertson's surgical publications have been dealt with in assorted chapters of this work where the chronological and geographical connections were important to understanding the background. They included contributions to scientific progress in the area of wound infection and hospital-acquired antibiotic-resistant infections, basic research on venous thrombo-embolism, and early beginnings of peri-operative fluid and electrolyte balance, along with surgical nutrition. Particularly noteworthy is that, in a very short surgical career, he delivered two of the most outstanding named lectures in medicine, namely the Moynihan and the Shattuck. Very few surgical leaders have ever achieved this recognition. From perspective of academic citations, the Moynihan Lecture probably stands out and is frequently quoted, even today, in connection with the recommended process for dealing with hospital-acquired infection. It has recently been invoked in the management of the vexing C-difficile problem in the Province of Quebec.

H. ROCKE ROBERTSON CHAIR IN SURGERY

On 8 June 1987 the Executive Committee of the Board of Governors of McGill University approved the establishment of the H. Rocke Robertson Chair in Surgery, the incumbent being the professor of surgery. Robertson wrote to then principal David Johnston on 16 June to say that he hoped the members of the Board of Governors would realize how grateful he was to be the recipient of what "for a person in my professional field and with my affiliations is the highest possible honour."[21]

MCGILL VISITING PROFESSORSHIP ON TRAUMA

January 18, 1996, was a special day at McGill. It was the first Annual H. Rocke Robertson Day, inaugurating a new visiting professorship on trauma, named in honour of Robertson and his achievements in trauma. The first visiting professor was Dr Kimball I. Maull, director of the Division of Trauma and Emergency Medical Service at the Stritch School of Medicine and Loyola University Medical Center. He delivered two lectures: "Missed Injuries, the Trauma Surgeon's Nemesis" and "Innovative Techniques in Controlling Liver Hemorrhage." The occasion was attended by Robertson, as well as current and former chairmen of the Department of Surgery, David S. Mulder, Lloyd MacLean, Alan G. Thompson, and Jonathan L. Meakins. Also present were many other surgeons who had worked with or been recruited by Robertson, including Doug McSweeney, E. John Hinchey, Harry L. Scott, E.D. Monaghan, Michael Laplante, Frank Guttman, Joseph Stratford, and Rea Brown.

DECLINE

By late 1992 and early 1993 Robertson began to withdraw from almost all of his activities and to get his affairs in order. His own health was declining. The diabetes that he had thought not to exist had become a real factor in his life, and he had symptoms of Parkinson's disease that interfered with his ability to write, without being debilitating. Roslyn was suffering increasingly from dementia, and he spent more of his time trying to care for her as she grew remoter and remoter from reality and more agitated by her condition.

By the mid-1990s they had to give up the wonderful farm, Struan, near Mountain, outside of Merrickville, that they had acquired in 1975, a few years after first moving to Ottawa. It was a lovely property, some eighty acres, with a stone house, a second house for the visiting family members and friends, and a large lawn, swimming pool, and rose garden. This had been a time to catch up with the family, enjoy the grandchildren, walk in the woods, and ski in the winters. They had a wonderful time, undoubtedly the most relaxing of their lives, and celebrated their fiftieth wedding anniversary there in 1987. Probably their closest friends during these years had been Arnold and Peggy Hart (retired chairman of the Bank of Montreal) and Robert and Mary Beattie (retired deputy governor of the Bank of Canada). They were simply no longer able to care for it themselves and had to move back into Ottawa, where they did not have the responsibilities of a large country estate. They moved to 200 Rideau Terrace, just on the edge of Rockcliffe Park.

In late 1997 the increasingly frail Robertson had a fall and broke his hip. He developed pneumonia – the Old Man's Friend – which led to his death in Ottawa on 8 February 1998. Roslyn would survive him for another three years, dying on 30 January 2001. Just over a month following his death, it was McGill's turn to gather the university community and other friends for a memorial service at the University Chapel in the William and Henry Birks Building on 9 March 1998.[22] Attendees were welcomed by Stanley Frost, and reflections were expressed by Dr David Mulder, Professor Helmut Blume, Ian Robertson, and Principal Bernard Shapiro.

It was the end of a particularly full and fulfilling life, in which the Robertson of his generation, far from "letting the side down," had instead added measurably to the legacy of public service idealized in his family. His contributions were significant on an international as well as national scale and had been recognized as such among the people who experienced them first-hand. He served his country during the war, the public as a respected doctor, the advancement of medicine as a clinician, teacher, and mentor, higher education as the principal of the leading university of his country, and the youth of the next generation by helping them to play a larger role in the design of their own futures. Few could match a record like this.

APPENDIX ONE

PRINCIPALS AND CHANCELLORS OF
MCGILL UNIVERSITY

YEARS	PRINCIPALS	CHANCELLORS
1824	George Jehoshapat Mountain	
1835	John Bethune	
1846	Edmund Allen Meredith	
1853	Charles Dewey Day	
1855	John William Dawson	
1864		Charles Dewey Day
1884		James Ferrier
1889		Donald A. Smith (Lord Strathcona)
1895	William Peterson	
1914		Sir William Macdonald
1918		Sir Robert Borden
1919	Sir Auckland Geddes	
1920	Sir Arthur Currie	Sir Edward Beatty
1934	Arthur Eustace Morgan	
1937	Lewis Williams Douglas	
1940	Frank Cyril James	
1943		Morris W. Wilson
1947		Orville S. Tyndale
1952		B.C. Gardner
1956		R.E. Powell
1962	Harold Rocke Robertson	
1964		Howard Irwin Ross
1970	Robert Edward Bell	Donald O. Hebb
1975		Stuart M. Finlayson
1976		Conrad F. Harrington

YEARS	PRINCIPALS	CHANCELLORS
1979	David Lloyd Johnston	
1984		A. Jean de Grandpré
1991		Gretta Taylor Chambers
1994	Bernard J. Shapiro	
1999		Richard W. Pound
2002	Heather Munroe-Blum	

APPENDIX TWO

CHRONOLOGY

1912   Born in Victoria on 4 August, the fourth child of Harold and "Dainty." The family lived at 510 Charles Street.

1921–25   Attended St Michael's School in Victoria.

1925–26   Attended École Nouvelle in Coppet, Switzerland.

1926–29   Attended Brentwood College on Vancouver Island. He graduated top of his class and head boy.

1929–32   Attended McGill University, earning his bachelor of science degree.

1932–36   Attended McGill Medical School, earning his MDCM and graduating first in his class.

1936–37   Rotating internship at Montreal General Hospital (MGH), from July to July.

1937   Married Beatrice Roslyn Arnold ("Rolly") on 28 June at the Arnold estate in Senneville, on the west end of Montreal Island.

1938   Son Thomas Rocke (Tam) was born in Montreal on 27 April.

1937–38   Pathology internship at the MGH, July to July.

1938–39　In September sailed with Roslyn and Tam to England, then travelled by train to Scotland, taking the position of clinical assistant in surgery, Royal Infirmary, Edinburgh, October to May.

1939　In September took up the position of demonstrator in anatomy at the Middlesex Hospital Medical School. Elected a Fellow of the Royal College of Physicians and Surgeons – FRCS (Edinburgh). With the outbreak of the Second World War, tried to join the British army but was told that he must return to Canada to enlist. Sailed back to Canada, landing in September, and moved into house on Montrose Avenue in Westmount.

1939–40　Junior assistant in surgery, MGH, October to June.

1940　In February joined the Royal Canadian Army Medical Corps, with the rank of lieutenant, staff, No. 1 Canadian General Hospital. Commissioned on 20 May. Son Ian Bruce was born on 20 June. In July sailed to England on the *Duchess of York*. In September promoted to captain.

1942　Promoted to major and appointed commander of No. 2 Canadian Field Surgical Unit.

1943–44　In July unit was assigned to join the Allied invasion of Sicily and Italy – Operation Husky.

1944　Unit returned to England in July to the No. 6 Canadian General Hospital at Farnborough. In November posted back to Canada, sailing on the *Queen Mary*. Promoted to the rank of lieutenant colonel. Posted to the Military Hospital in Vancouver; family moved immediately to Vancouver.

1945　Discharged from the army in October.

1945–59   Appointed director of surgery, Shaughnessy Hospital, Vancouver. In 1946 elected a Fellow of the Royal College of Physicians and Surgeons of Canada – FRCS (Canada).

1946   Daughter Beatrice Marian born on 7 September.

1947   Family moved to home at 1361 Minto Crescent, Vancouver. Son Stuart McGregor born on 3 November.

1950–59   Chief of surgery, Vancouver General Hospital. Professor of surgery, University of British Columbia.

1959   Moved with family (except Tam) to Montreal to take up the appointments of surgeon-in-chief, Montreal General Hospital, and professor of surgery and chairman of the Department of Surgery, McGill University.

1962–70   Principal and vice chancellor of McGill University.

1968–69   President of the Conference of Rectors and Principals of Quebec Universities.

1969   Appointed Companion of the Order of Canada on 19 December.

1970   Retired and moved to Ottawa. Continued with various directorships, studies, and other assignments, as well as with book collecting, for another twenty-five years.

1975   Moved to a farm near Mountain, Ontario, south of Ottawa.

1998   Died in Ottawa, 8 February.

2001   Roslyn died, 30 January.

APPENDIX THREE

AWARDS AND DISTINCTIONS

FELLOWSHIPS

1940   Fellow of the Royal College of Physicians and Surgeons,
        Edinburgh
1945   Fellow of the Royal College of Physicians and Surgeons of
        Canada; Fellow of the American College of Physicians and
        Surgeons
1968   Fellow of the Royal Society of Canada

MEDICAL SOCIETIES

American College of Surgeons (member, Board of Regents)
American Surgical Association
British Columbia Medical Association
British Columbia Surgical Society
Canadian Association of Gastroenterology
Canadian Medical Association
Canadian Society for Clinical Investigation
College of Physicians and Surgeons of British Columbia
College of Physicians and Surgeons of Quebec
International Surgical Group
James IV Association of Surgeons
Kidney Foundation of Canada
Montreal Medico-Chirurgical Society
Traffic Injury Research Foundation of Canada (president, 1967–73)
Royal College of Physicians and Surgeons, Edinburgh
Royal College of Physicians and Surgeons of Canada
Vancouver Medical Association

HONORARY DEGREES

1963	Bishop's University	DCL	
1964	University of British Columbia	DSC	
	University of Manitoba	LLD	
	University of Toronto	LLD	
	University of Victoria	LLD	
1965	Glasgow University	LLD	"Lister Centenary"
	Université de Montréal	D de l'U	
1967	Dartmouth College	LLD	
	University of Michigan	LLD	
1968	Memorial University, NF	DSC	
1969	Jefferson Medical College	DSC	
1970	McGill University	LLD	
	Sir George William University	LLD	

NON-MEDICAL

1964–68	Member, National Research Council of Canada
1964–70	Member, Executive Committee, National Conference of Canadian Universities and Colleges
1965–83	Director, Bell Canada
1983–85	Director, Bell Canada Enterprises
1972–81	President, Mont. Ste Hilaire Nature Conservation Centre. Honorary president thereafter.

HONOURS

Companion of the Order of Canada
Honorary Member of the Canadian Association of General Surgeons
Honorary Member of the American Osler Society
Commander of the Order of St John
Lister Prize for research in wound healing and treatment of antibiotic-resistant infections

For ease of reference, I have identified the principal sources of archival material in the possession of McGill University in general terms as parts of two different collections of documents, with particular references to subsets of these materials where appropriate. I am grateful to Gordon Burr for the proper technical identification of such materials and the description that follows.

The two chief archival sources utilized for this work on Robertson were the H. Rocke Robertson Private Fonds (McGill Archives reference number MG2001) and the McGill institutional records he created as principal, now held in the Principals' Fonds (McGill Archives reference number RG2). The fonds are described below. The citation for these records consists of two parts: the fonds number (either MG2001 or RG2) and the appropriate "c" reference for the container or box number within the fonds. For example, the reference for Robertson's private diaries is MG2001 c.4, 11–14, 18. His diaries can be found within these boxes in his private fonds by consulting a series-level finding aid with related file-by-file lists. The most frequently consulted archival series of records, the private diaries in the Robertson Private Fonds, are also arranged in chronological order.

H. Rocke Robertson Private Fonds (MG2001). Sources from these documents are identified in the notes by the abbreviation "MGHRR." This private fonds covers the period from 1912 to 2005 and consists of 4.6 metres of textual records, 314 photographs, and other materials. These archival records document H. Rocke Robertson's personal and family life, including his early education, athletic interests, and experiences during the Second World War in Britain, Sicily, and Italy, as well as some aspects of his professional life, including articles, speeches, and correspondence on his activities as a surgeon, surgeon-in-chief, professor of surgery, and McGill's principal.

In particular, his tenure as McGill's principal is revealed through personal diaries, correspondence files, newspaper and magazine clippings, photographs, and related ephemera reflecting his private views of his duties, including reflections on the changes he implemented at McGill, as well as his efforts to cope with radical student behaviour and the Quebec government's unwillingness to provide McGill with much needed financial assistance. Robertson's retirement activities are also reflected in these records.

The series consist of: (1) diaries, 1922–95 (c.4, 11–14, 18); (2) publications and research notes, 1945–88 (c.2, 4–5, 8, 16); (3) speeches, 1945–91 (c.4, 18–19); (4) personal and family related materials, 1912–2005 (c.1–4, 11, 15, 19–20); (5) student years at Brentwood College and McGill, 1925–36 (c.1, 47); (6) medical and professional activities, 1937–95 (c.1, 2, 4–6, 11, 15–16, 19); (7) McGill principal and administrative activities, 1937–95 (c.1, 3, 5–6, 10, 12, 15–16, 18–19); and (8) awards and honours, 1932–2005 (c.1, 2, 4, 6–8, 20).

Office of the Principal H. Rocke Robertson Fonds (MG2001). Sources from these documents are identified in the notes by the abbreviation "MGOP." This fonds consists of institutional records created in Robertson's official capacity as principal of McGill. The records cover the period from 1962 to 1970 and consist of 42.3 metres of textual records and 384 photographs. The chief series are: (1) academic matters and internal administration, 1962–70 (c.279–c.377); (2) outgoing correspondence, 1962–70 (c.378–c.380); (3) committees and organizations, 1962–70 (c.381–c.400); (4) subject files on student activism, the *McGill Daily* affair (1967–68), and the establishment of the CEGEP system (1970), 1967–70 (c.401–c.405, c.608–c.610); (5) annual reports, 1962–70 (c.540–c.549); and (6) addresses and writings, 1963–70 (c.568–c.569).

CHAPTER ONE

1 His father was James Robertson, born in Scotland in 1750, who studied medicine at the University of Edinburgh and thereafter joined the British East India Company as assistant surgeon of the Bengal Establishment in Calcutta, India, rising eventually to superintending surgeon. He married Elizabeth Tate in Scotland in 1799. There were six children, three boys and three girls. The boys studied in Scotland, while the girls lived with their parents in India, where their father died in 1817. Alexander Rocke Robertson was the eldest child.

2 See Arthur Herman, *To Rule the Waves: How the British Navy Shaped the Modern World* (New York: HarperCollins, 2004), 428–30. The British Navy had resisted the use of steam-powered ships as part of the fighting fleet, partly for good reasons (paddle-wheelers could not support the necessary guns for broadsides) and partly out of mere tradition, until it gradually began to convert in 1845, launching the first steam battleship, the *Ajax*.

3 Joseph Eberts (1785–1838) was the son of Herman Melchior Eberts (1753–1819) and Marie Françoise Hucques (1765–1813), who were married in Montreal in

1780. Herman was a descendant of Count Caspar Eberts and his wife, Maria Teresa Turr. Herman studied medicine at the University of Vienna and did postgraduate work at the University of Edinburgh. In 1774 he was commissioned assistant surgeon in the Landwehr and in 1776 accepted a commission as surgeon of the Hanau Regiment, part of the Brunswick contingent hired by the British government to suppress the rebellion in the American colonies, which arrived in Quebec on 1 June 1776. After serving fifteen months, he resigned his commission with the intention of settling in British North America. He commenced a successful medical practice in Montreal in the latter part of 1777. He ran into a serious problem a few years later when he contravened the law and religious edicts by exhuming and performing an autopsy on a body without first obtaining a court order. Apparently, a young woman from a prominent Montreal family had taken ill and died before a diagnosis could be made. Herman was one of the attending physicians and was determined to discover the cause of death with or without the permission of the family or the courts. Caught in the act, although the penalty for such crimes was normally death, his reputation and status in the community were so important that a lesser penalty – leaving the community – was imposed. He and his family settled in Detroit, at the time the westernmost British military post, where he practised medicine, kept a drug store, sold wine and spirits, and dabbled in the fur trade. He and his sons old enough to do so served with distinction on the side of the British in the War of 1812. Eberts himself became surgeon general in Brock's regiment. Both he and Marie died in Sandwich (now Windsor, Ontario). Marie Françoise Hucques was the daughter of Colonel Grégoire Hucques and Marie Judith Charbonneau. Hucques was an officer in the French army prior to the fall of Quebec in 1759 and subsequently remained in Canada. The Charbonneau family had settled in Quebec about a century earlier.

Joseph Eberts was born in Boucherville, Quebec, on 15 March 1785. He was employed by the Northwest Fur Company and was for a time in charge of the Wabash, or Indiana, region. Following their marriage, the couple settled in Moy, which later became part of Detroit. When the War of 1812 broke out, Joseph was commissioned an ensign in the Essex Regiment and was involved in several engagements during the conflict. After the war, the family moved up the Thames River, settling in Chatham, where he and his sons built up an extensive shipping and trading business. Joseph died in 1838 at the age of fifty-three as a result of an accident.

4   Ann Baker was the daughter of William Baker and Euphemia Bush of New York, who were married in 1785. In 1792 they moved with their two daughters to Detroit as part of the United Empire Loyalist migration. That same year, William re-entered the British service as a master builder and was put

in charge of the British dockyards, initially at Detroit and later at Sandwich (now Windsor) and Chatham. After the War of 1812, he was given the rank of captain and command of *Charlotte*, a sloop of war. Ann, as the daughter of a United Empire Loyalist, received a land grant in March 1834.

5 *The Chatham Planet*, 7 December 1881, quoted in Dr Edmond Urquhart Melchior Eberts, *The Eberts Family* (1944; reprint, Montreal: Boarish Press and Eberts Archives, 1987), 105.

6 Resolution of the Council of the Town of Windsor, Canada West, on the departure of A. R. Robertson, Junr. Esqr. to Vancouvers [*sic*] Island, 16 March 1864, in personal files of Stuart M. Robertson.

7 The official opening date of the Panama Canal was 15 August 1914.

8 The initial reaction of the United States Congress to the formation of the new Canadian confederation had been to declare that the existence of the confederation might contravene the Monroe Doctrine, probably not a considered resolution, or one that it would ever have dared to adopt while the British themselves were present.

9 The British government was initially not enthusiastic about allowing British Columbia to join Confederation and rejected a request to do so in November 1867. Undeterred by this initial rejection, the Legislative Council sent a request to Governor General Viscount George Stanley Monck asking that immediate steps be taken to bring the colony into Confederation. In response, a receptive Canadian Cabinet passed an order-in-council advocating the idea, and in March 1868 Monck requested that the colonial secretary commence the necessary proceedings. The British attitude evolved, and after the death in 1869 of British Columbia's governor, Frederick Seymour, the new governor, Anthony Musgrave, former governor of Newfoundland, arrived in office with a mandate to unite the colony with Canada. The following March the Legislative Council adopted terms of confederation, which included payment of the colony's debt and the establishment of a transportation link with the rest of Canada. Negotiations were successfully completed in June 1870. On 16 May 1871 an imperial order-in-council admitted British Columbia to Confederation, effective 20 July 1871. Musgrave, his mission accomplished, left the new province less than a week later, its last colonial governor. Completion of the promised rail link would be a contentious issue for many years, and as early as May 1878 a secessionist government was elected because of the delays, which was determined to secede from Canada if the construction of the Canadian Pacific Railway did not begin by May 1879. The last spike would be driven at Craigellachie, British Columbia, on 7 November 1885.

10 Calls to the provincial Bar are still required if a lawyer wishes to practise in a province's jurisdiction, but the western provinces of Alberta and British Columbia were very reluctant to allow any, even indirect, access to

their markets from outside the province and adopted rules that prohibited multi-jurisdictional firms from practising. These rules were initially challenged before the courts in Alberta and subsequently in British Columbia, and the legislation was held to be unconstitutional; see *Black* v. *Law Society (Alberta)*, [1989] S.C.R. 591. British Columbia also tried, unsuccessfully, to prevent non-Canadian citizens from practising in the province; see *Andrews* v. *Law Society (British Columbia)*, [1989] S.C.R. 143.

11 *British Columbian*, 9 November 1864.

12 By 1864 the gold rush fever was dying out. Some 25,000 miners, mostly from California, had passed through Victoria on their way to the Fraser River and the Cariboo fields, making the city very prosperous. As the rewards from the gold fields diminished, most of the prospectors returned home, leaving little of value behind them. The town was sprawling with wide dirt streets, wooden sidewalks, and few substantial buildings, making it a dust bowl in the summers and a mud hole in the winters. On the other hand, it remained the centre of West Coast commerce north of the Columbia River, and there had been an influx of European immigrants and capital, all intending to be there for the long term.

13 *British Colonist*, 9 November 1870.

14 *British Colonist*, 8 January 1867.

15 *British Colonist*, 19 March 1867.

16 The School Act was not passed until 19 May 1876 and provided for the establishment of public schools, the costs of which would be supported by a tax of three dollars per year on all male residents.

17 The British Columbia Legislature met for the first time following Confederation on 15 February 1872. The first premier was John Foster McCreight, whose government was defeated on a motion of nonconfidence on 23 December 1872. Lieutenant Governor Joseph William Trutch called on Amor De Cosmos ("Lover of the Universe," formerly William Alexander Smith, who had changed his name on 17 February 1854) to become premier and to form a government. It would be the first of a series of male governments comprising members who were mainly born and raised in North America and who had supported Confederation. De Cosmos had himself been one of the leading proponents of Confederation. Robertson declined to accept an appointment as attorney general in the De Cosmos government but continued to serve as a private member until the expiration of his term in 1875. In 1875 British Columbia became the first province to allow women to vote in municipal elections.

18 *Victoria Colonist*, 1 December 1880.

19 Robertson (the subject of this work) speculated that it might have been a malignant bone tumour, but neither the nature of the illness nor the type of operation performed has been definitively recorded.

20 The witnesses were A. Rocke Robertson and Ethel B. Barnard, both of Victoria.

21 His brother H.E.A. Robertson had been appointed a judge of the Cariboo Court several years earlier.

22 Telegram from Robertson to the Hon. G.H. Barnard, K.C., 14 April 1933, CN Telegraphs from Vancouver to the Chateau Laurier, Ottawa, in personal files of Stuart M. Robertson.

23 Personal files of Stuart M. Robertson.

24 *Vancouver Daily Province*, 7 May 1942, reprinted in *Saturday Night* magazine, 23 May 1942.

25 In his war diaries, for 21 June 1942, Robertson noted that he had received a copy of the editorial regarding the appointment of Farris as chief justice. "It re-opened the old sore, but I was awfully glad to read the truth of the matter stated so openly and clearly."

26 The Prince of Wales, later to be King Edward VIII prior to his abdication, undertook several official visits to Commonwealth countries at the behest of his father, George V. He toured Canada from 24 August to 10 November 1919. The CPR Royal Train arrived in Victoria on 28 September 1919.

27 Prohibition arrived in British Columbia in 1917, and store sales of liquor would not be allowed until 1921.

CHAPTER TWO

1 Rocke's grandfather would stay at Chenesiton House in London for several weeks each year with a bundle of legal files and work on arguments that would eventually be made before the Judicial Committee of the Privy Council, then the final court of appeal for Canadian legal disputes. (At the time, the Privy Council was the highest appeal court for Canada.) The pace of legal practice was obviously not as frenetic as it is today.

2 MGHRR.

3 The Victoria Cougars had won the Western Canada Hockey League championship and played the Montreal Canadiens for the Stanley Cup, 21–30 March, winning the first, second, and fourth games at Victoria's Patrick Arena, outscoring the Canadiens by a total of 16 goals to 8. For the Canadiens, Howie Morenz scored seven goals and assisted on the eighth. This is the only time, since the organization of the National Hockey League in 1917, that a non-NHL team has won the Stanley Cup.

4 The Olympic Games in the summer had been held in Paris, and the host country of the Summer Games was given the opportunity to host the Winter Games earlier in the same year. Holland, the 1928 summer host, had no

mountains for the alpine events, so the Winter Games were held in St Moritz. This joint responsibility was repeated in 1932 (Lake Placid and Los Angeles) and 1936 (Garmisch-Partenkirchen and Berlin) but fell out of favour following the Second World War.

5 It had clearly been less than a lark. The General Strike in the United Kingdom had occurred from 3–12 May 1926, brought about in large measure by the economic crisis in the British coalmining industry the previous year. The strike had been called by the General Council of the Trade Union Congress in a failed attempt to force the government to prevent wage reductions and worsening conditions for the coalminers. Even following the end of the strike, some miners remained resistant, but by October hardship had caused many to return to work, and by November most were back at work. Many were victimized and remained unemployed for many years, while those who went back to work faced longer hours and reduced wages.

6 Rocke would later, in 1937, spend part of his honeymoon at the Teepee Lodge.

7 Sir Arthur Currie had been appointed the eighth principal and vice chancellor of McGill University on 31 May 1920 and remained in this office until his death on 30 November 1933.

8 Note written by H.R.R., 10 January 1972, in MGHRR.

9 See chapter 1 at pages 10–11 and 16–17 for an initial discussion of the Barnards. Ethel is "Bonnie," and Ethel and Dainty were sisters.

10 Note written by H.R.R., 10 January 1972, in MGHRR.

11 In second year, his marks were: botany, 64%; chemistry, 76%, English, 65%; French, 75%; philosophy, 55%; zoology, 60%. In third year, the marks were: botany, 62%; chemistry, 50%; economics, 60%.

12 The names, a large number of which were well-known Westmount families, included: Webster, Price, Seagram, Henderson, Scott (F.R.), Ballantyne, Bolton, Cumyn, McConnell, Peters, Riordon, Cape, Bogert, Eakin, McLean, Meakins, Mackay, Birks, Kerrigan, McDougall, Carsley, and Dunn. Howard Webster was a particularly close friend, to whom he would turn regularly for both advice and financial support when he became principal of McGill.

13 The Alpha Delta Phi fraternity appeared on the McGill campus in 1897. The Memorial Chapter House on McTavish Street was designed by Harold Lee Fetherstonhaugh and occupied in 1930. It remained the location of the fraternity until 1960, when the McGill chapter moved to 3422 Peel Street, remaining there from 1960 to 1966, prior to moving to its present location at 3483 Stanley Street. The McTavish Street building was eventually destroyed to make way for the student building.

14 Leon Edel, a McGill graduate (BA 1927, MA 1928), was the biographer and editor of Henry James, a student of the Bloomsbury circle, and editor of

Edmund Wilson's diaries. He was one of the "Montreal Group" of critics and poets of the 1920s.

15 Dr Norman Bethune is best known for his work in China during the late 1930s. He had had general surgical training at the University of Toronto but had a particular interest in thoracic surgery as a result of suffering from tuberculosis and worked at McGill with a pioneer of thoracic surgery, Dr Edward Archibald, during which collaboration they developed a surgical program that enjoyed initial success but was eventually rejected in the mid-1930s by McGill. After this, Bethune became chief of thoracic surgery at Hopital du Sacré Coeur outside of Montreal. As a thoracic surgeon, he travelled to Spain during its vicious civil war (1936–37) and later to China (1938–39), where he performed battlefield surgical operations on casualties of these conflicts. The mobile medical units that he developed were an early model for the subsequent creation of Mobile Army Surgical Hospital (MASH) units, and he also developed the first practical method for supporting blood to accommodate the need for blood transfusions in battlefield circumstances.

16 Robert D. Murray was a law graduate in 1938 and played on the Canadian Davis Cup team against Japan the same year. He was inducted into the Canadian Tennis Hall of Fame in 1994. Malcolm Laird Watt (1913–2001) obtained a bachelor of arts degree from McGill in 1931 and a bachelor of commerce in 1934. He captained McGill to the 1933–34 Canadian intercollegiate tennis team championship and won the singles event in 1932 and 1933, as well as the doubles in 1931 and 1933. After graduation, he became the top-ranked Canadian tennis player in 1938 and 1939 and was on four Canadian Davis Cup teams, playing in 1934, 1938, and 1946 and acting as nonplaying captain in 1947.

17 Born in Dresden, Germany, in 1861, Horst Oertel emigrated to the United States at the age of fourteen. In 1894 he earned his medical doctorate from Yale University and continued with postgraduate studies in pathology at the Universities of Berlin, Leipzig, and Wurzburg until 1898. On his return to the United States, he was appointed director of the Russell Institute of Pathology in New York. He later undertook a period of study at Guy's Hospital, London. Oertel came to McGill in 1914 and retired as Emeritus Professor of Pathology in 1938. He died in 1956.

18 Harry Clifford Burgess was born in Sheffield Mills, Nova Scotia, and graduated from McGill University's Faculty of Medicine in 1905 with the degree of MDCM. He did a four-year internship at the Royal Victoria Hospital and thereafter at the Johns Hopkins Hospital in Baltimore. He later became medical superintendent at the Montreal Maternity Hospital for two years and then went on to postgraduate work in London, Vienna, and Berlin. In

1912 he was appointed demonstrator in obstetrics and gynaecology at McGill and, two years later, lecturer in the same subjects. Also in 1912, he was appointed assistant gynaecologist at the Royal Victoria Hospital, a position he held at the outbreak of the First World War. During the war he served with No. 3 Canadian General Hospital as captain and was later promoted to major and chief surgeon to No. 3 Canadian Casualty Clearing Station, with which he served during the battles of Messines and Passchendaele. After the war he resumed his service with the Royal Victoria Hospital as obstetrician and gynaecologist and as lecturer at McGill, holding these positions until his death on 1 January 1938 at the age of fifty-seven. He was widely regarded by fellow practitioners as one of the ablest of clinical surgeons and an extremely good teacher.

19 Born in Montreal in 1880 and educated at McGill University (BA 1901; MDCM 1905), Francis (Frank) Alexander Carron Scrimger served for two years at the Royal Victoria Hospital as house surgeon. In 1909 he went to Berlin and Dresden for advanced study. Upon his return he entered private practice and became an associate of the Royal Victoria Hospital. During the First World War he served with the Canadian Army Medical Corps. For his bravery in evacuating sick and wounded during the second battle of Ypres, he was awarded the Victoria Cross. Scrimger returned to medical practice at the Royal Victoria Hospital after the war and taught surgery in the Faculty of Medicine from 1931 to 1937. At the time of his sudden death at the age of fifty-seven from a heart attack in 1937, Scrimger was surgeon-in-chief of the Royal Victoria Hospital. In the newspaper accounts of his funeral on 11 February 1937, hardly a person of note in the Montreal, McGill, and medical communities was absent, and classes were suspended to enable professors and senior classes to be present.

20 Jonathan Campbell Meakins (1882–1959) joined the McGill medical faculty in 1909 as demonstrator in clinical medicine. He subsequently held a number of positions in pathology and experimental medicine before becoming dean of medicine, 1941–48. In addition, he was director of the Department of Experimental Medicine, 1918–19, 1924–48, and director of the University Medical Clinic, 1927–48. He was associated with the Royal Victoria Hospital and was at various times physician-in-chief and surgeon-in-chief. He was one of the early leaders calling for a system of compulsory health insurance in Canada, under the responsibility of the federal government (although he recognized the potential constitutional issues), which would allow citizens the free choice of their family doctors. He was the second Canadian (Charles F. Martin preceded him in 1928–29) to be elected president of the American College of Physicians in 1934–35. He was the first president of the Royal Canadian College of Physicians and Surgeons from 1929–31.

21 In first year, he had a C in anatomy, a C in histology and embryology, and a D in physiology. In second year, he got a C in physiology, a B in biochemistry, and a B in pharmacology. In third year, he failed pathology with an E and managed to scrape through a supplemental examination with a C. He got a C in medicine, a C in surgery, and a B in obstetrics and gynaecology.

22 Campbell Palmer Howard was a professor of medicine from 1924 to 1935.

23 Walter Linley Barlow had been a demonstrator in clinical surgery as early as 1904 and became an associate professor of surgery in 1937.

24 Edmond Melchior Eberts (1873–1945) was a first cousin of Robertson's father. He was the son of Herman Joseph Eberts (elder brother of Harold Robertson's mother, Margaret) and his first wife, Sarah Mary Gilbert. Herman Joseph Eberts was a barrister in the Northwest Territory who later moved with his family to Winnipeg. Edmond Eberts graduated in medicine from McGill in 1897 and took his fellowship with the Royal College of Surgeons in London and with the College of Physicians in London. He taught at McGill starting in 1905, becoming a full professor in 1929, and became the medical superintendent at the Montreal General Hospital.

25 Diary entry for 20 October 1934, in MGHRR.

26 MGHRR. He did apply for a Rhodes scholarship but was not successful. Had he been successful, it would have delayed marriage for the duration of the scholarship since at the time married men were ineligible.

27 MGHRR.

28 Diary entry for 8 August 1937, in which he recapped the period from 20 November 1935 to 7 August 1937, in MGHRR. Here, the particular reference was to the period from January to April 1936.

29 Robertson obviously wrote to Arnold on 10 November 1935 and must have outlined what he could do since this is referred to in Arnold's letter to him dated 18 November.

30 George Auld would die in service in 1940.

31 MGHRR.

CHAPTER THREE

1 For a splendid account of the post-First World War negotiations and decisions, see Margaret Olwen MacMillan, *Paris 1919: Six Months that Changed the World*, 1st US ed. (New York: Random House, 2002). Originally published as *Peacemakers: The Paris Conference of 1919* (London: J. Murray, 2001).

2 For an account of this remarkable man and his distinguished career, see James M. Graham, "Sir John Fraser and His Contributions to Surgery,"

Edinburgh Medical Journal 58, no. 3 (March 1951): 105–24. He was born on 23 March 1885 and died on 1 December 1947.

3 Letters referred to in this chapter are contained in MGHRR.

4 To distinguish between Rocke and his father in this portion of the book, I refer to the father as "Robertson" and use "Rocke" alone when referring to the son.

5 Eberts seems thereby to suggest that the Royal Victoria Hospital had higher standards than the Montreal General Hospital since it required the English fellowship as opposed to the Edinburgh qualification.

6 William Edward Gallie graduated from the University of Toronto in medicine in 1903. In 1906 he was appointed orthopaedic surgeon at the Hospital for Sick Children and in 1907 a junior surgeon on the staff of the Toronto General Hospital, but he left there three years later to devote his time to the Hospital for Sick Children, becoming its surgeon-in-chief in 1921. In May 1929 he was appointed professor of surgery and surgeon-in-chief at the Toronto General Hospital. His interests included clinical problems and their cures. He experimented on animals in order to develop or improve surgical procedures. As professor of surgery, he developed a systematic course of surgical training to enable residents to prepare themselves for examinations by the Royal College of Physicians and Surgeons of Canada. In 1941 he was elected president of the American College of Surgeons. Due to the Japanese attack on Pearl Harbor on 7 December of that year and the suspension of formal meetings of the college during the ensuing war, he held the office for a never-to-be-repeated six years.

7 Charles Ferdinand Martin was born in Montreal in 1868, educated at McGill in arts (BA) and medicine (MDCM 1892). After one year at the Montreal General Hospital he went to Europe for postgraduate study in pathology and medicine. Upon his return in 1894 he was appointed assistant demonstrator in pathology at McGill University and assistant physician at the Royal Victoria Hospital and in 1895 was appointed assistant demonstrator in medicine as well. He became professor of medicine in 1907. He retired as professor in 1936. He made many scientific contributions to medical literature, particularly concerning diseases of the blood and stomach, and to medical education. He was president of the Montreal Medico-Chiurgical Society, the Canadian Medical Association, the Association of American Physicians, and the Association of American Medical Colleges. He was the Canadian Open Tennis champion in 1890 and had donated a trophy for tennis at McGill, referred to above.

8 Trans Canada Airlines had introduced the transcontinental service on 1 March 1939.

9 Edward W. Archibald graduated from McGill with his MDCM in 1895, started his association with the Royal Victoria Hospital the same year, and apart from some specialized study in Europe and service overseas during the First World War, remained with the hospital until he retired at the end of the year in 1936 as surgeon-in-chief and director of the Department of Surgery at McGill University due to the mandatory retirement age of sixty-five. He was the first Canadian surgeon to be elected an honorary fellow of the New York Academy of Medicine. He was a past president of the American Surgical Association and an honorary member of the Royal Colleges in England and Australia and the Royal Academy of Medicine in Rome. Edwards was succeeded by Francis Scrimger, who died within days of his appointment.

10 McKenty had succeeded Scrimger in 1937 and remained as head of the Department of Surgery until 1945. Following graduation in medicine in 1904 with honours and two years of internship, he had studied in Germany, first stopping in London due to some health problems. While in London, he took both the primary and final examinations and became a Fellow of the Royal College of Surgeons of England, all in the space of only six months, a rare accomplishment, almost unknown at the time for a Canadian. For many years he was one of only four at the hospital (the others were T.G. Roddick, W.W. Chipman, and John McCrae) to hold a senior British diploma.

11 There was a difference between passing the examinations and becoming a Fellow, a distinction with which Robertson, later in his career, would become much involved as a member of the board of the Canadian accrediting body.

CHAPTER FOUR

1 Much of the detail in this chapter is derived from Robertson's diary entries during the war, all contained in MGHRR.

2 He and Frank Mills presented a study later in the war on their experience during the Sicilian and Italian campaigns with the use of penicillin in field surgical units.

3 A diary entry for 6 March 1941, assessing the day's work, observes: "Its war effort value was exceeding low, but that does not seem to matter much."

4 Frank Mills, from Toronto, received his medical degree from the University of Toronto, obtained a master of surgery in 1935, and was co-winner in 1938 of the Lister Prize in surgery. In 1944 he was promoted to lieutenant colonel and officer in charge of No. 18 Canadian General Hospital. After the war he returned to Toronto, where he was employed principally at the Toronto

General Hospital and also demonstrated in surgery at the University of Toronto.

5 There has long been speculation that the United States cryptographers had cracked the Japanese codes and knew there would be an attack on Pearl Harbor but that, *à la* Coventry, they allowed it to occur in order to have a reason to no longer be officially neutral. If true, the failure to get at least some portion of the Pacific fleet out to sea before the attack seems to have been particularly expensive.

6 Thirty or more years later Robertson would meet an Oxford scholar who claimed that he, personally, had delayed the invasion of Sicily by three weeks because he was not convinced that the dosage schedule of prophylactic repacrine had been properly established. Apparently, the Germans in Yugoslavia had run into difficulties with their regimen of two tablets twice a week, and many of the soldiers had developed severe allergic reactions when they took a third dose. The Allies decided to give the soldiers one tablet per day, which seemed to work satisfactorily.

7 Ottawa Civic Hospital, 2 September 1971, in MGHRR. In some respects the speech is "dated." Were he to be giving a similar address today, it would undoubtedly be amended to account for a more developed sensitivity to gender equity.

8 For a complete history of the medical aspects of the war, see W.R. Feasby, ed., *Official History of the Canadian Medical Services, 1939–1945* (Ottawa: Queen's Printer, 1956).

9 MacFarlane had received his appointment to the Canadian Army Overseas in 1941, having been chief surgeon of No. 15 Canadian General Hospital at the outbreak of the war, and would be named an Officer of the Order of the British Empire in recognition of his wartime services. As the consultant in surgery, he supervised all Canadian hospitals, field surgical units, and casualty clearing stations. After the war, he was appointed director of surgery at Christie Street and Sunnybrook Hospitals in Toronto and advisor to the director general of Treatment Services for the Department of Veterans Affairs. In 1946 he became the first full-time dean of medicine at the University of Toronto, until his retirement in 1961, following which he served as dean emeritus and as chairman of the university's Medical Sciences Council.

10 Although by no means a complete list, the Canadians included: W.H. (Bill) Mathews, pathologist-in-chief, Montreal General Hospital (MGH); James Shannon, orthopaedic surgeon-in-chief, MGH; Harold Elliott, neurosurgeon-in-chief, MGH; Campbell Gardner, senior general surgeon, MGH; Edward Mills, physician-in-chief, MGH; S. James Martin, senior general surgeon, MGH; John Gerrie, plastic surgeon-in-chief, MGH; Douglas G.

Cameron, physician-in-chief, MGH; Douglas Sparling, obstetrician and gynaecologist, MGH; J. Campbell Dickison, general trauma surgeon, MGH; Gerald Halpenny, senior physician, MGH, and president Canadian Medical Association; Sandy MacIntosh, Canadian thoracic surgeon; Gordon Copping, senior physician, MGH; and Lorne Montgomery, senior physician, MGH.

CHAPTER FIVE

1 All diary entries cited in this chapter are located in MGHRR.

2 I have chosen the more modern spelling rather than the older version, "interne." It is a peculiarly North American term for a recent medical graduate receiving supervised training in a hospital and acting as an assistant physician or surgeon.

3 This had been his bachelor of science degree at McGill in 1932, the MDCM in 1936, and a two-year internship at the Montreal General Hospital, which was heavily based in pathology, followed by the year's training at the Edinburgh Royal Infirmary under Sir John Fraser, during which he had successfully completed the requirements for the Edinburgh FRCS. Prior to the outbreak of the War, he had commenced study for the English FRCS, primarily studying anatomy and doing dissections under the direction of Professor John Tait at the Middlesex Hospital Medical School in London. During the war he had, of course, extensive exposure to surgery under circumstances and in conditions that were well short of optimal.

4 See A.W. Andison and J.E. Robichon, eds, *The Royal College of Physicians and Surgeons of Canada – Fiftieth Anniversary* (Ste Anne de Bellevue, QC: Harpnell's Co-operative Press, 1979).

5 The council had been founded by the British Columbia government in 1944 to operate laboratory facilities, conduct industrial research, and help develop technologies believed to be important to the province. It was reorganized as a nonprofit corporation in 1973, privatized as BC Research Inc. in 1993, renamed Vizon SciTech Inc. in 2004, and bought out in 2006 by Cantest Ltd.

6 H. Rocke Robertson and Fraser B. Gurd, "Water and Electrolyte Balance in Surgery," *Canadian Medical Association Journal* 43 (1943).

7 Douglas Waddell Jolly, *Field Surgery in Total War*, (London: Hamish Hamilton Medical Books, 1940).

8 H. Rocke Robertson, "Activities of a Field Surgical Unit," *Vancouver Medical Association Bulletin* 21 (May 1945).

9 See H. Bailey, *Surgery of Modern Warfare*, vol. 2 (Edinburgh: Livingstone, 1942), 9–17. Bailey classified hospitals according to their potential to provide

surgical care as either Class 1A, Class 1B, Class 2, or Class 3. Those in class 3 were essentially infectious disease units that were kept available for overflow from the peacetime hospitals. There was also a class of special hospitals, usually institutions related to maternity, children, and mental patients.

10 H. Rocke Robertson, "Vein Ligation in the Prevention of Pulmonary Embolus," *Canadian Medical Association Journal* 55 (1946).

11 These publications included: "Wounds and Infection," in William Richard Feasby, ed., *The Official History of the Canadian Medical Services, 1939–1945* (Ottawa: Queen's Printer, 1953), 175–87; "The Reaction of the Wall of a Vein to Intraluminal Blood Clot" (with T.S. Perrett, J.C. Colbeck, and P.D. Moyes), *Surgery, Gynecology and Obstetrics* 98 (1954): 705–9; "The Reaction of the Wall of a Vein to the Presence of Experimental Thrombus" (with T.S. Perrett, J.C. Colbeck, and J.T.M. Sandy), *Surgery, Gynecology and Obstetrics* 103 (1956): 323–6; and "The Reaction of Ligated Peripheral Veins to the Presence of Autogenous Clots and Thrombi" (with T.S. Perrett, J.C. Colbeck, J.R. Moore, and D.C. Blair), *Surgery, Gynecology and Obstetrics* 105 (1957): 727–32.

12 The lecture "Wound Infection" was published in *Annals of the Royal College of Surgeons of England* 23 (September 1958): 141–54.

13 H. Rocke Robertson, "Edward Archibald, 'The New Medical Science' and Norman Bethune," in David A.E. Shepard and Andrée Lévesque, eds, *Norman Bethune: His Times and His Legacy* (Ottawa: Bethune Foundation, Canadian Public Health Association, 1982), 71–9.

14 Milnes-Walker would later play an important role in the recruitment of Robertson by McGill University in 1959. See chapter 6.

15 The hospital itself had resulted from the benefaction of Peter Bent Brigham (1807–77), who left the residue of his estate to accumulate for twenty-five years from his death and then to be used for the founding of a hospital for the care of sick persons in indigent circumstances. Not unlike the controversy surrounding the will of James McGill, his immediate survivors were frustrated by being unable to get their hands on the money, and litigation took almost twenty-five years to be resolved. The ensuing time allowed for careful planning, including visits to Europe to study other hospitals, and the outcome was first-rate teaching, practice, and research from the very beginning, with the emphasis on academic opportunity, scientific advance, and community responsibility.

16 See H. Rocke Robertson, J.R. Moore, and W.A. Mersereau, "Observations on Thrombosis and Endothelial Repair Following Application of External Pressure to a Vein," *Canadian Journal of Surgery* 3 (1959): 5–16.

17 The occasion at Glasgow was the Lister Centenary. Also in 1965 the Université de Montréal conferred a doctorate of the university on Robertson.

18 It had been to Sir James that the young Christian Barnhard had come for advice on the ethical aspects of the transplant surgery upon which he was about to embark. Sir James came to visit the Montreal General Hospital and McGill University in 1960 or 1961 (see photograph of him with Robertson and David Wanklyn on page xix) and gave Robertson *Bibliotheca Osleriana: A Catalogue of Books Illustrating the History of Medicine and Science, Collected, Arranged and Annotated by Sir William Osler, and Bequeathed to McGill University*, ed. W.W. Francis, R.H. Hill, and Archibald Malloch (Oxford: Clarendon Press, 1929), which became one of his favourite books.

19 The hospital was steeped in tradition, founded in 1123 by one Rahere, a travelling *jongleur*, who earned his living as a nomadic public entertainer and who finally settled in the court of Henry I. On a pilgrimage to Rome, he fell sick and, thinking he would die, vowed that if he ever returned home he would found a hospital for poor men and, as far as possible, minister to their needs. He recovered and on his way home, in a vision, St Bartholomew appeared to him and bade him found both his hospital and his church in Smithfield, in London, just outside the walls of the city. With the authority of the king, Rahere set about to build both a hospital and church, completed six years after the visionary appearance of St Bartholomew, and the hospital is on the same site today. It was granted a royal charter in 1133.

20 Some of them included: Harvey Cushing (1922), Sir Berkeley Moynihan (1927), George Grey Turner (1929), Sir David Wilkie (1931), Henry Burgess (1933), Charles Max Page (1935), Robert Ernest Kelly (1935), Evarts A. Graham and Emile Holman (1952), and Fiorindo Simione (1956).

CHAPTER SIX

1 Terms of reference for the committee, as described in its report dated June 1958, in MGOP.

2 Report of the committee, recommendations 2 and 3, page 6, MGOP.

3 Report of the committee, page 2, MGOP.

4 The committee had concluded that Gurd did not have the necessary drive to fill the position. Years after they had both retired, Robertson sent Gurd the full reports of the special committee in which this assessment had been included; although Gurd had seen parts of it years before, he had never possessed a copy. He wrote to Robertson, returning the reports, on 30 October 1989, saying: "It was true that I was not ready for the top job in 1958. As I said, I needed a post-post-graduate course from you, and then I was ready. As for the comment that I lacked the necessary drive for the challenge, that does not bother me at all, since I have never tried to be a whiz-bang driving type!"

5 Fraser N. Gurd, *The Gurds, the Montreal General and McGill: A Family Saga* (Burnstown, ON: General Store Publishing House, 1976), 300. Much of the other factual background relating to the Montreal General Hospital has been gleaned from this work, Robertson's personal recollections, and those of others associated with both the hospital and McGill.

6 The letters referenced in this chapter are located in MGOP.

7 All diary entries cited in this chapter are located in MGHRR.

8 James Shannon started his career at McGill and the Montreal General Hospital as an assistant demonstrator in orthopaedic surgery (1939–45), lecturer in orthopaedic surgery (1946), assistant professor in general surgery (1948–60), and associate professor of surgery (1961–64).

9 David Angus Wanklyn had been elected a life governor of the Montreal General Hospital in 1929, became a member of the Board of Management in 1948, honorary treasurer in 1950, later vice president, and in 1961 president. In 1968 he was elected Honorary President. He had been president during the introduction of the Quebec Hospital Insurance Service and was influential in the management of the radical changes to hospital financing occasioned by the introduction of this regime. He died in Sidney, British Columbia, on 30 August 1988, in his eighty-eighth year. More important, for purposes of the call to Robertson, his family had roots in Senneville, and he had played golf with the Arnold family, so he know Roberston socially. He was a graduate of the Royal Military College and a close friend of many of the Montreal doctors. Serving overseas from 1940, he was the quartermaster of the No. 1 Canadian General Hospital, and he and Robertson spent time together while they were in England.

10 The importance and the quality of a good idea, especially in academic institutions, is no guarantee that it will be brought to early fruition. It had been clear to many leading academic physicians for some time that surgery was not progressing at the same rate as other branches of medicine. Jonathan Campbell Meakins made the point very forcefully in a letter dated 16 November 1943, addressed to Cyril James, pointing out that surgery as a professional pursuit was restrictively understood as a branch of therapeutics based to date almost entirely on an anatomical or pathologic anatomical foundation and that, with few exceptions, it was in the same position as therapeusis of a medical character had been forty years earlier. Medicine at the turn of the century rested almost entirely on the findings of the autopsy room and, dealing only with end results, had developed therapeutic nihilism. As long as surgery continued to restrict itself to purely reparative or extirpation procedures without a sound physiological basis for doing so, it would remain a spectacular, but often unreasoned, branch of therapeutics. The divergence in outlook had, in Meakins's view, a serious effect on the

mind of the undergraduate student, who was impressed by the dogmatic and spectacular environment of surgical practice, as compared to the positive but nonetheless dramatic successes of medicine. This confusion could be removed if there were, within the teaching and investigative pattern of a medical school, a full-time department of surgery that would exemplify experimental medicine with the recovery experiment as its basis but would use, he stressed, all the techniques employed by both physiological (including accurate techniques of biochemistry, biophysics, endrocrinology, pharmacology, physiology, and nutrition) and psychological medicine. This branch of medicine dominated by surgery was long overdue for a reformation or renaissance and needed to look to the medical schools of the universities to bring it about. It took, notwithstanding the position and reputation of Meakins, close to another twenty years for this idea to catch on, coinciding with the arrival of Robertson at the Montreal General Hospital.

11   Dr Fraser B. Gurd was appointed to serve as surgeon-in-chief at the Montreal General Hospital from 19 March 1947 until 31 August 1948, at which time he would retire as per the age limit. There was, therefore, a very short period between the appointment of Gurd and the opportunity for his replacement to be named. In the event, Gurd died suddenly while on a trip to Chicago at the end of February 1948. His successor, named in July 1948, was Ralph Richard Fitzgerald, a McGill graduate. Robertson would have been only thirty-six years old at the time of Gurd's death, and one can only speculate whether McGill and the Montreal General Hospital would have been willing to appoint someone so young to such important joint positions.

12   Gurd, *The Gurds, the Montreal General and McGill*, 237.

13   This was the estate of Alexander George Cross, born in Ormstown, Chateauguay County, on 12 August 1858, a graduate of McGill University, called to the Quebec Bar on 19 September 1881, who practised for many years prior to his appointment to the Court of King's Bench (now the Quebec Court of Appeal) on 11 March 1907 with a former minister of justice, Rodolphe Laflamme. Cross remained attached to McGill throughout his life, with a particular interest in the Debating Society, of which he was president for a decade. He was an alderman and later mayor (1903–04) of the City of Westmount. He died at Rideau Lake, Ontario, on 19 August 1919. The minutes of the Board of Management of the hospital dated 11 April 1945 indicate that the board had in mind an area of approximately 443,000 square feet, assessed at $450,000, but do not mention the location of the site. Three years later, on 12 May 1948, the Cross property was mentioned as unique for its proximity to the Children's Memorial Hospital and relative proximity to McGill, as well as for the fact that it could be purchased for only its land value. The Board of Management resolved to make an offer to the estate to purchase

part of lot 1724 of St Antoine Ward in the City of Montreal, lying between Cedar Avenue and Cote des Neiges Road and Pine Avenue West, for a price of $350,000 cash. On 19 May 1948 the president reported that the estate had accepted the offer. The 1948 Annual Report of the hospital reported that the area purchased was 305,000 square feet. The Children's Memorial Hospital at this time was located on the north side of Cedar Avenue, just to the west of where the Shriners Hospital (which opened 18 February 1925) is today. The Children's Hospital moved to its present quarters on Tupper Street in 1956. See MGOP and Montreal General Hospital Archives.

14 A total of $18 million was raised in a joint campaign involving the Montreal General Hospital, the Children's Memorial Hospital (now the Montreal Children's Hospital), and the Royal Edward Laurentian Hospital, of which the Montreal General was allocated 62 per cent.

Similar delays would occur a half-century later as another new McGill teaching hospital, the McGill University Health Centre, was contemplated and recontemplated for more than a decade as the Quebec government dithered about proceeding with a much-needed and more modern facility, its deliberations affected by the scope of the project, by the intra-Montreal rivalries between McGill University and the Université de Montréal (which had its own plans for a similar project and did not want to be seen to have been left behind by McGill), and by the general impecunious state of the Quebec government's finances.

15 MGOP.

16 McGill had a dramatic connection with the work, through the intervention of F.R. Scott, who defended it against the (criminal) charge that it was obscene, prevailing in the Supreme Court of Canada with a five-to-four decision that reversed a unanimous Quebec Court of Appeal, which held the work to have been obscene. The Supreme Court of Canada's decision is reported at 1962 S.C.R. 681 and that of the Quebec Court of Appeal at 1961 B.R. 681 (sub nom. Brodie et al v. The Queen). Scott also wrote a delightful poem about the case, entitled "A Lass in Wonderland," the first stanza of which is classic Scott:

> I went to bat for the Lady Chatte
> Dressed in my bib and gown.
> The judges three glared down at me
> The priests patrolled the town.

See F.R. Scott, Selected Poems (Toronto: Oxford University Press, 1962), 82.

17 His letter was not received until 31 December 1958. The day before, James had written to Ogilvie saying that he had not heard from Robertson and

that, if Ogilvie were to receive "any formal bit of paper" from him, he would appreciate a copy for submission to the university's Board of Governors.

18   On 2 January 1959 Robertson had written to N.A.M. MacKenzie, president of the University of British Columbia, to tender his resignation from the UBC position in view of his acceptance of the McGill offer, but he had expressed the wish, if it were agreeable to the university, to continue in his present position until 1 July, when he was to take up his duties at McGill.

19   The Montreal Children's Hospital is the successor to the Children's Memorial Hospital, which commenced operations on 30 January 1904 as a bilingual institution on Guy Street. It was the first hospital in Montreal with the sole mandate of caring for sick children. The growing number of patients prompted a move to Cedar Avenue in 1909. It became affiliated with McGill University as a teaching hospital in 1920. Continued growth in the services that were offered led to expansion and a move to the present location on Tupper Street in 1956 and a change of name to the Montreal Children's Hospital.

20   In the 1961 Annual Report of the Montreal General Hospital, the outcome was noted by the president in the following terms: "During the past year additional emergency facilities were provided in the out-patient department on the advice of the Surgeon-in-Chief, Dr. Rocke Robertson. A separate X-Ray room was established enabling emergency patients to have immediate X-Ray diagnosis with the minimum of movement. One thousand cases were treated in the new facilities during the first four months of operation and the decision to enlarge the Emergency Department has already been fully justified" (27–8). A copy of the report is included in MGOP.

21   Donald Robert Webster had come from Nova Scotia, having studied at Dalhousie University (BA 1922; MDCM 1925) and later at McGill (MSc 1930; PhD 1932). He had become surgeon-in-chief at the Royal Victoria Hospital and professor of surgery at McGill in 1953 and had made contributions in basic gastrointestinal physiology.

22   Ronald Christie (1902–86) came to McGill and the Royal Victoria Hospital in 1955 from Saint Bartholomew's Hospital in London, where he had developed a reputation for an innovative combination of clinical care and research. He had obtained his medical degree from the University of Edinburgh, pursuing a residency at Rockefeller University in New York and, in 1928, had trained as a resident under Dr Jonathan Campbell Meakins, physician-in-chief at the Royal Victoria Hospital, where he stayed for seven years. Following this, he returned to London, England, where he established himself as a lung specialist. Following the Second World War he demonstrated that penicillin could cure subacute bacterial endocarditis, a disease that, until then, had always proved fatal. Twenty years later, he was recruited back to

the Royal Victoria Hospital as physician-in-chief and director of the hospital's University Medical Clinic. He expanded the hospital's research capabilities, recruited department chiefs committed to both clinical care and research, and established the multidisciplinary Joint Cardio-Respiratory Service. In addition, Christie served as dean of medicine from 1964–67. As a result of his leadership, the Royal Victoria Hospital's reputation for excellence in academic medicine developed, particularly in relation to heart and respiratory diseases. The cardiology division eventually became an independent unit, and the respiratory group, named the Meakins-Christie Laboratories, moved to the new headquarters at the Montreal Chest Hospital.

23 The operation was performed by Drs H.J. Scott and A.R.C. Dobell.

24 Harris Schumacher was a prominent cardiac surgeon at the University of Indiana in Indianapolis. He had worked under Dr William Feindel for a time at the Montreal Neurological Institute and was fond of recounting an interesting experience he once had with United States Customs officials when entering the United States with some slides of brain tissue that he was studying. Having responded truthfully to the question of whether he was bringing anything with him, he was then regarded as a potential murderer until the scientific nature of his inquiries was established to the grudging satisfaction of the US officials.

25 Gurd appears to have had a bit more use for him than did Robertson, recognizing his special knowledge of electronics, general ability in physiological techniques, skill in regulation of arterial blood pressure, and knowledge of reflex cardiovascular responses to circulatory shock.

26 Robert Matthew Hay McMinn, *Tissue Repair* (New York and London: Academic Press, 1969), with a chapter by John Joseph Pritchard.

27 Joseph G. Stratford had come to McGill from Brantford, Ontario, in 1941 at the age of seventeen. He obtained a bachelor of science degree in 1945 and an MDCM in 1947. Working at the Montreal Neurological Institute under Hubert Jasper, he earned a master of science degree in surgery in 1951. Having finished his training in 1954, he joined the Central Division of the Montreal General Hospital in 1955, working with Harold Elliott, and stayed until May 1956, when he followed William Feindel, who had gone to Saskatoon the previous year.

28 Interview with David S. Mulder, Montreal, 27 July 2007.

29 Ibid.

CHAPTER SEVEN

1 It was not surprising that Stevenson would know this – he was a member of the McGill Senate advisory committee established to make recommenda-

tions to the search committee established by the McGill Board of Governors. As of 18 June 1962, when he spoke to him, Robertson was on the list of candidates being considered by the Senate advisory committee. The chairman of the Senate committee was Stanley B. Frost (acting dean of the Faculty of Graduate Studies), and the other members, in addition to Stevenson, were Maxwell Cohen (law), H.D. Woods (economics), and R.H. Common (agriculture).

2 All diary entries cited in this chapter are located in MGHRR.

3 MGOP.

4 Minutes of the Board of Management of the Montreal General Hospital, in MGOP.

5 Gurd notes that MacLean agreed to this arrangement but that some of the "elements" at the Royal Victoria Hospital thought MacLean should have put up a sterner fight. See Fraser N. Gurd, *The Gurds, the Montreal General and McGill: A Family Saga* (Burnstown, ON: General Store Publishing House, 1976), 315.

6 The letters referenced in this chapter are located in MGHRR.

7 For a brief account of the history of Mont. Ste Hilaire, see chapter 12, note 7.

8 This was only ten and a half years after commercial television had appeared in Montreal, with the first broadcast of CBFT (part of the CBC French-language broadcast system) on 6 September 1952.

9 Maurice Duplessis died on 7 September 1959 in Schefferville, Quebec. He was succeeded on 10 September by Joseph-Mignault Sauvé (1907–60), who died in early January 1960 and was replaced by Antonio Barrette (1899–1968). The Liberal government under Jean Lesage (1912–80) was elected on 22 June 1960. The campaign slogan was "It's time for a change" and spoke of the Quiet Revolution that followed. Cyril James had been particularly successful in obtaining funds from the federal government but only once Duplessis had died and the government had changed. While Duplessis had been in power, Quebec universities had been prohibited from accepting federal grants.

10 Gérin-Lajoie had been elected in the riding of Vaudreuil-Soulanges in 1960 and was re-elected in 1962 and 1966. From 1960 until 1964 he served as minister of youth and, in 1964, was the first person since 1875 to be appointed minister of education. He did not run in the 1970 election. At the very least, his statement seems to pre-empt what the Parent Commission, established the previous year, would conclude two and a half years later.

11 MGOP.

12 H.R.R. Speeches, 1962, in MGOP, original emphasis.

13 H.R.R. Speeches, 1965, in MGOP. This lecture was published in the *New England Journal of Medicine* 272 (1965).

14 H.R.R. Speeches, 1963, in MGOP.

15 MGOP.

16 This was one of four honorary degrees he received in 1964. The others were from the University of British Columbia, University of Manitoba, and University of Victoria. Bishop's University had been first to grant Robertson such a degree the previous year.

CHAPTER EIGHT

1 Laurendeau, an editor at *Le Devoir*, had suggested such an inquiry in January 1962, but the idea had been dismissed by the former Progressive Conservative prime minister and Saskatchewan native John G. Diefenbaker.

2 The report concluded that there was a "deep gulf of unawareness dividing French and English Canada, and this ignorance was pushing Canada" into "the greatest crisis" in its history. Two days later Quebec and France signed an entente dealing with educational and cultural exchanges. A second report from the Royal Commission, with proposals, would be tabled on 9 December 1968. Not to be completely outflanked by the Quebec government, on 3 September 1965 the federal government announced plans to spend $1 million in 1965 and 1966 on cultural exchanges with French-speaking countries, and on 17 November the first general cultural agreement was signed between Canada and France.

3 As time went on, the nature of the calculations made by the Quebec government were identified, and it became clear that there were different standards applied to the French-language system than to its English-language counterpart. These included, for example, separately counting the costs for the classical college system while lumping the corresponding figures into the grants made to the English universities and also separating the costs for teacher training in the French system (the Écoles normales) from those that were all borne by McGill and Bishop's University and appeared as grants to these universities.

4 H.R.R. Speeches, 1964, in MGOP.

5 During 2007 separatist elements have taken to objecting to the possibility that the queen might be invited to participate in the 400th anniversary of the founding of Quebec City, to be celebrated in 2008.

6 McGill was represented on the Parent Commission by David Climi Munroe (1905–76), who was vice chairman from 1961. He had served as the director of the School for Teachers, was a professor of education at McGill from 1949 to 1964, and was chairman of the Department of Education in 1954.

7 Robertson himself was not active in politics. His father's family had been Conservative, and for Quebec purposes, like most English-speaking people

in and around Montreal, he was more closely aligned with the Liberals than with any other party.

8 McGill's brief to the commission was dated 1 March 1965. The committee preparing the brief on behalf of McGill was chaired by Maxwell Chen and included Registrar Colin M. McDougall, Dean H.D. Woods, and Professors John W. Durnford, S.J. Frankel, Laurier La Pierre, J.R. Mallory, D.C. Munroe, Charles M. Taylor, and G.A. Woonton.

9 H.R.R. Speeches, 1965, in MGOP. This thought was eventually brought to a more formal status with the creation of the McGill Institute for the Study of Canada in 1994.

10 *Financing Higher Education in Canada, Being a Report of a Commission to the Association of Universities and Colleges of Canada, successor to the National Conference of Canadian Universities and Colleges and its Executive Agency, the Canadian Universities Foundation* (Toronto and Laval: University of Toronto Press and Les Presses de l'Université Laval, 1965). The Chairman was Vincent W. Bladen (University of Toronto) and the members were Louis-Paul Dugal (University of Ottawa), Senator Wallace M. McCutcheon, and Howard I. Ross (chancellor of McGill University). Its mandate had been to study, report, and make recommendations on the financing of universities and colleges of Canada, including: prospective financial requirements of universities and colleges for operation, research, physical facilities, and student aid; the proportion of the financial support of higher education that should be provided by tuition fees, contributions from governments, corporations, foundations, individuals, and other sources; policies regarding the allocation of funds for higher education and criteria by which institutions and students should be deemed eligible to receive such aid; organization for the financing of higher education, including the roles of appropriate agencies for the distribution of funds; and any other matter related to the financing of universities and colleges and university students.

11 H.R.R. Speeches, 1966, in MGOP.

12 He also received an honorary doctorate the same year from Dartmouth College in Hanover, New Hampshire, as part of the college's Canadian celebration.

13 H.R.R. Speeches, 1969, in MGOP.

14 On 24 March 1971 the report of the Quebec Police Commission that studied the police walkout recommended the formation of a contingency plan for emergencies and the separation of the Montreal Policemen's Brotherhood into separate units for officers and men.

15 The vote was 67 for, 5 against, and 2 abstentions.

16 See William Tetley, *The October Crisis, 1971: An Insider's View* (Montreal and Kingston: McGill-Queen's University Press, 2007), 4–16.

17 On 8 October 1970 Quebec medical specialists would go on strike to protest controls over physicians' service fees, returning to work on 18 October after the Quebec government passed legislation ordering them back.

18 The terrorist demands included a ransom of $500,000 in gold, the release and safe passage out of the country of twenty-three convicted FLQ "political prisoners," and publication of the FLQ manifesto.

19 Antifederal revisionists often claim that this had been federal interference in a Quebec matter, but the undisputable fact is that it was a Quebec decision.

20 Trudeau was a smart enough politician that he would not have acted unilaterally (at least based on what had happened to date) as the head of the federal government, knowing what political ammunition such an action would have provided for the separatists. Responding to requests from the governments in place was another matter altogether and politically defensible. Quebec premier Robert Bourassa was also sufficiently politically astute to know that it was better for him to have made the request than to have had the federal government act on its own initiative. See discussion in Tetley, *October Crisis*, 157–63.

21 In Montreal on 25 October 1970 Jean Drapeau's Civic Party won all fifty-two council seats in the civic election. This victory may have been helped by the fact that Drapeau's opponent from the Front d'Action Public (FRAP) was among those locked up under the War Measures Act.

22 Most of the FLQ members in exile eventually returned to Canada to face criminal charges. Jacques Cossette-Trudel and Louise Lanctot returned in December 1978; Jacques Lanctot, Michel Lambert, Alain Allard, and Pierre Charrette in 1979; Yves Langlois in 1982; and Raymond Villeneuve in 1984. The maximum sentence was three years' imprisonment.

23 Jacques Rose and Bernard Lortie were granted parole in 1978. Simard and Paul Rose were granted parole in 1982. Michel Viger was later (14 June 1971) sentenced to eight years imprisonment for his role in hiding Laporte's murderers.

CHAPTER NINE

1 All diary entries cited in this chapter are located in MGHRR.

2 H.R.R. Speeches, 1966, in MGOP.

3 The serious trend in this direction began to appear in 1964–65 and became alarming in 1965–66, a divergence pointed out to the minister and described to the McGill staff. It had been inferred, although not promised, that things would be better the next year, but, in fact, they were distinctly worse, which had led to the public statement.

4 A committee, chaired by the deputy minister of finance (Lesage was also minister of finance), was established, and a presentation was made to it in late February.

5 Statement of the McGill Association of University Teachers, 1966, in MGOP.

6 MGOP.

7 Ibid.

8 H.R.R. Speeches, 1966, in MGOP.

9 MGOP.

10 Kierans, then minister of health, had made public statements on 21 February 1966 to the effect that the treatment of McGill had come as a surprise to many members of the Cabinet and that the decision, which he called a misunderstanding and an inadvertent error, had come from the Ministry of Education. He was confident that the dispute over the amount of the grant would be resolved and said that the matter would be thoroughly reviewed and should not happen again since it gave rise to unfounded accusations as to unconscious or conscious discrimination. As to the error that had resulted in McGill getting only $98,000 of the $9 million increase in grants to education, he said the new statistical devices used in apportioning the reduced grants gave too much weight to assets and to projects under way. "If you start cutting down existing operations, then clearly the universities that are doing the most are going to be damaged the most." See *Montreal Gazette*, 21 February 1966, in McGill University Scrapbooks, vol. 17, MGOP.

11 One of the recommendations of the Parent Commission.

12 *Montreal Star*, 16 December 1966.

13 *Montreal Gazette*, 16 December 1966.

14 *Montreal Gazette*, 14 December 1966.

15 *Montreal Star*, 21 December 1966.

16 Laval and the Université de Montréal received $1,907 and $1,758 per student, respectively, while McGill received $1,020.

17 From 1961 to 1968 the staff had increased by 94%, the students by 69% (a favourable trend, although short of delivering a professor-student ratio that could have been regarded as ideal), and expenditures by 250%.

18 Subsequent McGill principals have continued to face the same difficulties as they attempt to achieve equitable financial treatment at the hands of the Quebec government, which acknowledges the existing inequities but refuses to act to solve the problem.

CHAPTER TEN

1 All diary entries cited in this chapter are located in MGHRR.

2 H.R.R. Speeches, 1965, in MGOP.

3 Referring to the recent troubles in California, he noted that at the height of the difficulties, it was estimated that there were 50 students who were active leaders of the cause. There were some 500 students who were strong supporters and who appeared at all occasions and some 5,000 who turned out to demonstrate only at the peaks of excitement. This out of a student body of 25,000.

4 This was a commission established jointly by the Association of Universities and Colleges of Canada and the Canadian Association of University Teachers to inquire into the Canadian models of university governance. The commissioners were Sir James Duff, from Great Britain, and Dr R.A. Berdahl of San Francisco State College, and they visited McGill in 1964. The commission's report would conclude (not surprisingly) that there was a need for greater democratization of university governance.

5 H.R.R. Speeches, 1967, in MGOP.

6 The particularly offensive paragraph read: "I'm telling you this for the historic records," she [Mrs Kennedy] said, "so that people a hundred years from now will know what I had to go through." She corroborated Gore Vidal's story, continuing: "That man [Lyndon Johnson] was crouching over the corpse, no longer chuckling but breathing hard and moving his body rhythmically. At first I thought he must be performing some mysterious symbolic rite he'd learned from the Mexicans or Indians as a boy. And then I realized – there is only one way to say this – he was literally fucking my husband in the throat. In the bullet wound in the front of his throat. He reached a climax and dismounted. I froze. The next thing I can remember, he was being sworn in as the new President."

7 H.R.R. Speeches, 1967, in MGOP.

8 The High Altitude Research Program had occupied much academic and administrative attention at McGill. Its premise was the launching of probes into high altitudes by firing them from an enormous cannon. Much research money was directed to it, but the nonmilitary utility began to fade over the years, and once the interest became solely military, McGill dropped its connection.

9 The letters referenced in this chapter are located in MGHRR.

10 "Participating in the publication of an obscene libel on the campus on or about the 3rd November 1967; namely an article in the column entitled 'Boll Weevils' appearing on page 4 of the supplement called 'Flux' of the McGill Daily of that date, the whole contrary to good order and incompatible with your status as a student of this University." It was this charge that had caused the rallies and occupation of administrative premises. A referendum was held among students, which showed a lack of support for Fekete – slightly

more than half of the students responded by saying that they did not want the charges withdrawn.

11 *Fekete* v. *Royal Institution for the Advancement of Learning et al.*, [1969] B.R. 1; [1968] C.S. 361.

12 The editors had also requested and obtained pre-publication advice from a well-known criminal lawyer in Montreal, Harvey Yarofsky, so they were well aware of the risks inherent in publishing the article.

13 The talk was given on 10 October 1978 and published in the *McGill Journal of Education* 15, no. 1 (Winter 1980): 7–22.

14 It was originally referred to as the "Corporation."

15 Student representation, in its own right, on the Board of Governors commenced in 1973. Students had already been given a back-door access to the board when the Senate decided to adopt the policy of naming a student as one of its five representatives to the board. Nonacademic staff got representational rights effective in 1975.

16 The attack would later extend even to the restricted endowments, and Quebec grants to McGill would be reduced by amounts that bore a suspicious (and statistically demonstrable) relationship to the rate of return from time to time on the capital of these endowments.

17 Meetings included one on 17 May 1967, which Robertson described as a "real exhauster." The MAUT salary committee, he noted, repeated ad nauseam the "old saws" about staff loyalty, their ready mobility, the absolute necessity of "keeping up with the Jones," and so forth. The bargaining process, he said, was a horrible thing, in which otherwise intelligent enough people lost all sense of balance and strove for more regardless of the reality of the situation.

18 See Marlene Dixon, *Things Which Are Done in Secret* (Montreal: Black Rose Books, 1976); and Stanley B. Frost, *McGill University*, vol. 2 (Montreal and Kingston: McGill-Queen's University Press, 1984), 456–8.

19 Gray's own take on the matter was expressed as: "In the middle of this McGill University fired me for protest activities including Operation McGill. I became an overnight celebrity. I ended up a spokesperson along with Michel Chartrand, the fiery president of the Montréal labour council of the CSN (Confédération des Syndicats Nationaux, or Confederation of National Trade Unions), and Raymond Lemieux, head of the French unilingualist movement. We toured the province speaking to cheering, overflowing auditoriums." See Stan Gray, "Stanley Gray: The Greatest Canadian Shit-Disturber," *Canadian Dimension* 38 (November–December 2004): 6.

20 H.R.R. Speeches, 1969, in MGOP.

21 MGOP.

22 Converted to 2007 dollars, this would be more than $340,000.

23 MGHRR, original emphasis.

24 He had even had the temerity to insist that he be paid for the ensuing year as an assistant professor, rather than as a lecturer, on the grounds that had he not been fired, he would have been promoted. Robertson noted in his diary entry for 25 August 1969 that, "in fact, he wouldn't and we shan't pay him." Gray threatened to appeal to the CAUT. Nothing came of it.

CHAPTER ELEVEN

1 All diary entries cited in this chapter are located in MGHRR.

2 Letters referenced in this chapter are contained in MGHRR.

3 This idea would eventually take root and lead to the formation of the McGill University Health Centre.

4 The KM *Admiral Graf Spee* (known more generally as the *Graf Spee*) was a German "pocket battleship," so named because it was built within the letter, although not the spirit, of the Treaty of Versailles, which limited Germany's right to vessels in excess of 10,000 tonnes and having armament in excess of 28 centimetres. It was effectively a large cruiser but with heavier armour and greater speed than any other ships. Its keel had been laid on 1 October 1932, and it was launched on 30 June 1934. Commissioned on 6 January 1936, it did service during the Spanish Civil War, and as the relentless progress toward the Second World War continued to a head, she was sent to cruise the South Atlantic in August 1939. After sinking considerable tonnage, she was engaged in a sea battle with forces of the British navy and, although successful in the exercise, nevertheless put in to the neutral port of Montevideo, Uruguay, for repairs on 14 December 1939, where permission was granted for a stay of three days only. Not fully repaired, although probably seaworthy, the *Graf Spee* then anchored in neutral waters in the Rio del Plata near Montevideo. Expecting to be met by a superior British force if it tried to escape, the ship was scuttled on 17 December 1939.

5 Records of the Senate, in MGOP.

6 Sir George Williams University conferred an honorary doctorate on Robertson the same year. In total, he received thirteen honorary degrees over the course of his career.

7 H.R.R. Speeches, 1970, in MGOP.

CHAPTER TWELVE

1 All diary entries cited in this chapter are located in MGHRR.

2 The artist was Lilias Torrance Newton, and the eventual outcome was a rather disappointing likeness.

3   A copy of the report is contained in MGHRR. The general terms of reference (established in September 1969) had been to inquire into the use of
science and technology in the Canadian Health Industry and, through this,
to examine the purpose and the priority of health science research, particularly to examine and make recommendations on: the overall level of research
activity in the health sciences considered in relation to national objectives
and priorities; the relative levels of research in the principal sectors of the
health field and their adequacy or appropriateness in terms of the particular needs and opportunities of the sectors concerned; the broad principles
and policies that govern the allocation of public funds for research in the
health sciences; and the organization and mechanisms for administering
these funds.

4   *The Report of the Committee to Enquire into and Report upon the Effect on
Human Health of Lead from the Environment* was delivered to Frank S.
Miller, the Ontario minister of health, on 29 October 1974. The committee
consisted of Robertson, Donald A. Chant, and Frank A. De Marco. A copy
of the report is contained in MGHRR.

5   The report, *Causes, Sites, Management and Outcome of Injuries in the Ottawa
Region*, was delivered in January 1977. A copy of the report is contained in
MGHRR.

6   Robertson had refused an invitation coming from his friend and colleague
Roger Gaudry to become executive director of the AUCC but did agree to
take on a study for the organization. The 23 May 1973 report, *Health Manpower Output of Canadian Educational Institutions*, was written by Robertson, J.F. Houwing, and L.F. Michaud. A copy of the report is contained
in MGHRR. The principal purpose of the study had been to determine the
output of the basic courses of studies at Canadian postsecondary institutions that lead to the first degree, diploma, or certificate required for practice in the various health disciplines.

7   One of the few confrontations that he had had as a director arose from a
proposed contract with the government of Saudi Arabia. The contract was
huge but involved some payments that Robertson had thought were inap-
propriate. The board voted in favour of the contract, and Robertson was the
sole dissident. On the occasion of his retirement, he noted that his participation on the board had been a great experience, with one obvious exception.

8   Mont. Ste Hilaire was bequeathed to McGill in 1959 by Brigadier A. Hamilton
Gault (1882–1958) as a memorial to his father, A.F. Gault, a former governor
of the university. It consists of approximately 1,000 hectares and has been
managed for conservation, scientific research, education, and recreation. It
was recognized by UNESCO in 1978 as Canada's first biosphere reserve and
is a migratory bird sanctuary. The site is the largest remaining remnant of

the primeval forests of the St Lawrence River Valley. The research set-up has laboratory and residence space for up to twenty-four, as well as conference facilities and dormitories for up to thirty-two participants.

9   See commentary by Faith Wallis, professor of history, who worked there, in MGHRR. There is, purportedly, a Rocke Robertson Rare Book Room at the Osler Library, but nothing exists where the sign indicates that it exists, and closer inspection leads the insistent investigator to a door, with no sign, that turns out to be nothing more than one of the stacks, a somewhat embarrassing state of affairs, given all the circumstances.

10 Other perhaps than the usual parental concern for the youngest child, there seems to have been little reason for worry regarding Stuart, who was by this time a graduate in honours English from Bishop's University, held a master of arts with distinction from Leeds University, and was enrolled in law at Queen's University.

11 The formal description of the work is H. Rocke Robertson and J. Wesley Robertson, *A Collection of Dictionaries and Related Works Illustrating the Development of the English Dictionary* (Vancouver: University of British Columbia Press, 1989), 74 pp.

12 See Peter F. McNally, "H. Rocke Robertson and J. Wesley Robertson, *A Collection of Dictionaries and Related Works Illustrating the Development of the English Dictionary* (Vancouver: University of British Columbia Press, 1989)," *Papers of the Bibliographical Society of Canada*, vol. 29, no. 1 (1991): 57–8; and Jaquelyn Lyman-Phillips, "Bibliographical Society of America, Short Notices," *Papers of the Bibliographical Society of Canada*, vol. 84, no. 2 (1990): 194–5.

13 David A.E. Shephard, *The Royal College of Physicians and Surgeons of Canada, 1960–1980: The Pursuit of Unity* (Ottawa: Royal College of Physicians and Surgeons of Canada, 1985).

14 James H. Graham was secretary of the Royal College of Physicians and Surgeons of Canada from 1953 to 1979 and director of specialties from 1980 to 1982. He also became Associate Honorary Archivist, working with David A.E. Shephard and Robertson in the production of the second volume of the history of the Royal College; see ibid.

15 MGHRR.

16 James A. Darragh was director of Fellowship Affairs for the Royal College of Physicians and Surgeons of Canada from 1977 to 1979 and executive director from 1980 to 1989, and he has been Honorary Archivist since 1992.

17 MGHRR.

18 In addition to works already noted, the collection includes: H. Rocke Robertson, *Quality of Case Assessment, Health Care Teaching and Research – Prospect and Retrospect, Symposium celebrating the twenty-fifth anniver-*

sary of the Faculty of Medicine, University of British Columbia, June 4-6, 1975 (Vancouver: University of British Columbia Press, 1975); and H. Rocke Robertson, J.F. Houwing, and L.F. Michaud, *Report on Health Manpower Output of Canadian Education Institutions* (Ottawa: Association of Universities and Colleges of Canada, 1973).

19 Osler Library, *Newsletter*, no. 88, June 1998.

20 Ibid.

21 MGHRR.

22 Robertson would doubtless have been amused to note from the program that his death had been anticipated and that the memorial service was, due to a misprint, apparently scheduled for 9 March 1997.

INDEX

homes of, 36, 86, 118, 239, 247,
254, 259; as Honorary Archivist-
Librarian of Royal College, 254–6;
honorary degrees, 103, 152, 164, 229,
243, 267, 283n17, 291n16, 292n12,
297n6; honours awarded to, 267;
as ideal principal for time, 197,
224; James's correspondence with,
111–13, 115, 117; leaves Vancouver,
118–19; and Lévesque, 165, 193–4;
in London, 48, 53–5, 58, 161–2; at
lycée, 23; and McGill University
(*see below*); meets and marries
Roslyn, 32–6; memorial service
for, 259; meniscectomy performed
on, 247–8; at Middlesex Hospital
Medical School, 54; Milnes-Walker
committee and, 107–8; and Mont.
Ste Hilaire, 249–50; *Montreal
Gazette* on, 134–5, 229–30, 232–4;
and Montreal General Hospital (*see
below*); *Montreal Star* on, 231–2;
moves to Ottawa, 243, 247; on
national unity, 182–3; networking
by, 99–101; on October Crisis, 171–
2; official portrait of, 246–7; and
open-heart surgery, 90–1; and Osler
Library, 256–7; and Parkinson's
disease, 259; on "parlous state" of
Quebec, 165–6; Penfield on, 235–6;
and penicillin, 59, 280n2; personality of, 99, 107; at Peter Bent
Brigham Hospital, Boston, 102–3;
on political engagement of universities, 164–5; politics of, 291–2n7;
post-retirement options, 235; post-
retirement years, 246–59; private
practice, 87; on prospects of Second
World War, 53–4; publications, 92–
6, 97–8, 149–50, 223, 248–9, 257–8,
298n6, 300n18; qualities of, 128,

224; and recognition in relationships, 28, 29; reputation of, 104, 116,
149; and research, 46, 90; retirement age, 225; return to Canada,
40–1, 55–6; Royal Victoria Hospital
and, 51; sabbatical for, 236, 237;
at Saint Bartholomew's Hospital,
103–4; and salary ceilings, 115; and
Schinbein, 82–3; scholarships for,
51; Science Council of Canada
and, 248–9, 251; and Second World
War (*see below*); on separation of
Quebec, 171–2, 173–4, 183, 237; at
Shaughnessy Veterans Hospital, 83,
87; Socratic method, 127; special
Convocation for, 243–5, 247; on
specialty training under aegis of
university program, 85–6; speeches
and lectures (*see below*); and sports,
30–1; and student demonstrations,
193, 194; studies completed by, 249;
surgical experience, 57, 59, 80–1, 83,
91–2, 98–9, 130, 149; in Switzerland,
23–4, 252; as teacher, 39, 52, 104, 127,
136; on teaching methods, 210–11;
at Teepee Lodge, Wyoming, 25–6,
275n6; and tensions in Quebec, 157;
and terrorism, 168; tour of medical schools, 87–9; and university
politics, 129; on university's role in
Canada, 148–9; and US surgeons,
85; at Vancouver General Hospital,
82–92; at Vancouver Military
Hospital, 82–3; as visiting professor, 97; visiting professorship on
trauma named in honour of, 258–9;
Wallis on, 257

MCGILL UNIVERSITY:
acceptance of principalship, 132–4;
and assistant professorship, 110–13;
becomes principal, 138–42; as can-